MINIMALLY INVASIVE SURGERY OF THE FOREGUT

MINIMALLY INVASIVE SURGERY OF THE FOREGUT

Edited by

JEFFREY H. PETERS, M.D.

Assistant Professor of Surgery, University of Southern California, and
Chief, Division of General Surgery, USC University Hospital,
Los Angeles, California

TOM R. DEMEESTER, M.D.

Professor and Chairman, Department of Surgery,
University of Southern California, Los Angeles, California

Illustrator

Corinne Sandone, M.A.

Quality Medical Publishing, Inc.

ST. LOUIS, MISSOURI

1994

Cover art:
Modified from Peters JH, DeMeester TR. Esophagus and hiatal hernia. In Schwartz SI, Shires GT, Spencer FC, eds. Principles of Surgery. New York: McGraw-Hill, 1994, p 1074.

Printed in the United States of America.

PUBLISHER Karen Berger
DEVELOPMENTAL EDITOR Carolita Deter
PROJECT MANAGER Carolita Deter
PRODUCTION Judy Bamert
BOOK DESIGN Susan Trail
COVER DESIGN Diane M. Beasley

Quality Medical Publishing, Inc.
11970 Borman Drive, Suite 222
St. Louis, Missouri 63146

LIBRARY OF CONGRESS CATALOGING-IN-PUBLICATION DATA

Minimally invasive surgery of the foregut / edited by Jeffrey H. Peters, Tom R. DeMeester ; illustrator, Corinne Sandone.
p. cm.
Includes bibliographical references and index.
ISBN 0-942219-62-7
1. Stomach—Endoscopic surgery. 2. Esophagus—Endoscopic surgery. 3. Intestine, Small—Endoscopic surgery. I. Peters, Jeffrey H., 1956- . II. DeMeester, Tom R., 1938- .
[DNLM: 1. Gastroesophageal Reflux—surgery. 2. Gastrointestinal Diseases—surgery. 3. Laparoscopy. 4. Thoracoscopy. WI 900 M665 1994]
RD540.5.M54 1994
617.5' 5059—dc20
DNLM/DLC
for Library of Congress 94-31703
CIP

TH/WW/WW
5 4 3 2 1

Contributors

James B. Atkinson, M.D.
Associate Professor of Surgery, Department of Surgery, University of Southern California/Childrens Hospital Los Angeles, Los Angeles, California

Romeo Bardini, M.D.
Associate Professor of Surgery, Department of Surgery, University of Padua, Padua, Italy

George Berci, M.D., F.A.C.S., F.R.C.S., Ed.(Hon.)
Former Director, Division of Surgical Endoscopy; Senior Consulting Surgeon, Cedars-Sinai Medical Center; Emeritus Clinical Professor in Surgery, University of California, Los Angeles, Los Angeles, California

Stefano Bona, M.D.
Staff Surgeon, Department of General and Oncologic Surgery, University of Milan, Milan, Italy

Luigi Bonavina, M.D.
Assistant Professor of Surgery, Department of General and Oncologic Surgery, University Of Milan, Milan, Italy

Cedric G. Bremner, M.B., B.Ch., Ch.M., F.R.C.S.(Eng), F.R.C.S.(Ed)
Professor of Clinical Surgery, Department of Surgery, University of Southern California, Los Angeles, Los Angeles, California

Ross M. Bremner, B.Sc., M.B., B.Ch.
Surgical Resident, Department of Surgery, University of Southern California, Los Angeles, California

Rudolf Bumm, M.D.
Professor of Surgery, Department of Surgery, Technical University of Munich, Munich, Germany

Geoffrey W.B. Clark, F.R.C.S.(Ed)
Research Fellow, Department of Surgery, University of Southern California, Los Angeles, California

Jean-Marie Collard, M.D.
Esophageal Surgeon, Digestive Surgery Unit, Louvain Medical School, Brussels, Belgium

Peter F. Crookes, M.D.
Assistant Unit Chief, Department of Surgery, University of Southern California, Los Angeles, California

Tom R. DeMeester, M.D.
Professor and Chairman, Department of Surgery, University of Southern California, Los Angeles, California

Carlos Eduardo Domene, M.D.
Assistant Professor, Department of Gastroenterology-Surgery, University of São Paulo, São Paulo, Brazil

Sherif G.S. Emil, M.D., C.M.
Resident Physician, Department of Surgery, Loma Linda University School of Medicine, Loma Linda, California

Mitsuo Endo, M.D.
Professor, First Department of Surgery, Tokyo Medical and Dental University, Tokyo, Japan

Charles J. Filipi, M.D.
Assistant Professor of Surgery, Department of Surgery, Creighton University, Omaha, Nebraska

Robert J. Fitzgibbons, Jr., M.D.
Professor of Surgery, Department of Surgery, Creighton University, Omaha, Nebraska

Eduardo T. Froes, M.D.
Fellow, Department of Surgery, University of Southern California, San Francisco, California, and Hospital Mater Dei and Socor, Belo Horizonte, Minas Gerais, Brazil

Keith E. Georgeson, M.D.
Professor of Surgery, The University of Alabama/The Children's Hospital of Alabama, Birmingham, Alabama

Johannes Heimbucher, M.D.
Department of Surgery, Würzburg University Hospital, Würtzburg, Germany

Ronald A. Hinder, M.D., Ph.D.
Harry E. Stuckenhoff Professor, Department of Surgery, Creighton University, Omaha, Nebraska

Arnulf H. Hölscher, M.D.
Professor of Surgery, Department of Surgery, Technical University of Munich, Munich, Germany

John G. Hunter, M.D.
Associate Professor of Surgery, Department of Surgery, Emory University School of Medicine, Atlanta, Georgia

Haruhiro Inoue, M.D.
Hospital Staff, First Department of Surgery, Tokyo Medical and Dental University, Tokyo, Japan

Leon G. Josephs, M.D.
Assistant Professor of Surgery, Division of Surgery, Boston University School of Medicine, Boston, Massachusetts

Namir Katkhouda, M.D.
Associate Professor of Surgery; Director, Minimally Invasive Surgery Program; and Chief, Division of Outpatient and Minimally Invasive Surgery, Department of Surgery, University of Southern California, Los Angeles, California

Werner K.H. Kauer, M.D.
Research Fellow, Department of Surgery, University of Southern California, Los Angeles, California

Tatsuyuki Kawano, M.D.
Research Associate, First Department of Surgery, Tokyo Medical and Dental University, Tokyo, Japan

Hilton Telles Libanori, M.D.
Fellow, Department of Gastroenterology-Surgery, University of São Paulo, São Paulo, Brazil

Marco Montorsi, M.D.
Associate Professor of Surgery, Department of General and Oncologic Surgery, University of Milan, Milan, Italy

G. Edward Morgan, Jr., M.D.
Associate Professor of Anesthesiology, Department of Anesthesiology, University of Southern California, Los Angeles, California

Jean Mouiel, M.D.
Professor of Surgery and Chief, Department of Surgery, University of Nice School of Medicine, Nice, France

Ary Nasi, M.D.
Assistant Professor, Department of Gastroenterology-Surgery, University of São Paulo, São Paulo, Brazil

Adrian E. Ortega, M.D.
Assistant Professor of Surgery, Department of Surgery, University of Southern California, Los Angeles, California

Dilip Parekh, M.D.
Associate Professor of Surgery and Associate Director of Surgical Oncology, Department of Surgery, University of Southern California, Los Angeles, California

Alberto Peracchia, M.D.
Professor of Surgery, Department of General and Oncologic Surgery, University of Milan, Milan, Italy

Jeffrey H. Peters, M.D.
Assistant Professor of Surgery, University of Southern California, and Chief, Division of General Surgery, USC University Hospital, Los Angeles, California

Henrique Walter Pinotti, M.D.
Professor of Surgery, Department of Gastroenterology, University of São Paulo, São Paulo, Brazil

Riccardo Rosati, M.D.
Assistant Professor of Surgery, Department of General and Oncologic Surgery, University of Milan, Milan, Italy

Marco Aurelio Santo, M.D.
Fellow, Department of Gastroenterology-Surgery, University of São Paulo, São Paulo, Brazil

Andrea Segalin, M.D.
Assistant Professor of Surgery, Department of General and Oncologic Surgery, University of Milan, Milan, Italy

J. Rüdiger Siewert, M.D., F.A.C.S.
Professor of Surgery, Department of Surgery, Technical University of Munich, Munich, Germany

Lee L. Swanström, M.D.
Assistant Clinical Professor, Department of Surgery, Oregan Health Sciences University, Portland, Oregon

Kimiya Takeshita, M.D.
Assistant Professor, First Department of Surgery, Tokyo Medical and Dental University, Tokyo, Japan

Thomas J. Watson, M.D.
Clinical Instructor in Surgery, Department of Surgery, University of Southern California, Los Angeles, California

Gerold J. Wetscher, M.D.
Research Fellow, Department of Surgery, Creighton University, Omaha, Nebraska

To our wives

Charlene and Carol

Preface

Minimally invasive surgical techniques have now expanded well beyond the initial innovation represented by laparoscopic cholecystectomy to encompass a broad range of procedures. Nowhere is the potential for this technology more evident than in its application to diseases of the foregut. Laparoscopic Nissen fundoplication will likely become the standard of care in the surgical treatment of patients with gastroesophageal reflux disease, a fact that may significantly increase the population of patients referred for surgical therapy. Esophageal myotomy for motor disorders of the esophagus, vagotomy for the treatment of peptic ulcer disease, and to some extent surgical palliation of esophageal and gastric malignancy have yielded to minimally invasive technology over the past several years. These advances have been met with increasing enthusiasm and the applications continue to unfold.

During an international symposium on minimally invasive surgery of the foregut held in Hong Kong in 1993, it became obvious that interest in this topic was intense and that there was a demand for comprehensive information on the current state of the art and evolving surgical technique. The idea for this book germinated from the excitement demonstrated at that meeting. We have drawn on the wisdom of an international group of experts in this rapidly developing surgical field. The authors of each chapter have been carefully chosen and include many practitioners who have pioneered these approaches. They are leading practitioners of esophageal and gastric surgery, not just "laparoscopic enthusiasts."

Our goal in writing was to produce a comprehensive book that transcends simple descriptions of surgical technique to encompass the broader physiologic principles of surgical therapy as well as the essentials of patient evaluation and selection so necessary for sound surgical decision making. To adequately assess the value of this new technology for surgery of the foregut, potential complications and results are discussed in detail as are corresponding benefits and risks. Organized into six sections, the first part focuses on fundamentals and includes major chapters on the physiologic and anesthetic considerations during laparoscopic and thoracoscopic surgery as well as a comprehensive review of ambulatory methods for evaluating foregut function. These topics are of critical importance in deciding which patients with foregut disease are appropriate candidates for limited access surgery. The remaining sections of the book, Parts II to VI, focus on specific diseases with corresponding treatment options. Thus Part II concentrates on esophageal motor disorders and outlines minimally invasive approaches in the treatment of esophageal achalasia and diverticula of the upper and lower esophagus. Part III thoroughly explores gastroesophageal reflux disease; it includes chapters on why patients reflux, selection of candidates for antireflux surgery, surgical treatment approaches, and lessons learned from failed antireflux repairs. The physiology and treatment of peptic ulcer disease and foregut neoplasms are detailed in Parts IV and V. Finally, Part VI reviews laparoscopic techniques for upper gastrointestinal perforations and discusses future applications for a new approach that has been termed "endo-organ" surgery.

An effort of this magnitude is, of course, not that of any individual but of many. We must express our appreciation for the highly professional and enthusiastic manner that characterized our interactions with the staff of Quality Medical Publishing. They have made the publication of this book a pleasure. Special thanks goes to Carolita Deter for her editorial assistance and to Julie Shepard who kept us on track in a timely fashion. We believe that the superb illustrations by Corinne Sandone is one of the most outstanding aspects of this book. Cory has worked tirelessly with us to depict the anatomic and technical details of each procedure. Her effort is reflected throughout the text. Finally, we would like to thank the authors of each chapter who have selflessly contributed their time and expertise to allow us to put together this comprehensive review of foregut disease.

Foregut surgery represents the new frontier for minimally invasive surgical treatment. We hope that this book will provide a foundation for clinical judgment and assist others in further investigation to expand the applications of minimally invasive surgery.

Jeffrey H. Peters
Tom R. DeMeester

Contents

Part III Gastroesophageal Reflux

Part IV Peptic Ulcer Disease

Part V Foregut Neoplasms

Part VI Acute Foregut Problems and New Therapeutic Approaches

MINIMALLY INVASIVE SURGERY OF THE FOREGUT

Part I

Fundamentals

Chapter

1

History of Endoscopic Examination of the Foregut

George Berci, M.D., F.A.C.S., F.R.C.S., Ed.(Hon.)

The possibility of inspecting organs located deep in a body cavity but connected through a passage to an external orifice has intrigued the more adventurous since ancient times. In contrast to other early primitive surgical procedures such as drainage of a bulging abscess, the more complex craniotomy, or the the so-called (bladder) stone cutters, endoscopic procedures required higher levels of skill, greater imagination, and the design of special instruments. The evolution of endoscopy parallels the development of specific instrumentation: the speculum, open tube with illumination, esophagoscope with a telescope, flexible esophagoscope, and video esophagoscope.

SPECULUM

The word *speculum* is derived from the Latin word "specular," which was defined in the second edition of the unabridged *Webster's Dictionary* as "a mirror, especially one of polished metal, used as a reflector" and "in medicine and surgery, an instrument for dilating a passage or cavity to facilitate its examination." This tool could be inserted into certain organs to minimal depths and provided poor visualization.

OPEN TUBE WITH ILLUMINATION

The initial breakthrough came when Philip Bozzini developed an open tube to reflect light into certain organs in 1806[1] (Fig. 1-1). This pioneer was born in 1773 in Mainz, Germany, the son of an Italian, Nicolas Maria Bozzini de Bozza, a member of an aristocratic Italian family who fled to Mainz after he killed another aristocrat in a duel. The medical faculty of the University of Mainz was dissolved by the French, who then occupied Mainz, and thus the younger Bozzini went to Jena, where he published his first report on the "light guide." He later moved to Frankfurt to avoid becoming a French citizen. The naturalization process and procurement of a medical license proved difficult. Having been in the Austrian army, he had letters of commendation from His Highness Karl von Osterreich, which helped him obtain his naturalization papers. However, despite the fact that he was an experienced general practitioner, the medical authorities insisted that he take the examinations. After repeated

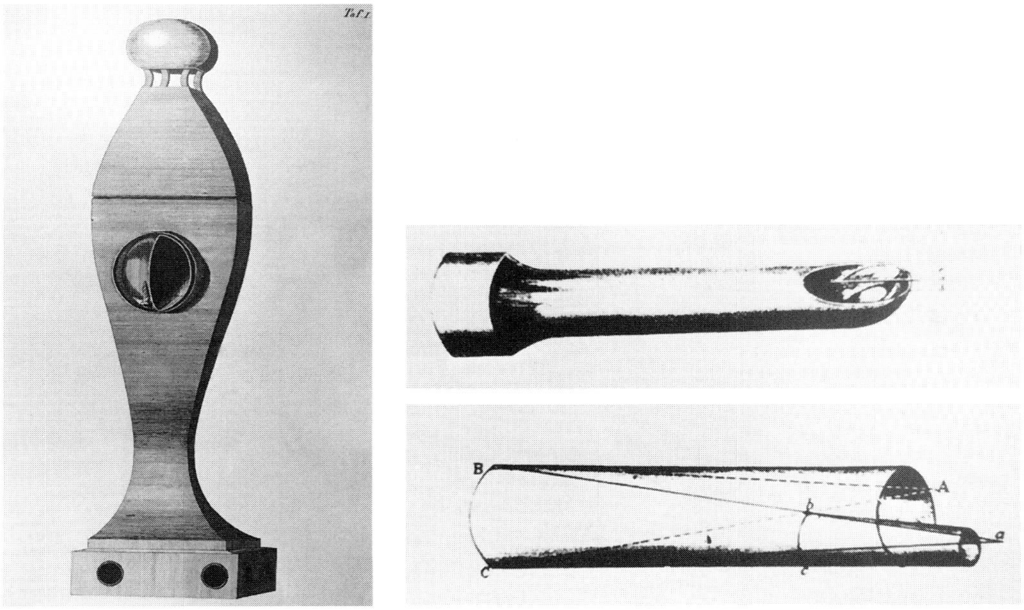

A

B

Fig. 1-1. A, Bozzini's light carrier. A candle was placed in a special housing. The opening was half covered to keep the reflected light from entering the human eye. The other half of the opening was the visual path. Various tubes with a highly polished interior could be attached to the other end of this illuminator. In other words, the human eye saw only the reflected light at the tip of the introduced instrument. **B,** Bozzini's tubes. Top: To examine the larynx a mirror was placed at a 45-degree angle to reflect the light and the image. Bottom: Various tubes with inserts could be used depending on the orifice to be examined.

attempts to pass, he was finally granted a license to practice medicine. His "friendly" colleagues ridiculed his invention as "laterna magica in corpore humano," an abortive attempt. Bozzini saved the lives of 42 patients during the typhus epidemic that many thought was spread by Napoleon's army. Eventually he became infected and died at the age of 35 years from this disease.

In Boston in 1827 Fisher and Hays[2] published an article describing an open-tube system in a Z configuration with a reflecting mirror (Fig. 1-2). The examiner could look through a hole in the deflecting system after the instrument was introduced into various cavities.

In 1865 Desormeaux, a French physician, designed a burner that used a mixture of alcohol and turpentine with a siphoning thread (wick) to provide continuous illumination.[3] He was one of the first to discover that if the beam of a light source is condensed by a lens the intensity is increased because the illuminated area is smaller and the object appears brighter. He also built a deflecting mirror into this unit, which was attached to a side arm where a straight metal tube could be connected to serve as an endoscope. By use of a semipermeable reflecting material (coated mirror), he could view internal organs through this deflector and direct the beam of the light to the appropriate area (Fig. 1-3). He was one of the pioneers in designing a tube to

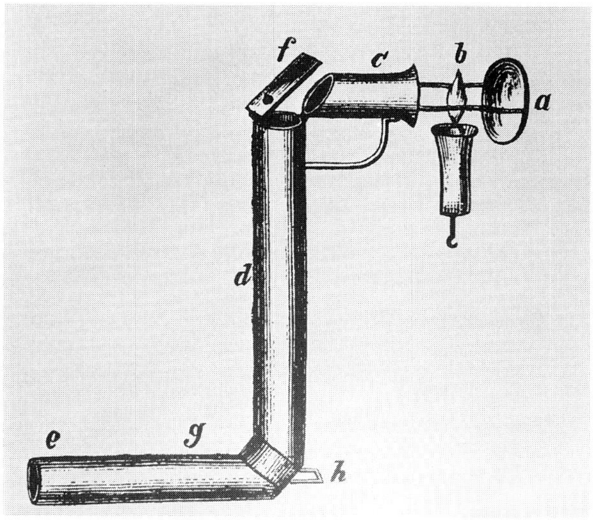

Fig. 1-2. Fisher and Hays' open-tube endoscope. A concave mirror *(a)* reflected the light of a candle *(b)* through a tube *(c)* into a reflecting mirror *(f)* with a hole for observation. This continued to a vertical tube *(d)* and a joint *(h)*, where another reflecting mirror was inserted for the horizontal examining tube (*g* to *e*).

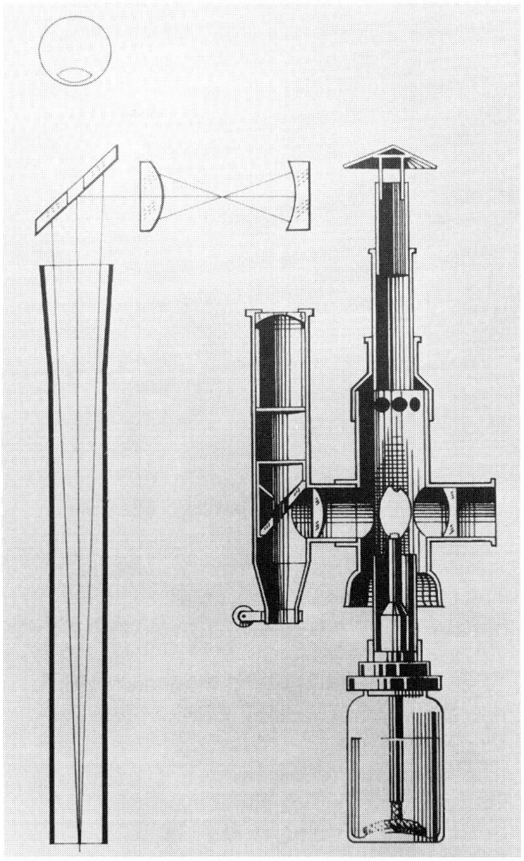

Fig. 1-3. Desormeaux's illuminator used an alcohol-turpentine mixture with a wick. This burner with a variety of concave and reflecting mirrors and attachable tubes was designed to examine the esophagus. This "light unit" proved to be too cumbersome and created smoke, a noxious odor, and significant heat in the housing. It was not widely accepted.

examine the esophagus. These initial examinations caused such discomfort and pain that the use of this technique was limited until topical anesthesia (2% cocaine) and heavy sedation (morphine) became available.

Bevan from Guy's Hospital, in a short letter to the editor of *Lancet* published in 1868, described a simple instrument that substituted for the tube. This instrument consisted of four wires with a hinge that were introduced into the upper third of the esophagus[4] (Fig. 1-4). No manufacturer was identified.

In 1870 Waldenburg reported the case of a 40-year-old woman with an 8-month history of pressure symptoms in the left side of the neck during swallowing.[5] She complained that chewed and swallowed food got stuck and that she could palpate a bulging lump in this area. She learned how to massage these areas proximally to cause regurgitation or distally so that the food entered the stomach. Albert von Zenker, the German pathologist, described pharyngoesophageal diverticulum before Waldenburg's time, and Waldenburg wanted to to observe this anatomic anomaly. Therefore he devised an esophagoscope consisting of two tubes, the lower one slightly conical in shape, 8 cm long with a 1 cm diameter at the distal end, that connected to a second proximal telescoping tube. A movable handle for easier introduction was added later (Fig. 1-5). The material used for this tubing was pure silver. A slot milled into the inner tube held the position of the outer tube during advancements by a screw placed in the outer tube. Waldenburg later used a three-tube system, again with the telescopic arrangement, permitting examination of the more distant part of the esophagus. He performed this examination only in bright sunlight with a reflecting ENT head mirror.

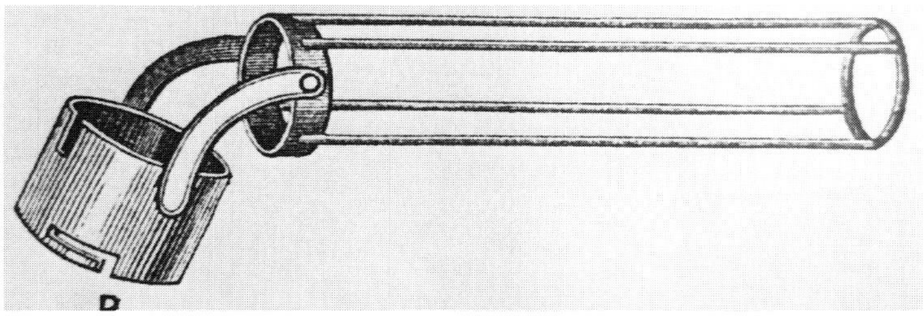

Fig. 1-4. Bevan used a four-wire system with a hinge to facilitate extraction of foreign bodies in the upper third of the esophagus.

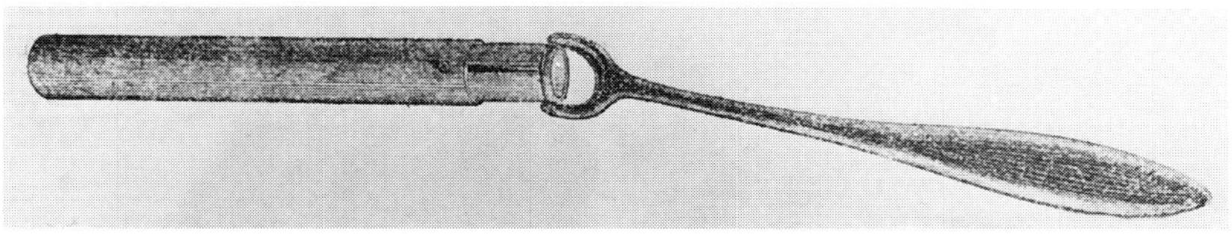

Fig. 1-5. Waldenburg devised a telescopic two-tube system made from pure silver that had a handle to facilitate introduction into the esophagus. Reflected sunlight (head mirror) was used for illumination. He later developed a three-tube telescopic system.

Mikulicz, a professor of surgery at the University of Vienna, described the use of esophagoscopy for treatment of foreign bodies, inflammations, and tumors. He performed his first esophagoscopy with an open tube and stylet in 1881.[6] For illumination he introduced a platinum wire with a separate cooling system connected to a battery (Fig. 1-6). This was later replaced by miniature globes. Using the Stoerk esophagoscope that he had modified, he treated 30 patients in his first year, defining the indications and contraindications. Patients fasted and their stomachs were lavaged. A bougie was introduced first to make sure that the tube could be passed without great resistance. Mikulicz used a syringe with an attached, bent metal tube that had side holes to spray a 1% to 1.5% cocaine solution in the upper third of the esophagus. The instrument had a rubber-tipped, malleable stylet and a variety of tubes with diameters of 11.5 to 13 mm and lengths ranging from 25 to 40 cm. These sizes had been determined after anatomic studies of the esophagus in 60 cadavers.

Stoerk was one of the early endoscopists who had long advocated esophagoscopy.[7] In 1887 he invented a right-angled system in which the telescoping tubes could be extended by slow advancement of the various portions after the patient was given a topical anesthetic. The stylet consisted of small pieces of metal jointed to the instrument and was advanced as a unit (Fig. 1-7).

In 1893 Lowe developed an apparatus consisting of four wires and a joint with a device at the distal end to collect secretions (Fig. 1-8). The diameter of the instrument was 15 mm and the lower part was 9 cm in length. Allegedly, a rubber cup at the proximal part decreased the secretions to be collected in the lower esophagus. The string attached to the proximal part was to protect the patient from swallowing the

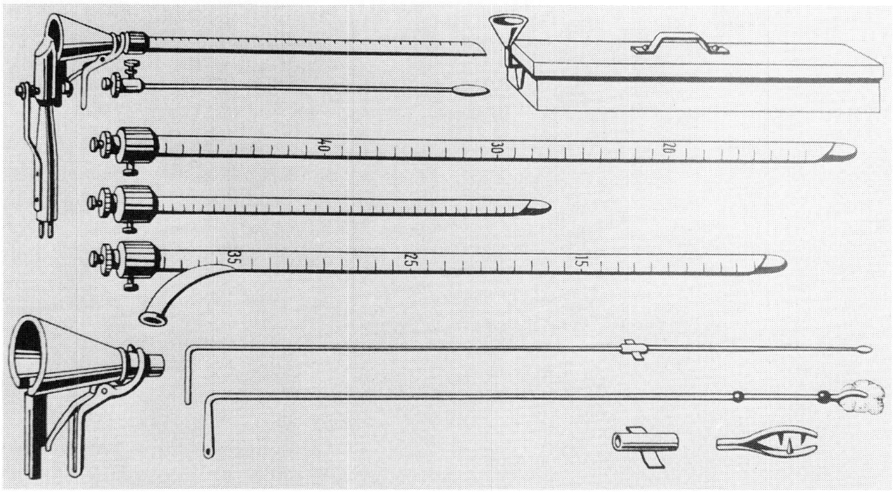

Fig. 1-6. Mikulicz modified the Nitze telescopic system for gastroscopy. He also developed an esophagoscope that consisted of a rigid tubing system with an obturator and a funnel-shaped eyepiece that was used to conduct an attachable proximal reflected light source. The tubes were of various lengths and diameters. The design of a cotton-wool holding forceps is depicted on the bottom. A closed container with a lid held the disinfectant solution, which was poured through an attached funnel.

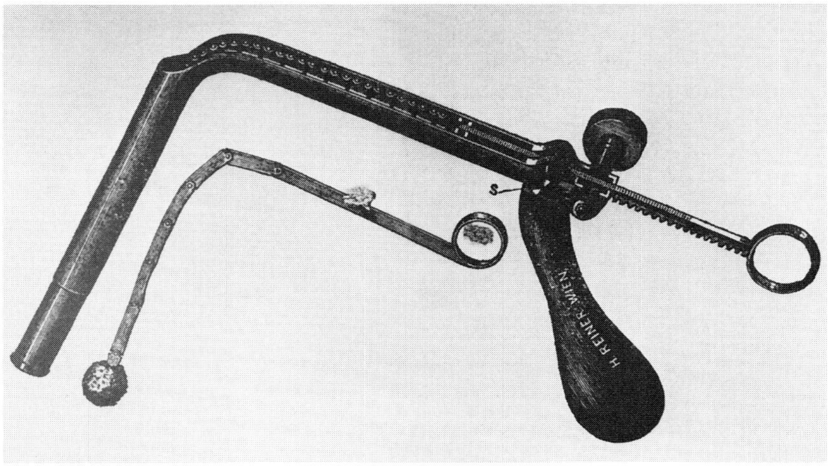

Fig. 1-7. Stoerk developed a right-angled esophagoscope. The part introduced through the mouth consisted of a two- or three-tube telescopic system that was advanced by a cock-and-wheel system attached near the handle. A multiple-joint flexible obturator made introduction easier.

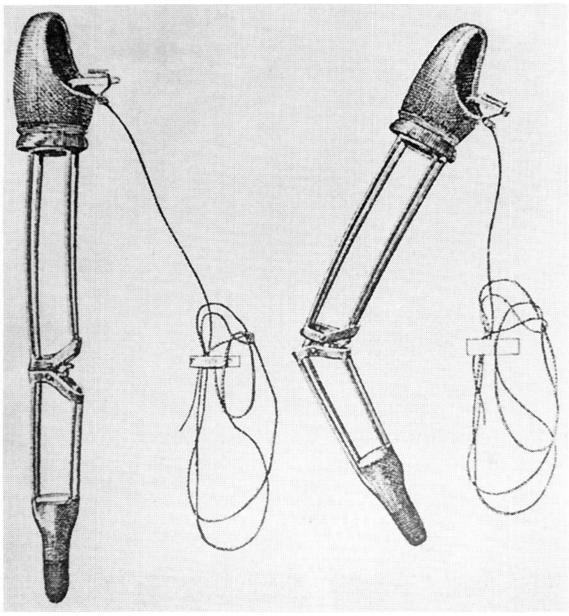

Fig. 1-8. Lowe's esophagoscope was similar to Bevan's system. It consisted of a speculum with a four-wire system to expand the esophagus and was introduced in a bent position (see joint). The distal tip incorporated a device for collecting secretions. A cutout rubber part at the upper end was supposed to prevent secretions from entering the esophagus.

instrument.[8] Lowe preferred to use a head mirror and reflected sunlight, but he acknowledged that an electric globe could be used if needed.

A year later Hacker described in great detail the removal of foreign bodies (coins, bone, etc.).[9] He also preferred reflected light. To avoid the side effects of morphine sedation, he used only 20% cocaine for topical anesthesia. After the tube was introduced, the patient's head was positioned over the edge of the table to gain deeper extension and was held at that angle by an assistant. He even performed the procedure in children 6 to 8 years of age but limited the duration to 10 minutes in this age group. Hacker described in detail the changes in the appearance of the mucosa, strictures, and carcinomas. He had an excellent referring source (The Billroth Clinic). By 1894 he had treated 100 patients with carcinomas (10 in the upper third, 40 in the middle third, and 30 in the lower third of the esophagus and 20 at the cardia). His esophagoscope consisted of interchangeable tubes in lengths of 19, 30, 40, 45, and 50 cm with diameters of 10 to 15 mm (Fig. 1-9). The most commonly used diameters were 11 and 14 mm. The stylet had a protruding, soft, flexible rubber tip. A graduation on the outside wall was used to record the depths of the findings as measured from the teeth. Examinations were always performed on fasting patients late in the afternoon. Hacker preferred that patients have a glass of good wine or tea in the early morning. He recommended slow movements and patience during the examination and noted the importance of slow and systematic application of cocaine as a topical anesthetic. In exceptional cases chloroform anesthesia was used, but extreme caution was recommended to avoid respiratory complications. He never mentioned using suction to remove accumulated secretions. Perhaps, given the patient positioning, secretions were wiped from the patient's mouth by the assistant. He advised lubricating the tube and using gentle manipulations when removing

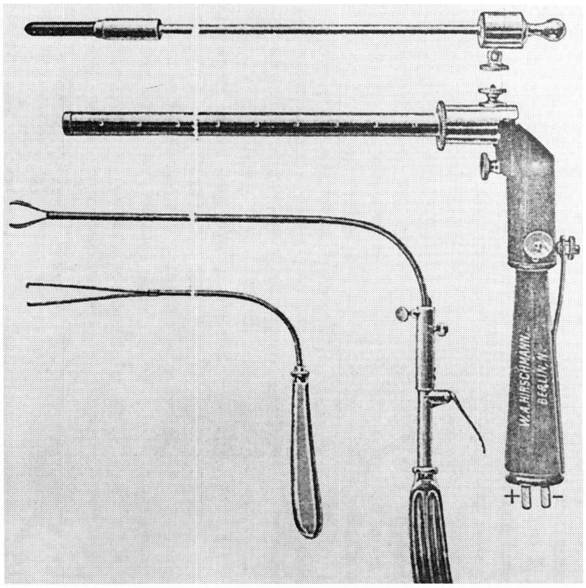

Fig. 1-9. Hacker developed a variety of instruments. The one shown is a rigid tube with an elegantly designed reflecting light, which is incorporated into a right-angled handle. The rigid tube is introduced with an obturator. Various graspers are shown below.

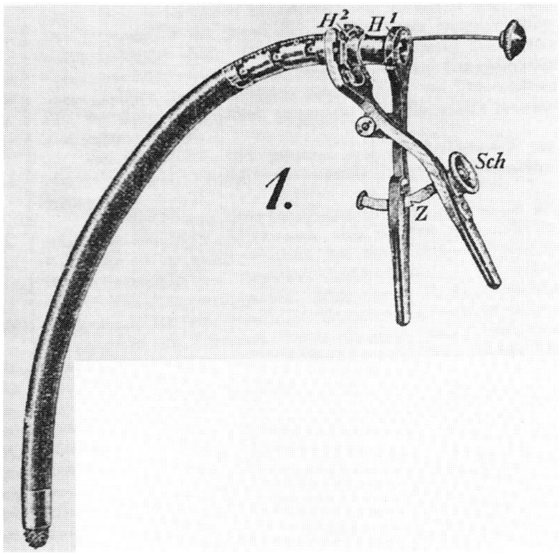

Fig. 1-10. Kelling, who was interested in many other endoscopic applications, developed a flexible esophagoscope consisting of several members of a chain. It was advanced in a flexed position with the obturator. When it was in position, the handle was closed to straighten the tube.

foreign bodies. In one case he had to convert the procedure to an open esophagotomy although he safely removed a partial denture consisting of five teeth. Some of his patients were referred from mental institutions, and he spoke of the problems involved in treating this group of patients. Of 19 patients in whom foreign bodies were removed, 10 had a normal esophagus and nine had a narrowed esophagus.

Rosenheim, another well-known esophagoscopist of this period, preferred Stoerk's tubular formed speculum. He used an ENT head mirror with reflected light for illumination.[10] In 1896 he reported the case of a 24-year-old laborer who swallowed his dentures. Several unsuccessful attempts were made to remove the dentures with a bougie at other institutions. After 1 hour of intermittent unsuccessful attempts, Rosenheim performed an esophagotomy and removed the dentures. The patient developed an infection and bilateral recurrent nerve paralysis.

Kelling introduced an interesting design in 1897.[11] He used a tube made from small segments of chain. In the flexible position the tube could be introduced into the esophagus and then, by pulling wires connected to a handle, it could be made rigid or straight. Reflected light was employed for illumination (Fig. 1-10).

Esophagoscope With a Telescope

In 1879 Nitze developed a telescope to transmit an image from the inside of a deeply located organ to the naked eye.[12] In his first model, developed before the discovery of the electric globe, a platinum wire was connected to an external battery to provide illumination. The heat was eliminated by a separate cooling device. Immediately after Edison's discovery, Nitze replaced the platinum wire with a miniature globe.

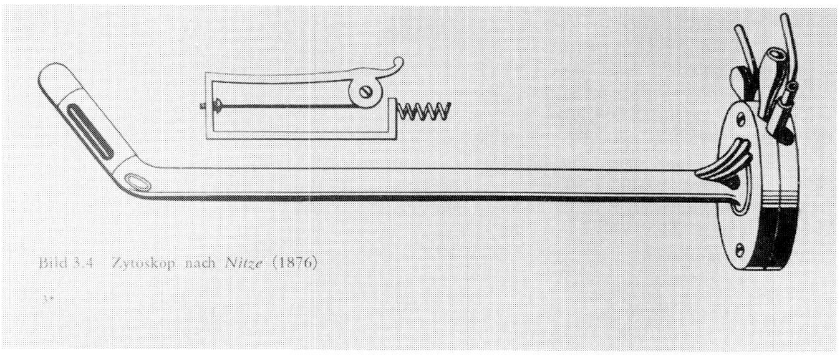

Fig. 1-11. Nitze invented the first telescope to be used as a cystoscope. Originally a platinum wire was heated by a battery until it glowed, thus providing illumination. The same telescopic system was later used in open-tube esophagoscopes. Enlarged view of the platinum wire built in the oblique position to illuminate the urinary bladder.

This telescope was introduced into a cystoscope and the bladder was examined (Fig. 1-11). Mikulicz immediately ordered an esophagoscope with this telescope as well as an angulated one to use as a gastroscope. These telescopes contained tiny handmade lenses that were placed at certain air interspaces; because of the great amount of light absorption, the images were extremely dim. Although the system was improved during the ensuing decades, the basic principle remained much the same.

In 1932 Henning developed an optical esophagoscope in which the tube diameter was only 7.3 mm and its usable length 42 cm.[13] A telescope with a distal light carrier was introduced after the esophagoscope was in position and the organ was observed. The direction of view was not straightforward but rather 135 degrees (forward oblique). The wall of the esophagus could be examined in greater detail, and the area in question scanned by rotating the telescope. Following Nitze's development of the telescope, this system became the standard for rigid telescopes.

Hopkins, an English physicist, introduced the rod lens system in 1954.[14] In principle, this system replaced the air interspace with glass rods. This was a major improvement and provided the following distinct advantages:

1. The smaller degree of light absorption produced a brighter and more visible image.
2. A larger viewing angle provided better orientation.
3. Improved resolution showed smaller detail.
4. Natural color could be seen.
5. The diameter could be made smaller without interfering with the image quality, leading to broader applications.
6. Documentation through still and movie films and videotape was made possible.

The Hopkins system stimulated the development of pediatric endoscopes, including a newborn and infant esophagoscope.[15] Optical foreign body forceps facilitated the simple and successful removal of swallowed materials in young children.

Savary and Miller published their first monograph on the use of the modern esophagoscope with the Hopkins telescope in 2563 cases in 1978.[16] This monograph documented their excellent results with illustrations depicting the radiologic and endoscopic appearance of benign and malignant changes in the foregut. They developed a large number of the modern instruments used in a closed esophagoscopic system. Questionable areas were distended via insufflation to obtain more information about the extent or infiltration of tumors.

FLEXIBLE ESOPHAGOSCOPE

In 1954 two physicists, Hopkins from the United Kingdom[14] and Heel from Holland,[17] published in the same issue of *Nature* articles detailing the advantages of a flexible image and light-transmitting system.

Hirschowitz et al. described the first fiberoptic gastroscope in 1958.[18] Originally a lateral view device with a continuous focusing system, the instrument was rapidly improved to offer a straightforward view.

Examination of the esophagus using a flexible esophagoscope became the method of choice for the examiner and the patient. Mild intravenous sedation and/or topical anesthesia could be used. The improved fiber technology provided an excellent image quality. Instrument channels allowed precise biopsy specimens to be obtained under direct visual control.

VIDEO ENDOSCOPE

Despite the improved telescopic lens, examination was sometimes difficult because of the monocular view through a small dim pupil. The interpretation of findings was all too often subjective, and the observed abnormality was difficult to reproduce. The potential of an enlarged image on a video screen that could be viewed by the entire operating team simultaneously had enormous significance.

The first bronchoesophagoscopy was televised in France by Soulas in 1956.[19] The patient was in effect brought to a television studio where an Orthicon studio camera weighing 150 pounds was connected to an esophagoscope and telescope. Later Montreynaud used a 20-pound hand-held video camera attached to an esophagoscope.[20] My team at the the University of Melbourne developed the first endoscopic miniature television camera in 1962.[21] It weighed 300 gm and used a half-inch Vidicon tube attached to an endoscope. During the Asian Pacific Congress in Melbourne, broncho- and esophagoscopies were televised from the hospital "live" to the conference center. Despite the monochromatic nature of the reproduction, it was obvious to those attending that this was the wave of the future.

Further improvements and innovations in electronic imaging permitted the use of heavier color television cameras that required more light. The introduction of the charged coupling device "chip" cameras created a breakthrough in television endoscopy. These small cameras, weighing 300 to 400 gm, provided an improved image quality, greater light sensitivity, and good color reproduction. They provided a means of communication between the assistant and the entire surgical team, which is crucial in therapeutic endoscopy. The television screen ushered in a new era in endoscopic surgery.

Further refinements include the "super-miniaturization" of the charged coupling device chip. This has resulted in flexible esophagoscopes with chips so small that they can be incorporated into the distal tip of the instrument and introduced into the esophagus or stomach directly. The image is enlarged and of exceedingly good quality, which has enhanced our diagnostic abilities and improved therapeutic maneuvers. Today these instruments are crucial for the examination, assessment, and precise tissue sampling of esophageal disorders.

It has been a long journey of progress from the Bozzini esophagoscope with a candle for illumination and the Waldenburg telescopic silver tubes that used reflected sunlight. Most impressive, however, are the surgeons and physicians of a century ago who sought to explore the esophagus with crude self-made instruments. It was through their efforts and vision that endoscopic examination of the foregut became a reality.

I am most indebted to Professor med. Reuter, President of the Max Nitze Museum, Stuttgart, for supplying pertinent historical data and to Ms. Marilyn Ragsdale for her assistance in preparing the manuscript.

REFERENCES

1. Bozzini P. Lichtleiter. Eine Erfindung zur Anschaung innerer Teile und Krankheiten. J Prak Arznk 24:107-124,1806.
2. Fisher J, Hays I. Instruments for illuminating dark cavities. J Med Phys Sci 14:409-411, 1827.
3. Desormeaux AJ. De l'Endoscope et des ses Applications an Diagnostic des Affections de l'Urethre et de la Vessie. Paris: Bailliere, 1865.
4. Bevan JA. Oesophagoscope. Lancet 1:470-471, 1868.
5. Waldenburg L. Oesophagoscopie. Berl Klin Wochenschr 48:578-579, 1870.
6. Mikulicz J. Ueber Gastroskopie und Oesophagoskopie. Wien Med Presse 45:1406-1408, 1881.
7. Stoerk. Ein neues Oesophagoskope. Wien Med Wochenshr 34:1118-1119, 1887.
8. Loewe L. Beitraege zur Oesophagoskopie. Dtsch Med Wochenschr 12:271-273, 1893.
9. Hacker V. Ueber Technik der Oesophagoskopie. Wien Klin Wochenschr 6:91-94, 1894.
10. Rosenheim T. Ueber Oesophagoskopie. Berl Klin Wochenschr 12:247-252, 1895.
11. Kelling G. Endoskopie fur Speiserohre und Magen. Munch Med Wochenschr 34:934-937, 1897.
12. Nitze M. Eine neue Beobachtungs und Untersuchungsmethode fur Harnrohre, Harnblase und Rectum. Wien Med Wochenschr 24:651-652, 714-716, 1879.
13. Henning N. Ueber ein neues Oesophagoskope fur den Gebrauch der inneren Klin. Dtsch Klin Wochenschr 11:1673-1676, 1932.
14. Hopkins HH. The rod lens system. Patents: Great Britain: 954629, 1954; United States: 3257902, 1955.
15. Gans SL, Berci G. Advances in endoscopy of infants and children. J Pediatr Surg 6:199-233, 1971.
16. Savary M, Miller G. The esophagus. Solothurn, Switzerland: Glassman, 1978.
17. Heel ACS. A new method for transporting optical images without aberrations. Nature 173:39, 1954.
18. Hirschowitz BS, Curtis LE, Peters CW. The fibergastroscope. Gastroenterology 35:50-54, 1958.
19. Soulas A. Televised bronchoscopy. Presse Med 64:97, 1956.
20. Montreynaud JM. Television endoscopy. In Montreynaud JM, ed. Traite de Photographie et de Cinematography Medicales. Paris: Montel, 1960, pp 192-193.
21. Berci G, Davids J. Endoscopy and television. Br Med J 1:1610-1613, 1962.

Chapter

2

Anesthetic Considerations

G. Edward Morgan, Jr., M.D.

The physiologic changes associated with laparoscopic and thoracoscopic surgery have multiple anesthetic implications. The unusual patient positioning and one-lung ventilation required also influence the anesthetic management. Since there is a paucity of information on anesthesia in the literature for these foregut surgical techniques, much of this chapter is based on experience with more conventional, less invasive procedures such as laparoscopic cholecystectomy or thoracoscopic lung biopsy. Laparoscopic and thoracoscopic surgeries are discussed separately because their anesthetic implications are so different.

ANESTHESIA FOR LAPAROSCOPIC SURGERY

Physiologic Effects of Pneumoperitoneum

Pulmonary Function. The hallmark of laparoscopy is the creation of a pneumoperitoneum with pressurized CO_2. The resulting increase in intra-abdominal pressure displaces the diaphragm cephalad, causing a decrease in lung compliance and an increase in peak inspiratory pressure. Atelectasis, diminished functional residual capacity, ventilation-perfusion mismatch, and pulmonary shunting contribute to a decrease in arterial oxygenation.[1] These changes are exaggerated in patients with underlying pulmonary disease or morbid obesity, during extended periods of insufflation, or by use of high insufflation pressures (greater than 25 cm H_2O or 18 mm Hg).[2]

Although the nonflammability and high solubility of CO_2 lessen the risks of explosion or gas embolism, its relatively high diffusibility increases systemic absorption. This absorption into the vasculature of the peritoneum combined with smaller tidal volumes because of poor lung compliance leads to increased arterial CO_2 levels and decreased pH.[2] Extraperitoneal insufflation (e.g., pelviscopy) appears to be associated with greater CO_2 diffusion than intraperitoneal insufflation (e.g., cholecystectomy).[3]

Cardiac Function. Pneumoperitoneum also affects cardiac function. Moderate insufflation pressures seem to leave heart rate, central venous pressure, and cardiac output unchanged or slightly elevated.[4,5] This would appear to result from increased effective cardiac filling because blood tends to be forced out of the abdomen and into the chest. However, higher insufflation pressures tend to collapse the major abdominal veins (particularly the inferior vena cava), which compromises venous return and leads to a drop in preload and cardiac output in some patients.[5]

Hypercarbia, if allowed to develop, will stimulate the sympathetic nervous system and thus increase blood pressure, heart rate, and the risk of dysrhythmias. Attempting to compensate by increasing the tidal volume or respiratory rate will increase the mean intrathoracic pressure, further hindering venous return and increasing mean pulmonary artery pressures. Although these effects are usually well tolerated in healthy patients, they can prove quite challenging in patients with impaired baseline cardiac function, restrictive lung disease, or intravascular volume depletion.

Physiologic Effects of Trendelenburg and Reverse Trendelenburg Positions

Trendelenburg Position. The head-down position causes a cephalad shift in abdominal viscera and the diaphragm. Functional residual capacity, total lung volume, and pulmonary compliance are thus decreased. Atelectasis may occur during spontaneous ventilation. Although these changes are usually well tolerated by healthy patients,[6] obesity or preexisting lung disease increases the risk of episodes of hypoxemia.[7] The head-down position also tends to shift the trachea upward. An endotracheal tube that is anchored at the mouth may migrate into the right mainstem bronchus.[8] Insufflation of the abdomen can further shift the tracheobronchial tree in relation to an endotracheal tube.[9,10] Although gravity would favor an increased incidence of passive regurgitation of gastric contents in the head-down position, aspiration is less likely since the regurgitated material tends to flow out the mouth rather than "up" the trachea.

The Trendelenburg position has gained an undeserved reputation for being beneficial in patients with hypotension and shock. Although preload often increases markedly, mean arterial pressure and cardiac output usually remain unchanged or decrease. These seemingly paradoxical responses may be explained by carotid and aortic baroreceptor-mediated reflexes.[7] Increased venous pressure in the head results in a corresponding increase in cerebrospinal fluid pressure, whereas a decrease in venous pressure in the abdomen increases the risk of venous gas embolism.[7]

Reverse Trendelenburg Position. In some respects the physiologic effects of a head-up position are the opposite of those of a head-down position. The reverse Trendelenburg position increases functional residual capacity and decreases the work of spontaneous ventilation. Preload is decreased and baroreceptors increase sympathetic tone, heart rate, and peripheral vascular resistance. However, general anesthesia blunts these compensatory mechanisms, causing a decrease in cardiac output and mean arterial pressure. Thus the reverse Trendelenburg position may attenuate some of the respiratory embarrassment induced by a pneumoperitoneum, but it may exacerbate circulatory impairment. Trendelenburg and reverse Trendelenburg positions necessitate proper anchoring to prevent the patient from falling off the table.[10]

Anesthetic Management

Anesthetic approaches to laparoscopic surgery include infiltration of local anesthetic with an intravenous sedative,[11] epidural or spinal anesthesia,[12] and general anesthesia.[13]

Local Anesthesia. Experience with local anesthesia has been largely limited to brief gynecologic procedures (particularly laparoscopic tubal sterilization and intrafallopian transfers[14]) in a relatively young, healthy, and motivated patient population. The primary advantage of this technique, rapid postoperative recovery, is of greatest importance in ambulatory patients. Disadvantages include patient discomfort, suboptimal visualization of intra-abdominal organs, and conversion to general anesthesia should open laparotomy become necessary.

Epidural Anesthesia. Epidural anesthesia is another alternative for laparoscopic surgery. However, a high level is required to achieve complete relaxation of abdominal muscles and to prevent the diaphragmatic irritation caused by insufflation of CO_2. Healthy patients were able to increase their spontaneous ventilation to maintain a normal $PaCO_2$ during high (T2 level) epidural anesthesia despite a 20-degree Trendelenburg position.[15] Older patients, particularly those with lung disease or those requiring sedation, might not be able to compensate by increasing minute ventilation sufficiently. Likewise, a high sympathetic block may result in significant hypotension in patients with limited cardiovascular reserve or volume depletion.

General Anesthesia. Because of the considerations discussed earlier, most laparoscopic surgery is performed under general anesthesia. Although the choice of a specific technique or drug regimen often depends on the patient's preexisting medical problems, some general guidelines apply. First, endotracheal intubation with positive pressure ventilation is usually favored. Reasons include (1) the risk of regurgitation from increased intra-abdominal pressure during insufflation (see following discussion of complications); (2) the necessity for controlled ventilation to prevent hypercarbia in the anesthetized patient; (3) the relatively high peak inspiratory pressures required because of the pneumoperitoneum; and (4) the need for muscle paralysis during surgery to allow lower insufflation pressures, provide better visualization, and prevent unexpected patient movement. Although some investigators have advocated spontaneous or assisted ventilation with a face mask or Brain laryngeal mask, these techniques are not recommended for laparoscopic procedures lasting longer than 30 minutes or in patients at risk for aspiration.[16,17] Furthermore, insertion of a nasogastric tube and gastric decompression are usually performed to reduce the risk of visceral perforation during trochar introduction and to optimize visualization.

A variety of induction and maintenance drugs have been used successfully during laparoscopic surgery, including desflurane,[18] isoflurane,[19,20] propofol,[19] and alfentanil.[20] The most important considerations are adequate muscle relaxation and stable hemodynamics. Halothane is probably best avoided because of its dysrhythmogenic tendency should the patient become hypercarbic. The use of nitrous oxide is controversial. Critics point out that nitrous oxide produces bowel distention[21,22] and may increase the incidence of postoperative nausea and vomiting. However, a recent prospective double-blind study of 50 patients undergoing laparoscopic cholecystectomy failed to demonstrate any significant differences in operating conditions, bowel distention, or postoperative nausea and vomiting whether or not 70% nitrous oxide was used.[13]

Insufflation with CO_2 leads to varying degrees of systemic absorption and the potential for hypercarbia.[3] Monitoring end-tidal CO_2 levels can provide a guide for increasing minute ventilation to maintain normocarbia. This assumes a constant gradient between arterial CO_2 and end-tidal CO_2. Although this assumption appears generally valid in healthy patients undergoing laparoscopy,[1,23] it does not apply in instances of increased alveolar dead space. For example, any significant reduction in lung perfusion increases alveolar dead space, dilutes expired CO_2, and thereby lessens end-tidal CO_2 measurements. This may occur during laparoscopy if cardiac output drops because of high insufflation pressures, reverse Trendelenburg position, or gas embolism. Furthermore, abdominal distention lowers pulmonary compliance. Large tidal volumes are usually avoided because they are associated with high peak inspiratory pressures and can cause considerable movement of the surgical field. The resulting choice of lower tidal volumes and higher respiratory rates may lead to poor alveolar gas sampling and erroneous end-tidal CO_2 measurements. In fact, end-tidal CO_2 values have been found to be particularly unreliable in patients with significant cardiac or pulmonary disease undergoing laparoscopy.[2] Thus placement of an arterial catheter should be considered in patients with cardiovascular disease or if large changes in cardiac output or high airway pressures are anticipated. A Foley catheter should be placed for all but brief procedures.

Complications

Gas Extravasation. The use of pressurized gas introduces the possibility of extravasation of CO_2 along tissue planes, resulting in subcutaneous emphysema, pneumomediastinum, or pneumothorax.[24] An increase in peak inspiratory pressure may signal a developing pneumothorax, inadequate muscle relaxation, endotracheal tube obstruction, or endobronchial intubation. Although subcutaneous emphysema is often obvious clinically, arterial blood gases, end-tidal CO_2, and chest x-ray films are helpful in establishing the diagnosis of pneumomediastinum or pneumothorax. Possible causes of these complications include misplacement of the insufflating cannula in the subcutaneous tissues,[25] instrumental rupture of the pleura,[26] and dissection of gas through a defect in the diaphragm.[10] Nitrous oxide should be discontinued if it is being utilized as part of the anesthetic technique, and insufflating pressures should be decreased as much as possible. Residual deposits of CO_2 are usually absorbed uneventfully postoperatively but may stress the ventilatory capabilities of patients with preexisting pulmonary disease or metabolic acidosis. These patients may benefit from the continuation of mechanical ventilation into the immediate postoperative period.

Gas Embolization. Venous CO_2 embolism resulting from unintentional insufflation of gas into an open vein may lead to hypoxemia, pulmonary hypertension, pulmonary edema, and cardiovascular collapse.[27] However, because of the relatively high solubility of CO_2, a larger volume of gas is required and the effects are more transient compared to air embolism. As opposed to the diagnosis of air embolism, end-tidal CO_2 increases during CO_2 gas embolism, assuming gas bubbles are able to gain access to the pulmonary circulation. Treatment includes immediate release of the pneumoperitoneum, discontinuation of nitrous oxide, insertion of a central venous catheter for gas aspiration, and placement of the patient in a head-down left lateral decubitus position.[28]

Gastric Reflux. Whether patients undergoing laparoscopic surgery are at particularly high risk for gastric reflux is controversial. It seems logical that insufflation of the peritoneal cavity and a head-down position would increase the likelihood of regurgitation; however, reflux has been reported to be a rare finding, as measured by changes in intraoperative esophageal pH.[29] Obviously patients at risk for aspiration (e.g., those with hiatal hernia, morbid obesity, and gastric outlet obstruction) must be managed accordingly.

Cardiovascular Instability. Vagal stimulation during trochar insertion, peritoneal insufflation, or manipulation of viscera can result in bradycardia and even sinus arrest.[10] Although this usually resolves spontaneously, elimination of the stimulus (e.g., disinflation of the peritoneum) and administration of a vagolytic drug (e.g., atropine sulfate or glycopyrrolate) should be considered. Routine premedication with atropine sulfate has been recommended by some authors.[30] The cardiac effects of laparoscopic surgery have been described previously. One review reported a higher incidence of intraoperative hypotension during laparoscopic cholecystectomy compared with cholecystectomy by laparotomy despite a younger and healthier patient population.[31] Preoperative fluid loading has been recommended to avoid this complication.[31] Hypotension due to hemorrhage following perforation of a major abdominal vessel by the pneumoperitoneum needle or trochar is rare, but the number of such complications can be deceptive given the potential for a large retroperitoneal hematoma[30] and the difficulty in estimating blood loss during laparoscopic procedures. Conversion to an open surgical procedure may be required.

Pulmonary Dysfunction. Even though laparoscopic procedures are associated with less muscle trauma and incisional pain than open surgery, pulmonary function can be significantly altered for at least 24 hours postoperatively.[32] For example, forced expiratory volume, forced vital capacity, and forced expiratory flow are reduced by approximately 25% following laparoscopic cholecystectomy as opposed to a 50% reduction following open cholecystectomy.[33,34] The cause of this dysfunction may be partially related to diaphragmatic tension during the pneumoperitoneum.[31]

Pain. Following laparoscopic surgery, incisional pain and pain from diaphragmatic irritation referred to the neck and shoulders are common. Strategies for pain control include local anesthetic infiltration into puncture sites and peritoneal instillation,[35] activation of a thoracic epidural with a local anesthetic,[34] parenteral ketorolac,[36] and bilateral intercostal nerve blocks.[37] Large doses of systemic opioids are generally avoided because of their potential for causing nausea and vomiting.

Nausea and Vomiting. Nausea and vomiting are common postoperative complications of laparoscopic surgery. Interestingly, they occur despite routine emptying of the stomach with a nasogastric or orogastric tube. Possible causes include peritoneal distention, splanchnic manipulation, or celiac axis traction.[38] The following preventive measures have been suggested: avoidance of opioids,[38-40] intraoperative droperidol (0.625 mg) or metoclopramide (10 to 20 mg),[38] replacement of volatile anesthetics with propofol infusions,[39,41] acupoint injection,[42] and electroacupuncture.[43]

ANESTHESIA FOR THORACOSCOPIC SURGERY

Physiologic Effects of Pneumothorax During Spontaneous Ventilation

Mediastinal Shift. Whereas laparoscopy requires establishing a pneumoperitoneum by introducing pressurized CO_2 into the abdomen, thoracoscopy creates a pneumothorax by allowing air at atmospheric pressure to enter the chest (i.e., an open pneumothorax). Normally the lungs are kept expanded during spontaneous ventilation by the negative pleural pressure that results from the opposing tendencies of lung elastic recoil and chest wall expansion. When air enters the pleural space, the negative pleural pressure on that side of the chest is lost. This allows the ipsilateral lung (the "up lung" or "nondependent lung" when the patient is in the lateral decubitus position) to collapse from its unopposed elastic recoil. Negative pleural pressure is maintained on the contralateral side (the "down lung" or "dependent lung"). In fact, during spontaneous inspiration the pleural pressure on the dependent side becomes increasingly negative and shifts the mediastinum toward that side. This mediastinal shift decreases the tidal volume in the dependent lung and in extreme cases may lead to circulatory shock.[44]

Paradoxical Respiration. Besides causing mediastinal shift, the increasingly negative pleural pressure surrounding the dependent lung during spontaneous inspiration draws gas into that lung. In fact, because the gas in the nondependent lung is at atmospheric pressure, it tends to cross the carina and pass into the dependent lung. Thus the already collapsed lung becomes smaller during inspiration, whereas the dependent lung expands. This paradoxical respiration is reversed during expiration. During general anesthesia, mediastinal shift and paradoxical respiration are prevented by positive pressure ventilation.[44]

Physiologic Effects of the Lateral Decubitus Position

Awake Patients. The lateral decubitus position alters lung ventilation and perfusion. Specifically, dependent lung ventilation is increased because of more efficient contraction of the diaphragm and greater lung compliance compared with the nondependent side. Since gravity increases perfusion in the dependent lung, normal ventilation-perfusion matching is preserved.

Anesthetized Patients. General anesthesia decreases functional residual capacity and alters the relative compliance of the lungs so as to favor ventilation of the nondependent lung. Because the dependent lung still receives greater perfusion, a ventilation-perfusion mismatch results. Positive pressure ventilation and muscle paralysis further increase ventilation to the nondependent lung and worsen the ventilation-perfusion mismatch.[44] The end result may be hypoxemia in patients with severe preexisting lung disease.

Anesthetic Management

Local and Regional Anesthesia. Infiltration with local anesthetic or intercostal nerve blocks at the level of the incision and two levels above and below can provide adequate anesthesia for simple thoracoscopic procedures (e.g., chemical pleurodesis[45] or needle biopsy[46]). Despite the effects of mediastinal shift and paradoxical respiration described previously, these techniques are usually well tolerated and produce minimal changes in $PaCO_2$ and PaO_2. However, the increased time and multiple incisions required for most thoracoscopic foregut surgery preclude anything but general anesthesia.

General Anesthesia. Routine administration of positive pressure ventilation will expand the nondependent lung and prevent good visualization and surgical exposure. This problem is usually solved with one-lung anesthesia administered through a double-lumen endobronchial tube or bronchial blocker tube.[47] Of course, intentional collapse of the nondependent lung results in perfusion without ventilation on that side. The ensuing intrapulmonary shunt and widened PaO_2 gradient can result in hypoxemia. However, perfusion of the nonventilated lung is often decreased by hypoxic pulmonary vasoconstriction, surgical compression, or increased vascular resistance due to atelectasis. If the patient becomes hypoxemic despite an FiO_2 of 1.0, several interventions can be attempted, including confirmation of correct tube position with a fiberoptic bronchoscope, periodic inflation of the collapsed lung, continuous insufflation of oxygen into the collapsed lung, administration of continuous positive airway pressure to the collapsed lung, or administration of positive end-expiratory pressure to the ventilated lung.[48,49] CO_2 elimination is usually not greatly affected by one-lung ventilation if minute ventilation is unchanged or slightly increased. The potential wide swings in oxygenation are ideally monitored by continuous arterial blood gas measurement.

Alternatives to one-lung ventilation include high-frequency jet ventilation or apneic oxygenation. Although pressure-controlled insufflation of the chest with CO_2 at 4 to 11 mm Hg improves visualization,[49-51] it is generally unnecessary if a double-lumen tube can be successfully placed and can exaggerate the effects of mediastinal shift.

Complications

Cardiovascular instability is not uncommon during thoracoscopy. Causes of hypotension include surgical compression of cardiac structures, inadequate venous return and filling pressures, gas embolization, and dysrhythmias. Indwelling arterial catheters and central venous pressure or pulmonary artery catheters can prove quite useful in patients at high risk for these complications.[49] Some patients may benefit from mild inotropic support during one-lung ventilation.[49]

REFERENCES

1. Puri GD, Singh H. Ventilatory effects of laparoscopy under general anaesthesia. Brit J Anaesth 68:211-213, 1992.
2. Wittgen CM, Andrus CH, Fitzgerald SD, Baudendistel LJ, Dahms TE, Kaminski DL. Analysis of the hemodynamic and ventilatory effects of laparoscopic cholecystectomy. Arch Surg 126:997-1001, 1991.
3. Mullet CE, Viale JP, Sagnard PE, Miellet CC, Ruynat LG, Counioux HC, Motin JP, Boulez JP, Dargent DM, Annat GJ. Pulmonary CO_2 elimination during surgical procedures using intra- or extraperitoneal CO_2 insufflation. Anesth Analg 76:622-626, 1993.
4. Marshall RL, Jebson PJR, Davie IT, Scott DB. Circulatory effects of carbon dioxide insufflation of the peritoneal cavity for laparoscopy. Brit J Anaesth 44:680-684, 1972.
5. Kelman GR, Swapp GH, Smith I, Benzie RJ, Gordon NLM. Cardiac output and arterial blood-gas tension during laparoscopy. Brit J Anaesth 44:1155-1162, 1972.
6. Scott DB, Slawson KB. Respiratory effects of prolonged Trendelenburg position. Brit J Anaesth 40:103-107, 1968.
7. Wilcox S, Vandam LD. Alas, poor Trendelenburg and his position! A critique of its uses and effectiveness. Anesth Analg 67:574-578, 1988.
8. Heinonen J, Takki S, Tammisto T. Effect of the Trendelenburg tilt and other procedures on the position of endotracheal tubes. Lancet 1:850-853, 1969.
9. Burton A, Steinbrook RA. Precipitous decrease in oxygen saturation during laparoscopic surgery. Anesth Analg 76:1177-1178, 1993.

10. Shantha TR, Harden J. Laparoscopic cholecystectomy: anesthesia-related complications and guidelines. Surg Laparosc Endosc 1:173-178, 1991.
11. Bordahl PE, Raeder JC, Nordentoft J, Kirste U, Refsdal A. Laparoscopic sterilization under local or general anesthesia? A randomized study. Obstet Gynecol 81:137-141, 1993.
12. Edelman DS. Laparoscopic cholecystectomy under continuous epidural anesthesia in patients with cystic fibrosis. Am J Dis Child 145:723-724, 1991.
13. Taylor E, Feinstein R, White PF, Soper N. Anesthesia for laparoscopic cholecystectomy. Is nitrous oxide contraindicated? Anesthesiology 76:541-543, 1992.
14. Milki AA, Hardy RI, Danasouri I, Giudice LC, Lamb EJ. Local anesthesia with conscious sedation for laparoscopic intrafallopian transfer. Fertil Steril 58:1240-1242, 1992.
15. Ciofolo MJ, Clergue F, Seebacher J, Lefebvre G, Viars P. Ventilatory effects of laparoscopy under epidural anesthesia. Anesth Analg 70:357-361, 1990.
16. Goodwin APL, Rowe WL, Ogg MA. Day case laparoscopy. A comparison of two anaesthetic techniques using the laryngeal mask during spontaneous breathing. Anaesthesia 47:892-895, 1992.
17. Brimacombe J, Shorney N. Laparoscopy and the laryngeal mask airway? Anaesth Intensive Care 20:245-246, 1992.
18. Van Hemelrijck J, Smith I, White PF. Use of desflurane for outpatient anesthesia. A comparison with propofol and nitrous oxide. Anesthesiology 75:197-203, 1991.
19. Marshall CA, Jones RM, Bajorek PK, Cashman JN. Recovery characteristics using isoflurane or propofol for maintenance of anaesthesia: A double-blind controlled trial. Anaesthesia 47:461-466, 1992.
20. Karp KB. Anesthetic recovery after ambulatory laparoscopy: A comparison of isoflurane and alfentanil infusion. AANA J 58:83-88, 1990.
21. Verheecke G. Nitrous oxide and laparoscopy. Anaesthesia 46:698, 1991.
22. Thomas DV. Nitrous oxide should not be used during laparoscopy nor during other abdominal operations. Anaesthesia 47:80-81, 1992.
23. Brampton WJ, Watson RJ. Arterial to end-tidal carbon dioxide tension difference during laparoscopy: Magnitude and effect of anaesthetic technique. Anaesthesia 45:210-214, 1990.
24. Hasel R, Arora SK, Hickey DR. Intraoperative complications of laparoscopic cholecystectomy. Can J Anaesth 40:459-464, 1993.
25. Lew JKL, Gin T, Oh TE. Anaesthetic problems during laparoscopic cholecystectomy. Anaesth Intensive Care 20:91-92, 1992.
26. Biswas TK, Smith JA. Laparoscopic total fundoplication: Anaesthesia and complications. Anaesth Intensive Care 21:127-128, 1993.
27. Clark CC, Weeks DB, Gusdon JP. Venous carbon dioxide embolism during laparoscopy. Anesth Analg 56:650-652, 1977.
28. Hasnain JU, Matjasko MJ. Practical anesthesia for laparoscopic procedures. In Zucker C, ed. Surgical Laparoscopy. St. Louis: Quality Medical Publishing, 1991, pp 77-86.
29. Roberts CJ, Goodman NW. Gastro-oesophageal reflux during elective laparoscopy. Anaesthesia 45:1009-1011, 1990.
30. Nord HJ. Complications of laparoscopy. Endoscopy 24:693-700, 1992.
31. Rose DK, Cohen MM, Soutter DI. Laparoscopic cholecystectomy: The anaesthetist's point of view. Can J Anaesth 39:809-815, 1992.
32. Cunningham AJ, Brull SJ. Laparoscopic cholecystectomy: Anesthetic implications. Anesth Analg 76:1120-1133, 1993.
33. Frazee RC, Roberts JW, Okeson GC, Symmonds RE, Snyder SK, Hendricks JC, Smith RW. Open versus laparoscopic cholecystectomy: A comparison of postoperative pulmonary function. Ann Surg 213:651-654, 1991.
34. Rademaker BM, Ringer J, Odoom JA, de Wit LT, Kalkman CJ, Oosting J. Pulmonary function and stress response after laparoscopic cholecystectomy: Comparison with subcostal incision and influence of thoracic epidural analgesia. Anesth Analg 75:381-385, 1992.
35. Helvacioglu A, Weis R. Operative laparoscopy and postoperative pain relief. Fertil Steril 57:548-552, 1992.
36. Ding Y, White PF. Comparative effects of ketorolac, dezocine, and fentanyl as adjuvants during outpatient anesthesia. Anesth Analg 75:566-571, 1992.
37. Hanley ES. Anesthesia for laparoscopic surgery. Surg Clin North Am 72:1013-1019, 1992.
38. Parris WCV. Anaesthesia for laparoscopic cholecystectomy. Anaesthesia 46:997, 1991.

39. Stanton JM. Anaesthesia for laparoscopic cholecystectomy. Anaesthesia 46:317, 1991.
40. Okum GS, Colonna RP, Horrow JC. Vomiting after alfentanil anesthesia: Effect of dosing method. Anesth Analg 75:558-560, 1992.
41. Raftery S, Sherry E. Total intravenous anaesthesia with propofol and alfentanil protects against postoperative nausea and vomiting. Can J Anaesth 39:37-40, 1992.
42. Yang LC, Jawan B, Chen CN, Ho RT, Chang KA, Lee JH. Comparison of P6 acupoint injection with 50% glucose in water and intravenous droperidol for prevention of vomiting after gynecological laparoscopy. Acta Anaesthesiol Scand 37:192-194, 1993.
43. Ho RT, Jawan B, Fung ST, Cheung HK, Lee JH. Electro-acupuncture and postoperative emesis. Anaesthesia 45:327-329, 1990.
44. Morgan GE, Mikhail MS. Clinical Anesthesiology. East Norwalk, Conn.: Appleton & Lange, 1992, pp 404-418.
45. Rusch VW, Mountain C. Thoracoscopy under regional anesthesia for the diagnosis and management of pleural disease. Am J Surg 154:274-278, 1987.
46. Menzies R, Charbonneau M. Thoracoscopy for the diagnosis of pleural disease. Ann Intern Med 114:271-276, 1991.
47. Doyle DJ. Univent tube for thoracoscopic procedures. J Cardiothorac Vasc Anesth 7:374-375, 1993.
48. Barker SJ, Clarke C, Trivedi N, Hyatt J, Fynes M, Roessler P. Anesthesia for thoracoscopic laser ablation of bullous emphysema. Anesthesiology 78:44-50, 1993.
49. Hasnain JU, Krasna MJ, Barker SJ, Weiman DS, Whitman GJR. Anesthetic considerations for thoracoscopic procedures. J Cardiothorac Vasc Anesth 6:624-627, 1992.
50. Millar FA, Hutchison GL, Wood RAB. Anaesthesia for thoracoscopic pleurectomy and ligation of bullae. Anaesthesia 47:1060-1062, 1992.
51. Toy FK, Smoot RT. Preliminary experience with thoracoscopic surgery. J Laparoendosc Surg 2:303-309, 1992.

Chapter

3

Physiologic Alterations of Endosurgery

Adrian E. Ortega, M.D. • Jeffrey H. Peters, M.D.

An understanding of the physiologic effects of endoscopic surgery is essential since it is distinctly different from that encountered in traditional open surgery. Historically, laparoscopic surgery was performed predominantly in young, healthy women undergoing gynecologic procedures. Little is known of the physiologic consequences of laparoscopic surgery. The precise physiologic alterations associated with endoscopic surgery become even more critical as more complex procedures are being performed in patients with cardiopulmonary deficits and other systemic comorbid conditions. Differences have been described in terms of hemodynamic and pulmonary function. In addition, stress responses and immunologic alterations may differ significantly.

HEMODYNAMIC AND CARDIOVASCULAR PHYSIOLOGY

Most endoscopic surgery is performed in the abdomen and pelvis after gas is insufflated into the peritoneal cavity. Exceptions include the use of double-lumen endotracheal tubes without gas insufflation in the thorax and the use of abdominal wall-lifting devices to facilitate exposure in the abdominal and pelvic cavities. The dynamics of the pneumoperitoneum are central to understanding hemodynamic and any cardiovascular physiologic changes in endoscopic surgery.

Factors Influencing Hemodynamic Changes During Endoscopic Surgery Requiring Pneumoperitoneum

- Mechanical effects of increased intra-abdominal pressure
- Systemic effects of the absorbed gas
- Control of hypercarbia/minute ventilation
- Intravascular volume status
- Absolute level of intra-abdominal pressure
- Body positioning
- Anesthetic technique
- Cardiovascular comorbidity

The cardiovascular changes associated with pneumoperitoneum represent a complex balance between the mechanical effects of increased intra-abdominal pressure and the systemic effects of the absorbed gas. A variety of other factors mitigate the effects of these two fundamental processes, including control of hypercarbia through augmentation of minute ventilation, intravascular volume status, absolute level of intra-abdominal pressure, body positioning, anesthetic technique, degree of surgical or pain stimulus, and cardiovascular comorbidity.

Mechanical Effects of Increased Intra-Abdominal Pressure

Insufflation of the abdominal cavity and elevation of intra-abdominal pressure have three predominant mechanical effects: increased afterload, increased venous resistance, and increased mean systemic pressure (Fig. 3-1).

Isolated elevation of intra-abdominal pressure produces compression of the splanchnic circulation, resulting in increased afterload and depression of cardiac function. Kashtan et al.[1] demonstrated that intra-abdominal hypertension produced by infusion of saline solution into the peritoneal cavity resulted in increased cardiac afterload and a downward shift of the left ventricular function curve so that similar left atrial filling pressures resulted in lower cardiac output (Fig. 3-1).

Depressed cardiac function as a result of increased afterload can be either ameliorated or exacerbated by the effects of intra-abdominal hypertension on venous return through the inferior vena cava. Venous return is influenced by augmentation of both mean systemic pressure and venous resistance. The mean systemic pressure is the pressure at the level of capillaries, small veins, and venules. It therefore constitutes the "pump," or pressure head, driving venous return and reflects "preload" in the broadest sense. It is determined by blood volume, vascular tone, and pressure of tissues surrounding the capacitance vessels. Its effect as a pump driving venous return is opposed by venous resistance or the hydraulic resistance of the veins between the site of highest mean systemic pressure and the right atrium. In the context of endoscopic surgery using pneumoperitoneum the greatest venous resistance will be located in the intra-abdominal inferior vena cava. Intra-abdominal hypertension, therefore, results in two opposing factors on venous return: increased mean systemic pressure, which promotes venous return, and increased venous resistance, which impedes venous return (Fig. 3-1).

Kashtan et al.[1] demonstrated that in hypovolemic and normovolemic states the relative effect of increased venous resistance predominates over the increased mean systemic pressure. Venous return is diminished with intra-abdominal hypertension, and cardiac output is reduced by Starling mechanisms (Fig. 3-2). Conversely, in relatively hypervolemic subjects the increased mean systemic pressure produces increased hydrostatic pressure within the inferior vena cava, which is minimally compressed. The pump effect of increased mean systemic pressure therefore influences venous return to a greater degree than the increased venous resistance in hypervolemia. The net effect is increased venous return and increased cardiac output as mediated by Starling mechanisms (Fig. 3-2).

Cardiac performance in terms of the mechanical effects of the pneumoperitoneum is therefore most dependent on the patient's volume status but is also influenced by the level of intra-abdominal pressure applied. Diamant et al.[2] found that an intra-abdominal pressure of 5 mm Hg in dogs was associated with increased flow through the inferior vena cava, increased cardiac output, and mean arterial pressure. At an intra-abdominal pressure of 40 mm Hg, caval flow, cardiac output, and mean arterial

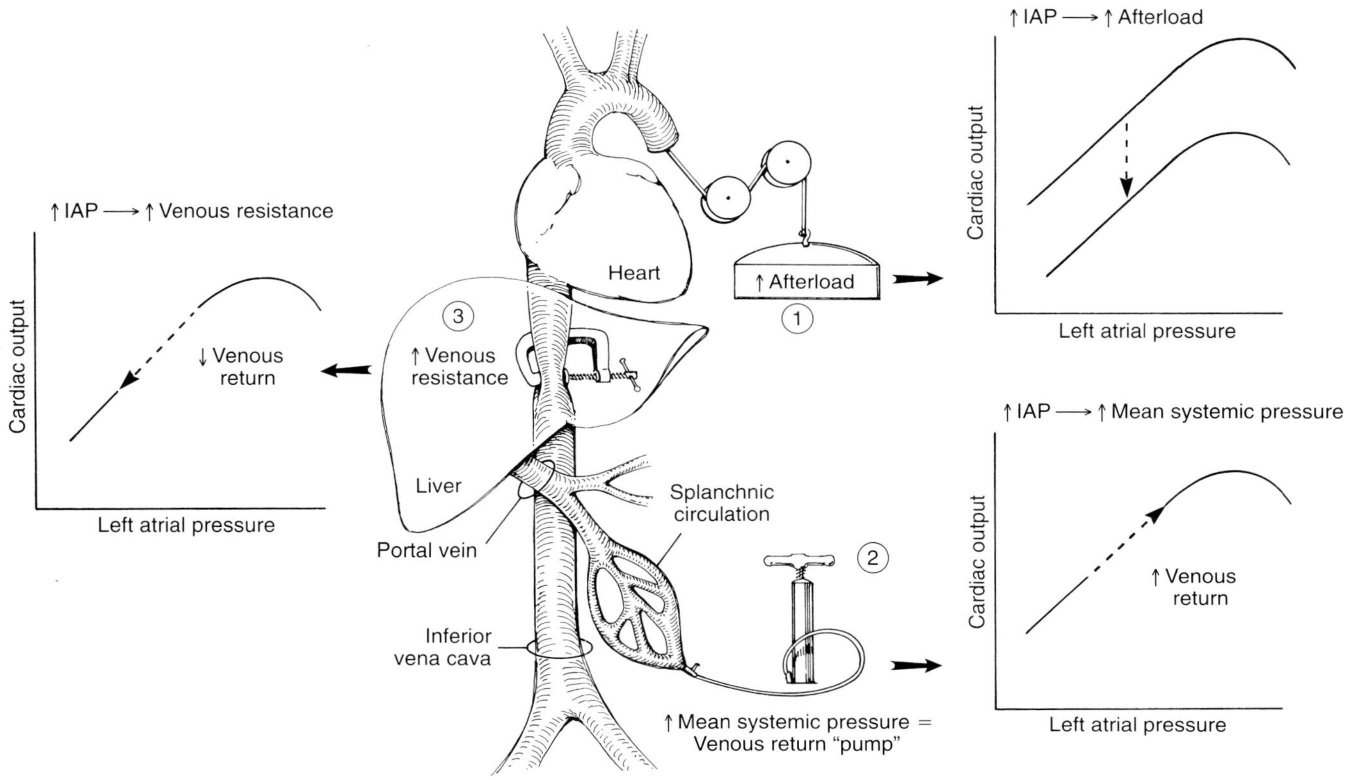

Fig. 3-1. Hemodynamic effects of increased intra-abdominal pressure (IAP). *1*, Increased afterload increases the work of the heart as well as myocardial oxygen consumption. *2*, Intra-abdominal hypertension increases venous resistance at the level of the intra-abdominal inferior vena cava, which impedes venous return. *3*, Increasing mean systemic pressure augments the "pump" effect around capacitance vessels, tending to drive venous return toward the heart. The isolated impact of these effects is depicted in each Starling curve.

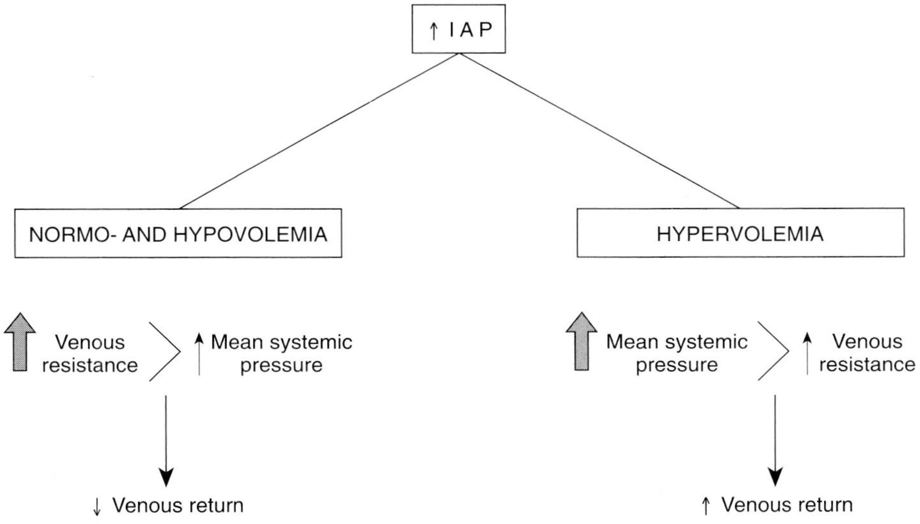

Fig. 3-2. Hemodynamic effects of increased intra-abdominal pressure on venous return (volume dependence). Increased intra-abdominal pressure in normovolemic and hypovolemic subjects produces an elevation of venous resistance that is greater than the concomitant increase in mean systemic pressure. The net result is decreased venous return during insufflation in normo- and hypovolemic patients. Conversely, relatively hypervolemic subjects experience an increased mean systemic pressure that is greater than the elevation in venous resistance. Hypervolemic patients experience increased venous return during insufflation.

pressure were diminished. Similarly, Kelman et al.[3] reported that intra-abdominal pressures up to 20 mm Hg were associated with increased central filling pressures and cardiac output. Elevations of intra-abdominal pressures to 40 mm Hg were associated with decreased central venous pressure and cardiac output.

Physiologic Effects of Gas Absorption During Pneumoperitoneum

Since the inception of laparoscopy a variety of gases have been used to induce pneumoperitoneum, including air, nitrous oxide, carbon dioxide, and more recently helium and argon. In 1924 Zolikollifer suggested that carbon dioxide may be the gas of choice.[4] Unlike air or nitrous oxide, carbon dioxide does not support combustion. It is clear, colorless, widely available, and rapidly absorbed from the abdominal cavity.

Absorption from the abdominal cavity of an insufflated gas depends on net diffusion and perfusion of the peritoneum. Net diffusion can be expressed as a single formula:

$$D = \frac{\Delta P \times A \times S}{d \times \sqrt{MW}}$$

in which D is the diffusion rate, ΔP is the partial pressure difference between the abdominal cavity and the bloodstream, A is the cross-sectional area between the two, S is the solubility of the gas, d is the distance across which diffusion takes place, and MW is the molecular weight of the gas. The two properties unique to each gas are its solubility and its molecular weight. This ratio of $S/\sqrt{MW}$ is the diffusion coefficient. If oxygen is arbitrarily assigned a diffusion coefficient of 1, the relative plasma diffusion coefficients of a variety of gases are as follows:

Oxygen	1.0
Carbon dioxide	20.3
Nitrogen	0.53
Helium	0.95
Nitrous oxide	11.8

Carbon dioxide is 20 times as diffusible as oxygen or helium and 40 times as diffusible as nitrogen. The principal determinants of gas absorption from a body cavity are therefore the difference in partial pressures between the two compartments (peritoneum and bloodstream) and the diffusion coefficient of the gas. Because of its high solubility, carbon dioxide reaches rapid equilibrium with the blood circulating at the surface of the peritoneal cavity. Absorption is also influenced by the rate of blood flow to the peritoneum. Increases in cardiac output will also increase gas absorption from the peritoneal cavity (Fig. 3-3).

Once absorbed into the bloodstream, only a small fraction of carbon dioxide is carried in solution. Most is bound by hemoglobin and ultimately eliminated by the lungs. Not all carbon dioxide is eliminated by the lungs during periods of hypercarbia. The body responds by moving carbon dioxide into various storage sites.[5] The total carbon dioxide storage capacity of the body is estimated to be 120 L. In addition to the hemoglobin-buffering system, other storage facilities for carbon dioxide include bone and visceral stores such as skeletal muscle. Bone constitutes the largest potential reservoir.

The net effect of carbon dioxide storage is to lower the circulating levels of

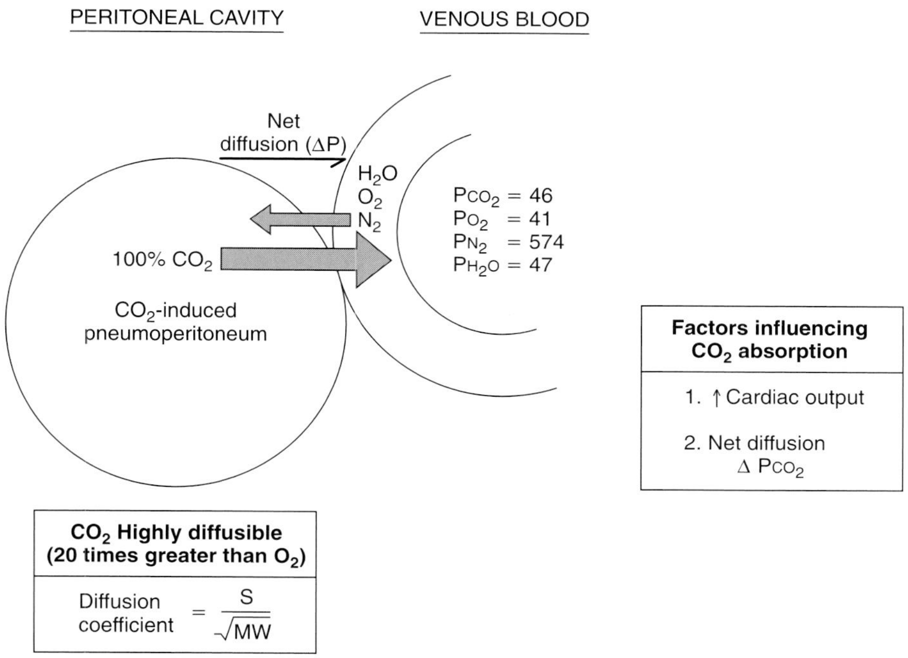

Fig. 3-3. Systemic absorption of insufflated carbon dioxide. Differences in pressures of carbon dioxide in the peritoneal cavity and the bloodstream favor its absorption. This process is rapid for carbon dioxide given its high solubility in comparison to other gases. Increased cardiac output also favors increased absorption.

carbon dioxide. Short periods of hypercarbia such as that produced by a Valsalva maneuver may only result in increased alveolar and blood carbon dioxide. Longer periods (20 to 60 minutes) such as those seen during insufflation for endoscopic procedures may result in recruitment of skeletal muscle and other visceral storage sites. Periods of hypercarbia of several weeks' duration result in significant storage of carbon dioxide by bone. These storage dynamics explain why patients in chronic carbon dioxide retentive states show precipitously increased and exaggerated plasma levels of carbon dioxide and why patients exposed to long periods of insufflation may have elevated arterial carbon dioxide ($PaCO_2$) for extended periods of time following desufflation.

Hypercarbia and acidosis are well-documented sequelae of the carbon dioxide–induced pneumoperitoneum used in endoscopic surgery. Liu et al.[6] studied 16 healthy patients undergoing laparoscopic cholecystectomy, observing a 10 mm Hg rise in both the mean arterial and end-tidal carbon dioxide concentrations. Eighty percent of patients required increased minute ventilation to maintain safe levels of carbon dioxide. In these otherwise healthy patients there was excellent correlation between the end-tidal carbon dioxide ($PetCO_2$) and arterial blood gas measurement of carbon dioxide ($PaCO_2$).

The correlation of $PetCO_2$ and $PaCO_2$ diminishes in patients with pulmonary disease and other comorbid conditions. Witgen et al.[7] compared a group of healthy American Society of Anesthesiologists (ASA) class I patients undergoing laparoscopic cholecystectomy with ASA class II and III patients. They observed more pronounced hypercarbia and acidosis in the ASA class II and III than in healthy ASA class I patients. Moreover, in those patients with additional comorbidity, the $PetCO_2$ may differ widely from arterial blood gas analysis of carbon dioxide. This latter observation is because end-tidal capnography measures carbon dioxide at the end of expiration and contains both dead space air and alveolar air. Chronic lung diseases increase the dead space component of expired air, resulting in an underestimation of the $PetCO_2$ in comparison to arterial blood gas measurements.

Work by Leighton et al.[8] and Bongard et al.[9] should dispel any misconceptions that hypercarbia and acidosis are the results of mechanical impairment of pulmonary function resulting from the pneumoperitoneum. They compared the effects of carbon dioxide– and helium-induced pneumoperitoneum on cardiopulmonary function in both animal models and human subjects undergoing laparoscopic cholecystectomy. In the latter study, carbon dioxide–induced pneumoperitoneum was associated with a 15 mm Hg rise in $PaCO_2$. The arterial carbon dioxide concentration did not change with helium-induced pneumoperitoneum.[9] They also noted a significant corresponding acidosis in the carbon dioxide–induced pneumoperitoneum, with the mean pH falling from 7.43 to 7.29.

Because of differences in partial pressures between the peritoneal cavity and the bloodstream in carbon dioxide–induced pneumoperitoneum and the high solubility of carbon dioxide, a steady state is established rapidly, producing elevations in $PaCO_2$. Unlike an inert gas such as helium, carbon dioxide exhibits potent effects on the heart and vasculature mediated through the direct effects of both hypercarbia and acidosis and indirect effects mediated through the sympathetic nervous system (Fig. 3-4).

The direct effects of hypercarbia and acidosis on the myocardium and blood vessels are generally opposite those mediated through increased sympathetic activity.[10,11] Hypercarbia and acidosis are myocardial depressants. The predominant effect on denervated blood vessels appears to be vasodilation. The relative importance of increasing $PaCO_2$ vs. decreasing pH is unknown. Moreover, the greatest effect of hypercarbia and acidosis appears to be on the capacitance blood vessels, that is, the postarteriolar capillaries and veins.

Paradoxically, the aortic and carotid body chemoreceptors are exquisitely sensitive to hypercarbia. Chemoreceptor afferent impulses stimulate the posterior hypothalamus, the mesencephalic reticular substance, as well as respiratory and vasomotor centers to produce hyperventilation, cortical activation, increased sympathetic outflow, and increased skeletal muscular activity. The overall effects of these "centrally mediated" actions of hypercarbia coupled with increased adrenomedullary discharge are responsible for the production of tachycardia, enhanced myocardial contractility, vasoconstriction, and arterial hypertension. In effect, the centrally mediated actions of carbon dioxide antagonize its direct effects on the myocardium and the peripheral vascular system. In healthy normal subjects breathing carbon dioxide–rich air the net effects include elevation in circulating levels of epinephrine and norepinephrine as well as hyperventilation. Carbon dioxide "breathing" also produces greater increases in cardiac output relative to the arterial hypertension. Overall, there is a decrease in systemic vascular resistance because the local vasodilatory effects of carbon dioxide are greater than the neurologically or sympathetically mediated vasoconstriction.[10]

Rasmussen et al.[12] examined the effects of hypercarbia and cardiac function in 12 ASA class II and III patients undergoing carotid endarterectomy. Anesthesia was maintained with a combination of oxygen, nitrous oxide, and methoxyflurane. Eleva-

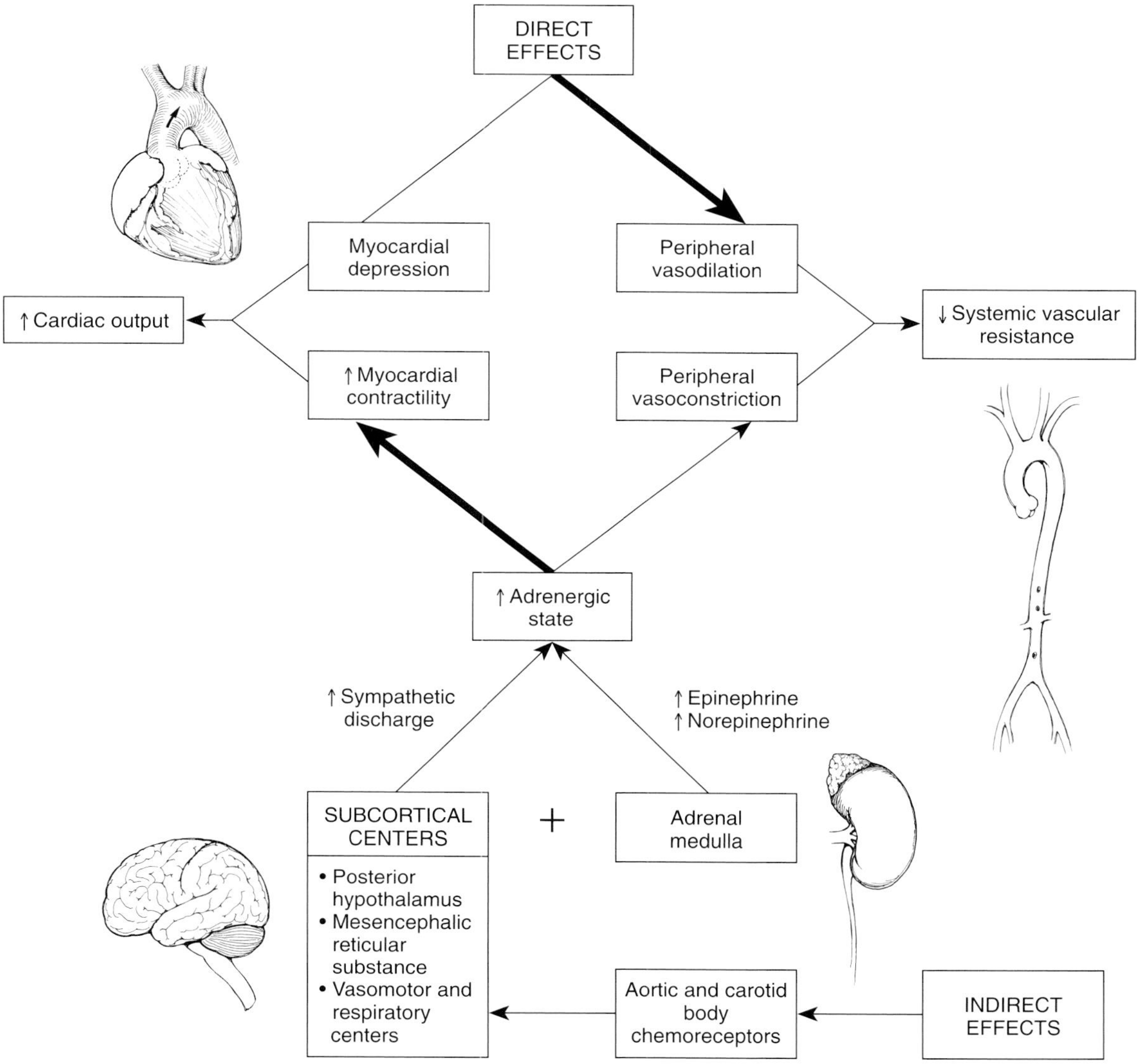

Fig. 3-4. Hemodynamic effects of hypercarbia. Increased $PaCO_2$ and acidosis produce hemodynamic alterations through their direct actions on the heart and vasculature as well as indirect effects mediated through the sympathetic nervous system. The direct and indirect effects generally oppose one another. Overall, hypercarbia produces increased cardiac output with diminished systemic vascular resistance.

tions in the $PaCO_2$ to 56 to 65 mm Hg, a range not uncommonly seen in laparoscopy, produced significant elevations in cardiac output and stroke volume coupled with decreased systemic vascular resistance. Plasma catecholamines were increased two to three times above the baseline.

Extreme hypercarbia adversely affects myocardial contractility. The attendant acidosis interferes with the ability of cells to respond to the chemical stimulus of sympathetic nerves. Moreover, acidosis stimulates parasympathetic nervous activity, potentially manifest as increased cardiac vagal tone.

Other Factors Affecting Hemodynamic Function

An analysis of the literature on hemodynamic function in laparoscopic surgery reveals confounding and confusing results. Studies reporting increased, decreased, or unchanged cardiac output and every other hemodynamic parameter during insufflation can be found in the literature.[3,13-21] These discrepant results suggest that a variety of cardiovascular manifestations are possible and depend on a number of factors. The importance of intravascular volume status and control of hypercarbia have been described. Several other factors may contribute to the net hemodynamic effects observed in any given procedure and patient, including body positioning, anesthetic technique, and underlying cardiopulmonary disease (Fig. 3-5).

Body positioning in the horizontal, Trendelenburg, and reverse Trendelenburg stations influences venous return and cardiac output (see Chapter 2). Pentecost et al.[22] demonstrated that a 20-degree Trendelenburg position could increase cardiac output by 20%. Kelman et al.[3] studied hemodynamic changes in patients undergoing laparoscopy in the horizontal vs. Trendelenburg positions. Central filling pressures and cardiac outputs were significantly greater in the patients tilted head down.

The importance of anesthetic techniques in determining the direction of hemodynamic changes associated with laparoscopic surgery is self-evident. Inhalational agents such as halothane produce myocardial depression, whereas others such as isoflurane produce enhanced myocardial contractility. Alterations of the sympa-

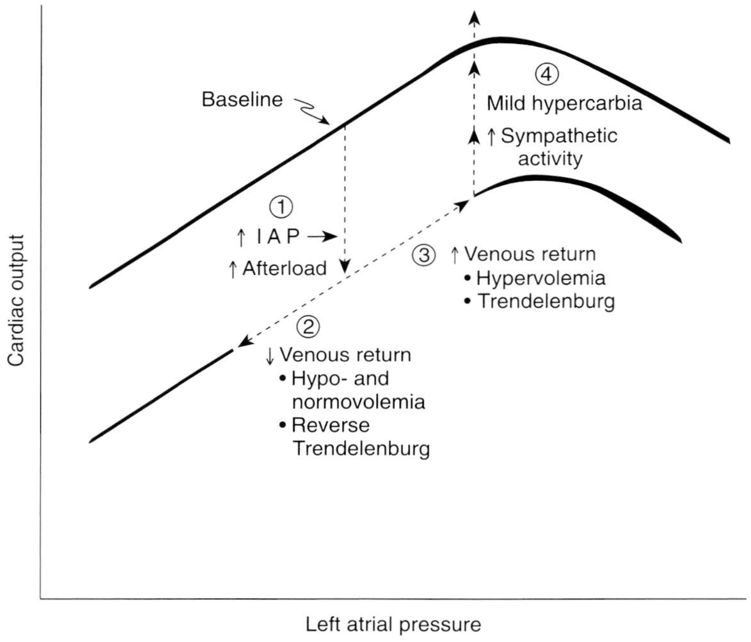

Fig. 3-5. Summary of cardiac function after carbon dioxide insufflation. *1*, Increased intra-abdominal pressure increases afterload, downshifting the Starling curve. *2*, Venous return is diminished in hypo- and normovolemia as well as in the reverse Trendelenburg position. *3*, Relative hypervolemia results in increasing venous return that drives the Starling curve higher. *4*, Mild to moderate degrees of hypercarbia shift the Starling curve up via the net effects of enhanced sympathetic activity. Other factors modulating these responses include anesthetic technique and underlying cardiac disease.

thetic activity from surgical stimuli with narcotic agents may also be important. Although there are no comparative studies of the effects of anesthetic regimens or the difference in hemodynamic effects during endoscopic surgery, such investigations may be warranted.

Patients with significant cardiopulmonary comorbidity deserve special mention. Because of the association of pulmonary disease with cardiovascular disease and vice versa, patients in both disease groups may be at risk for intraoperative hypercarbia and acidosis with the attendant alterations in hemodynamic function. Safran et al.[16] examined the cardiopulmonary responses in 15 high-risk cardiac patients (ASA class III and IV) undergoing laparoscopy. They reported significant elevations in central filling pressures, systemic vascular resistance, and mean arterial pressure. Cardiac output was reduced on average. However, risk class per se was not predictive of the degree of hemodynamic compromise. They concluded that pneumoperitoneum increased mean arterial pressure and systemic vascular resistance as well as decreased cardiac output in patients with poor cardiac reserve. These investigators suggested that preload augmentation may offset the stress of increased afterload, helping to avoid left ventricular decompensation. This approach counters the more common practice of reducing preload in patients with left ventricular failure. It does, however, seem reasonable given the dynamics of increased intra-abdominal pressure and its effects on venous return. This study underscores the importance of careful and invasive monitoring of high-risk patients during minimally invasive procedures.

Organ-Specific Perfusion

Organ-specific or regional blood flow may be acutely altered during abdominal insufflation. Ishizaki et al.[18,23] demonstrated in a canine model that insufflation to 16 mm Hg diminished cardiac output as well as flow through the portal vein and superior mesenteric artery. Hepatic arterial flow was not significantly altered.

Pneumoperitoneum may also diminish renal perfusion. Iwase et al.[24] compared renal blood flow in patients undergoing laparoscopic and minilaparotomy cholecystectomy by measuring urine output and clearance of *p*-aminohippurate. Although no significant differences in blood pressure, pulmonary artery pressure, central venous pressure, or cardiac index were detected in the two groups, transient oliguria and decreased renal plasma flow calculated from clearance of *p*-aminohippurate were noted.

The mechanisms responsible for these alterations in organ-specific blood flow remain obscure. One possible explanation invokes Poiseuille's law:

$$\text{Flow} \propto \text{Radius}^4$$

Blood flow through any given vessel is proportional to its radius to the fourth power. Minor diminution in vessel diameter may dramatically decrease flow. Other mechanisms invoked include humorally mediated vasoconstriction by carbon dioxide as well as intrinsic myogenic control of vascular tone produced by increased intra-abdominal pressure.

Venous Stasis

Femoral venous hypertension and venous stasis are associated with the pneumoperitoneum and exacerbated by positioning in the reverse Trendelenburg position.

Millard et al.[25] demonstrated a 37% reduction in peak systolic velocity in the common femoral vein measured by Doppler ultrasonography in patients undergoing laparoscopic cholecystectomy. Intermittent sequential pneumatic compression reversed the effect, returning the peak systolic velocity to normal. Clear documentation of an increased risk of venous thrombosis and pulmonary embolism following laparoscopic surgery is lacking. Anecdotal evidence supports prophylactic measures whenever possible.

PULMONARY FUNCTION

It has been recognized since the early part of this century that laparotomy, in particular upper abdominal surgery, results in a self-limited (5 to 7 days) but significant decrease in pulmonary function when preoperative and postoperative measurements are compared.[26]

Standard spirometric pulmonary function is derived from the rate of flow measured by having the patient inspire maximally to total lung capacity and then exhale as forcefully and as rapidly as possible to residual volume. The rate of airflow measured during this period indirectly reflects the flow resistance properties of the airways. Airway obstruction can be detected by calculating flow rates during certain time intervals along the forced vital capacity (FVC) curve, most commonly the volume exhaled in the first second, or the FEV_1. The FEV_1, expressed as a percentage of the FVC (FEV_1/FVC, termed the FEV%), is an alternative measure of airway obstruction. Normal patients can exhale 75% to 80% of the FVC in the first second. Obstructive diseases (such as asthma) tend to impair expiratory flow rates and cause a decline in FEV_1 and the FEV%. Restrictive conditions (such as postoperative pain) result in decreased FVC. Although the absolute volume of the FEV_1 may decline as well, the FEV_1 as a percentage of FVC is usually normal.

The pulmonary consequences of abdominal surgery are complex. Physiologic changes are related to anesthesia as well as the magnitude and type of the surgical procedure. Abdominal surgery generally results in a restrictive pattern of pulmonary physiologic change, with reduction of both vital capacity and function residual capacity.[27,28] Historically, investigators have measured decreases in tidal volume and FVC averaging 40% to 50% after an upper midline incision.[26] More recently, transcutaneous oxygen saturation monitoring has identified a 30% to 35% incidence of hypoxemia (O_2 saturation <85%) following laparotomy.[29]

A number of factors account for these observed changes.[27,30] Pulmonary volumes are markedly altered after upper abdominal surgery as a result of incisional pain, muscular dysfunction, and diaphragmatic alterations. Intercostal nerve blockade and epidural analgesia only partly return pulmonary measurements to their preoperative levels.[31-34] Careful study has found fluid accumulation in the pleural space in a large percentage of patients, which may also account for some of the observed changes.[35]

Investigations into the decrement in pulmonary function after open cholecystectomy have documented declines averaging 50%. Lattimer et al.[27] studied 46 patients after upper abdominal surgery and noted a 59% decline in FVC on postoperative day 1, which slowly improved to 27% by postoperative day 7. Similar changes were seen in the measured FEV_1. Patel et al.,[34] interested in the effects of incisional infiltration of bupivacaine, found a 49% decline in FVC immediately after open cholecystectomy, which improved to 21% with the use of a local anesthetic. Frazee et al.[36] reported that laparoscopic cholecystectomy diminishes pulmonary function by approximately one

Table 3-1. Pulmonary function after open and laparoscopic surgery*

Tests	Preop.	Postop.	%Diff.	$p^\dagger$
Forced vital capacity (L)				
Open (n = 9)	3.52 ± 0.32	2.24 ± 0.24	35.8	0.09
Laparoscopic (n = 31)	3.56 ± 0.18	2.67 ± 0.17	22.9	
Forced expiratory volume (L)				
Open (n = 9)	2.86 ± 0.33	1.81 ± 0.21	35.0	0.15
Laparoscopic (n = 31)	2.76 ± 0.15	2.01 ± 0.12	24.3	
Forced expiratory flow (L)				
Open (n = 7)	3.3 ± 0.47	1.98 ± 0.35	40.2	0.67
Laparoscopic (n = 31)	2.59 ± 0.21	1.83 ± 0.14	24.4	

Note: Results are given as the mean ± SEM.
*From Peters JH, Ortega A, Lehnerd SL, et al. The physiology of laparoscopic surgery: Pulmonary function after laparoscopic cholecystectomy. Surg Laparosc Endosc 3:370, 1993.
†Student's *t* test.

fourth. Peters et al.[37] compared FVC, FEV, and forced expiratory flow (FEF) in patients undergoing laparoscopic and open cholecystectomy (Table 3-1). Pulmonary function was less impaired following the laparoscopic procedure.

Putensen-Himmer et al.[38] reported a prospective randomized trial in 20 healthy (ASA class I) patients undergoing elective open and laparoscopic cholecystectomy. FVC and FEV were reduced by 57% and 54% in the open cholecystectomy patients 24 hours postoperatively. The laparoscopic patients experienced decrements from preoperative FVC and FEV_1 values of 30% and 15%, respectively. When measured 72 hours postoperatively, these values were more nearly normal in the laparoscopic patients than in those undergoing the open technique (FVC = 91% vs. 77% and FEV_1 = 92% vs. 77%).

The adequacy of postoperative pain control certainly influences the magnitude of change observed in postoperative pulmonary function but is difficult to control and measure. Schauer et al.[39] examined this issue in a comparative study of patients undergoing laparoscopic and open cholecystectomy. Pulmonary complications, including atelectasis and hypoxia, were less frequent in patients following laparoscopic cholecystectomy. They noted an eightfold decrease in postoperative pain medication delivered via patient-controlled analgesia devices in patients undergoing laparoscopic cholecystectomy.

Although the above studies highlight differences in postoperative pulmonary function in patients undergoing laparoscopic vs. conventional open surgery, preoperative pulmonary function tests continue to play an important role in identifying patients susceptible to extreme hypercarbia and acidosis during abdominal insufflation with carbon dioxide. Witgen et al.[40] examined over 80 demographic, laboratory, and perioperative parameters in 31 patients undergoing laparoscopic cholecystectomy. Preoperative arterial blood gas analysis and pulmonary functions tests were performed in an effort to identify patients at risk for intraoperative acidosis (pH < 7.35). Neither age nor preoperative arterial blood gas analysis predicted the development of acidosis. Preoperative pulmonary function tests demonstrating FEVs <70% and diffusion defects <80% of predicted values did identify patients at risk for intraoperative hypercarbia and acidosis.

METABOLIC AND STRESS HORMONAL RESPONSES

Injury and surgery are associated with metabolic and stress hormonal responses. Cuthbertson[41] defined two phases of the metabolic response to injury—an ebb or shock phase and a flow phase. Moore[42] later divided the flow phase into catabolic and anabolic stages. The ebb phase takes place in the first several hours following injury. It is characterized by hyperglycemia and restoration of circulatory volume and tissue perfusion. Once circulatory volume and tissue perfusion are restored, the flow phase begins. Catabolism pervades the early phases of injury. Eventually, once fluid deficits are corrected, infection and pain are controlled, oxygenation is restored, and wounds are closed, anabolism may begin.

The early metabolic alterations of injury include increased lipolysis, hyperglycemia secondary to gluconeogenesis and insulin resistance, and net proteolysis with negative nitrogen balance. These metabolic responses as well as other physiologic alterations induced by injury are mediated by complex interactions between a variety of systems, including the hypothalamic-pituitary axis, autonomic nervous system, endocrine system, mediators that have local and systemic actions such as cytokines, vascular endothelial cell products, and intracellular products of single cells.

Immediately after injury there is a rapid increase in the secretion of catecholamines. Because catecholamines rapidly disappear from blood, increased levels are not readily demonstrable following injury. An increase in urine catechols is much more readily apparent. Catecholamines increase lipolysis as well as promote gluconeogenesis and glycogenolysis.

Plasma cortisol is also transiently elevated, usually 24 to 48 hours following injury. It plays a permissive role in the actions of catecholamines. Growth hormone

Stress Hormonal Responses to Injury or Surgery*

Increased Release		Decreased Release or Unchanged
Epinephrine	Beta-endorphin	Insulin
Norepinephrine	Growth hormone	Estrogen
Dopamine	Prolactin	Testosterone
Glucagon	Somatostatin	Thryroxine
Renin	Eicosanoids	Triiodothyronine
Angiotensin	Histamine	Thyroid-stimulating hormone
Arginine vasopressin	Kinins	Follicle-stimulating hormone
ACTH	Serotonin	Luteinizing hormone
Cortisol	Interleukin-1	Immunoglobulin F
Aldosterone	Tumor necrosis factor	
	Interleukin-6	

*Adapted from Gann DS, Foster AH. Endocrine and metabolic responses to injury. In Schwartz SI, ed. Principles of Surgery, 6th ed. New York: McGraw-Hill, 1994, pp 3-59.

aids in the mobilization of lipids. Glucagon is also involved in glycogenolysis, gluconeogenesis, and lipolysis.

The stress hormonal responses are primarily tailored to the magnitude, duration, and nature of the injury. A variety of other factors mitigate the injury response, including gender, age, pain, nutritional status, and infection. For example, females have less of a metabolic and endocrine response than males.

The differences in metabolic and stress hormonal responses in endoscopic and open surgery are just beginning to be explored. Dominioni et al.[44] prospectively randomized patients to either laparoscopic or open cholecystectomy and observed greater elevations in cortisol, prolactin, and C-reactive protein in the patients having the open procedure. They concluded that laparoscopic cholecystectomy was less traumatic than open surgery. Mealy et al.[45] also noted greater elevations in sedimentation rates and C-reactive protein in patients undergoing open cholecystectomy than in those having laparoscopic cholecystectomy. Vanillylmandelic acid was higher in the laparoscopic group, suggesting a greater adrenergic response in these patients. Finally, McMahon et al.[46] reported very similar stress hormonal and acute-phase responses among patients undergoing either laparoscopic or minilaparotomy cholecystectomy. These investigators suggest that factors other than metabolic responses may be important in determining postoperative recovery. Further studies in broader operative settings, including more extensive procedures than cholecystectomy, are necessary to more fully understand potential differences in metabolic and stress responses during endoscopic and conventional surgery.

IMMUNOLOGIC RESPONSES

Despite the overlap between stress hormone and immunologic alterations in the postoperative period, more readily appreciable differences in immune function between endoscopic and open surgery are emerging. Harmon et al.[47] found greater elevations in interleukin-6 in patients undergoing open colectomy compared to those resected laparoscopically. Other investigators have demonstrated that early and exaggerated interleukin-6 responses are associated with significant subsequent postoperative morbidity.[48,49] Significantly greater depressions of lymphocyte counts (CD3 and OKDR) and T-cell proliferation (assayed by phytohemagglutinin-A) in patients undergoing laparoscopic vs. open cholecystectomy have been reported.[44,50] These studies suggest potentially fewer alterations of immune function following endoscopic than open surgery. Further study is needed to determine if minimally invasive procedures confer clinical advantages in terms of fewer infectious complications and benefits in oncologic surgery.

REFERENCES

1. Kashtan J, Green JF, Parsons EQ, Holcroft JW. Hemodynamic effects of increased abdominal pressure. J Surg Res 30:249, 1981.
2. Diamant M, Benumof JL, Saidman LJ. Hemodynamics of increased intra-abdominal pressure: Interaction with hypovolemia and halothane anesthesia. Anesthesiology 48:23, 1978.
3. Kelman GR, Swapp GH, Smith I, Benzie RJ, Gordon LM. Cardiac output and arterial blood-gas tension during laparoscopy. Br J Anaesth 44:1155, 1972.
4. Nadeau OE, Kampmeier OF. Endoscopy of the abdomen: Abdominoscopy. A preliminary study, including a summary of the literature and description of the technique. Surg Gynecol Obstet 41:259, 1925.
5. Farhi LE, Rahn H. Gas stores of the body and the unsteady state. J Appl Physiol 7:472, 1955.

6. Liu S-Y, Leighton T, Davis I, Klein S, Lippmann M, Bongard F. Prospective analysis of cardiopulmonary responses to laparoscopic cholecystectomy. J Laparendosc Surg 1:241, 1991.
7. Witgen CM, Andrus CH, Fitzgerald SD, Baudendistel LJ, Dahms TE, Kaminski DL. Analysis of hemodynamic and ventilatory effects of laparoscopic cholecystectomy. Arch Surg 126:997, 1991.
8. Leighton TA, Liu S-Y, Bongard FS. Comparative cardiopulmonary effects of carbon dioxide versus helium pneumoperitoneum. Surgery 113:527, 1993.
9. Bongard FS, Pianim NA, Leighton TA, Dubecz S, Davis IP, Lipmann M, Klein S, Liu SY. Helium insufflation for laparoscopic operation. Surg Gynecol Obstet 177:140, 1993.
10. Price HL. Effects of carbon dioxide on the cardiovascular system. Anesthesiology 21:652, 1960.
11. Richardson DW, Wasserman AJ, Patterson JL. General and regional circulatory responses to change in blood pH and carbon dioxide tension. J Clin Invest 90:31, 1961.
12. Rasmussen JP, Dauchot PJ, DePalma RG, Sorensen B, Regula G, Anton AH, Gravenstein JS. Cardiac function and hypercarbia. Arch Surg 113:1196, 1978.
13. Hodgson C, McClellan RMA, Newton JR. Some effects of peritoneal insufflation of carbon dioxide at laparoscopy. Anaesthesia 25:382, 1970.
14. Smith I, Benzie RJ, Gordon NLM, Kelman GR, Swapp GH. Cardiovascular effects of peritoneal insufflation of carbon dioxide for laparoscopy. Br Med J 3:410, 1971.
15. Lenz RJ, Thomas TA, Wilkins DG. Cardiovascular changes during laparoscopy: Studies of stroke and cardiac output using impedance cardiography. Anaesthesia 31:4, 1976.
16. Safran D, Sgambati S, Orlando R. Laparoscopy in high-risk cardiac patients. Surg Gynecol Obstet 176:598, 1993.
17. Johannsen G, Anderson H, Juhl B. The effects of general anaesthesia on hemodynamic events during laparoscopy with CO_2 insufflation. Acta Anaesthesiol Scand 33:132, 1989.
18. Ishizaki Y, Bandai Y, Shimomura K, Abe H, Ohtomo Y, Idezuki Y. Changes in splanchnic blood flow and cardiovascular effects following peritoneal insufflation of carbon dioxide. Surg Endosc 7:420, 1993.
19. Westerband A, Van De Water JM, Amzallag M, Lebowitz DW, Nwasokwa ON, Chadavoyne R, About-Taleb A, Wang X, Wise L. Cardiovascular changes during laparoscopic cholecystectomy. Surg Gynecol Obstet 175:535, 1992.
20. Marshall RL, Jebson DJR, Davie IT, Scott DB. Circulatory effects of carbon dioxide insufflation of the peritoneal cavity for laparoscopy. Br J Anaesth 44:680, 1972.
21. Motew M, Ivankovich AD, Bieniarz J, Albrecht R, Zahed B, Scommegna A. Cardiovascular effects and acid-base and blood gas changes during laparoscopy. Am J Obstet Gynecol 115:1002, 1973.
22. Pentecost BL, Irving DW, Shillingford JP. The effects of posture on the blood flow in the inferior vena cava. Clin Sci 24:149, 1963.
23. Ishizaki Y, Bandai Y, Shimomura K, Abe H, Ohtomo Y, Idezuki Y. Safe intra-abdominal pressure of carbon dioxide pneumoperitoneum during laparoscopic surgery. Surgery 114:549, 1993.
24. Iwase K, Takenaka H, Oshima S, Ohata T, Ishizaka T, Yagura A. Serial changes in renal function during laparoscopic cholecystectomy—A comparison with mini-laparotomy cholecystectomy [abst]. Presented at the International Society of Surgery, Hong Kong, August 1993.
25. Millard JA, Hill BB, Cook PS, Fenoglio ME, Stahlgren L. Intermittent sequential pneumatic compression in prevention of venous stasis associated with pneumoperitoneum during laparoscopic surgery. Arch Surg 128:914, 1993.
26. Beecher HK. The measured effect of laparotomy on respiration. J Clin Invest 12:63, 1993.
27. Latimer RG, Dickman M, Day WC, Gunn ML, Schmidt CD. Ventilatory patterns and cardiopulmonary complications after upper abdominal surgery determined by preoperative pulmonary spirometry and blood gas analysis. Am J Surg 122:622, 1971.
28. Gal TJ. Physiologic basis and rationale for pulmonary function testing in patients undergoing head and neck surgery. Otolaryngol Clin North Am 14:723, 1982.
29. Aldren CP, Barr LC, Leech RD. Hypovolemia and postoperative pulmonary complications. Br J Surg 78:1307, 1991.
30. Ford GT, Whitelow WA, Rosenal JW, Cruse PJ, Cuenter CA. Diaphragm function after upper abdominal surgery in humans. Am Rev Respir Dis 127:431, 1983.
31. Vadeboncover TR, Riegler FX, Gautt RS, Weinberger. A randomized, double blind comparison of the effects of interpleural bupivacaine and saline on morphine requirements and pulmonary function after cholecystecotmy. Anesthesiology 71:339, 1989.

32. Hendolin H, Lahtinene J, Tuppurainen T, Partanen K. The effect of thoracic epidural analgesia on respiratory function after cholecystecotmy. Acta Anaesthesiol Scand 31:645, 1987.
33. Ross WB, Tweedic JH, Leong YP, Wyman A, Smithers BM. Intercostal blockage and pulmonary function after cholecystecotmy. Surgery 105:166, 1989.
34. Patel JM, Lanzofome RJ, Williams JS, Muller BV, Hinshaw JR. The effects of incisional infiltration of bupivacaine hydorchloride upon pulmonary functions, atelectasis and narcotic need following elective cholecystectomy. Surg Gynecol Obstet 157:378, 1983.
35. Light RW, George RB. Incidence and significance of pleural effusion after abdominal surgery. Chest 69:621, 1976.
36. Frazee RC, Roberts RW, Okeson GC, Symonds RE, Snyder SK, Hendricks JL, Smith RW. Open versus laparoscopic cholecystectomy: A comparison of postoperative pulmonary function. Ann Surg 213:651, 1991.
37. Peters JH, Ortega A, Lehnerd SL, Campbell AJ, Schwartz DC, Ellison EC, Innes JT. The physiology of laparosopic surgery: Pulmonary function after laparoscopic cholecystectomy. Surg Laparosc Endosc 3:370, 1993.
38. Putensen-Himmer G, Putensen C, Lammer H, Lingnau W, Aigner F, Benzer H. Comparison of postoperative respiratory function after laparoscopy or open laparotomy for cholecystectomy. Anesthesiology 77:675, 1992.
39. Schauer PR, Luna J, Ghiatas AA, Glen ME, Warren JM, Sirinek KR. Pulmonary function after laparoscopic cholecystectomy. Surgery 114:389, 1993.
40. Witgen CM, Naumheim KS, Andrus CH, Kaminski DL. Preoperative pulmonary function evaluation for laparoscopic cholecystectomy. Arch Surg 128:880, 1993.
41. Cuthbertson DP. Observations on the disturbance of metabolism by injury to the limbs. Q J Med 1:233, 1932.
42. Moore FD. Bodily changes in surgical convalescence. Ann Surg 137:289, 1953.
43. Gann DS, Foster AH. Endocrine and metabolic responses to injury. In Schwartz SI, ed. Principles of Surgery, 6th ed. New York: McGraw-Hill, 1994, pp 3-59.
44. Dominioni L, Cuffari S, Giudice G, Nicora L, Dionigi R. The acute phase response after laparoscopic cholecystectomy and after open cholecystectomy [abst]. Presented at the International Society of Surgery, Hong Kong, August 1993.
45. Mealy K, Gallagher H, Barry M, Lennon F, Traynor O, Hyland J. Physiologic and metabolic responses to open and laparoscopic cholecystectomy. Br J Surg 79:1061, 1992.
46. McMahon AJ, O'Dayer PJ, Cruikshank AM, McMillan DC, O'Reilly DSJ, Lowe GDO, Rumley A, Logen RW, Baxter JN. Comparison of metabolic responses to laparoscopic and minilaparotomy cholecystectomy. Br J Surg 80:1255, 1993.
47. Harmon G, Senagore A, Kilbride M, Luchtefeld M, MacKeigan J, Warzynksi M. Cortisol and IL-6 response attenuated following laparoscopic colectomy [abst]. Presented at the Society of American Gastrointestinal Endoscopic Surgeons, Phoenix, Arizona, April 3, 1993.
48. Baigrie RJ, Lamont PM, Kwiatknowsli D, Dallman MJ, Morris PM. The cytokine response to major surgery. Br J Surg 79:757, 1992.
49. Roumen RM, Hendriks T, Van der Meer JWM, Garis RJA. Cytokine patterns in patients after major vascular surgery, hemorrhogic shock, and severe blunt trauma relation with subsequent adult respiratory syndrome and multiple organ failure. Ann Surg 218:769, 1993.
50. Griffith J, Everett N, Corley P, McMahon M. Laparoscopic versus "open" cholecystectomy—Reduced influence upon immune function and the acute phase response [abst]. Presented at the Society of American Gastrointestinal Endoscopic Surgeons, Phoenix, Arizona, April 3, 1993.

Chapter

4

Diagnostic Evaluation of Foregut Function

Peter F. Crookes, M.D. • Geoffrey W.B. Clark, F.R.C.S.(Ed)
Tom R. DeMeester, M.D.

The physician who undertakes surgical treatment of foregut disorders has traditionally relied on a gastroenterologic colleague to perform the necessary workup and refer the patient for surgery. This practice was perpetuated by the rather nonselective nature of many operations for benign diseases of the upper gastrointestinal tract and failure to understand why they sometimes failed. This situation is changing. The rapid expansion of minimally invasive surgical techniques has increased the referrals for surgical treatment of patients with benign foregut disease, sometimes at the insistence of the patients themselves. Although this may be gratifying to those who possess the necessary technical skills, it also places a considerable burden on surgeons to understand the disease process sufficiently to make informed decisions about appropriate treatment and to understand the effects of the proposed surgical procedure. It is our conviction that the best operative decisions will be made by surgeons who perform their own examinations and interpret their own physiologic studies.

Benign diseases of the foregut—the portion of the gastrointestinal tract within the reach of the gastroscope—may be classified as either structural or functional. The distinction is important because progress in understanding the disease begins with observation of visible lesions and advances with exposure and quantification of the underlying pathophysiologic defects. Common structural lesions include diverticula, benign tumors, and mucosal lesions such as peptic ulcer, gastritis, esophagitis, or their complications, for example, esophageal stricture or pyloric stenosis. They are usually diagnosed by barium roentgenography or endoscopy. Functional abnormalities of the foregut are usually disorders of either secretion or propulsion. Examples include gastroesophageal reflux, achalasia, primary esophageal motility disorders, gastroparesis, acid hypersecretion, and duodenogastric reflux. Functional abnormalities may exist in isolation, but often they coexist with, or are the underlying cause of, a structural abnormality. Examples of this are the severe peristaltic defect in the esophageal body that often accompanies peptic strictures and the peptic ulceration that may complicate acid hypersecretion. Failure to consider defects of function may have serious consequences when no structural abnormality is observed, leading to the erroneous conclusion that the patient is suffering from "stress" or a psychosocial disorder. Similarly, to ignore the functional defect because a structural lesion is seen on endoscopy may lead to inappropriate therapy, for example, when a fundoplication is performed in a patient whose underlying problem is impaired esophageal clearance or delayed gastric emptying. This chapter provides an overview of the investigation of benign foregut disease and will emphasize the physiologic aspects of testing.

SYMPTOMS OF FOREGUT DISEASE

The common symptoms arising from the foregut include:

1. Pain, discomfort, or difficulty in swallowing (i.e., dysphagia and odynophagia). It is usually easy to distinguish "transfer" dysphagia (difficulty in getting food from the mouth into the pharynx) from "transport" dysphagia (food can be swallowed but is delayed in entering the stomach). Transfer dysphagia is often neurologic or muscular in origin and may be associated with aspiration, nasal regurgitation, hoarseness, or dysarthria. Transport dysphagia may be associated with regurgitation of swallowed food and saliva that tastes bland because it has not entered the stomach.
2. Epigastric pain, nausea, bloating, fullness, early satiety, or vomiting all suggest a stomach disorder. These symptoms are very nonspecific and may also be the result of disease of the heart, gallbladder, pancreas, liver, small bowel, or colon.
3. Heartburn with acid or alkaline (bitter) regurgitation suggests gastroesophageal reflux disease.
4. Atypical symptoms unrelated to eating and suggestive of diseases in other organ systems such as chest pain mimicking angina pectoris; wheezing, recurrent pneumonia, and pulmonary disease; and hoarseness and laryngeal disease. These may all be due to gastroesophageal reflux disease or esophageal motility disorders.

Many studies have emphasized the low sensitivity and specificity of all these symptoms, whether singly or in combination.[1] Thus a careful history directs the focus of the clinician to the correct sequence of investigations. Once a clear identification of the underlying pathophysiologic defect has been made, the surgeon can plan a rational surgical approach with anticipation of a successful outcome for the patient.

STRUCTURAL STUDIES

Endoscopy is generally the first step in the investigation of patients with foregut symptoms. The exception is when the patient's chief complaint is dysphagia; in this situation a barium study should be obtained to provide a "road map" prior to endoscopy. Modern flexible endoscopes are usually video endoscopes that display the image on a screen. Not only is this ideal for teaching, but the images may be digitalized for later printout and inclusion in the patient's record or the entire study may be recorded on videotape for subsequent demonstration to colleagues or patients.

In most patients a topical local anesthetic spray and sedation with intravenous administration of a short-acting benzodiazepine are required. Monitoring of heart rate and pulse oximetry must be carried out, and resuscitation equipment must be available. The scope is introduced through a mouth guard placed between the patient's teeth. It is passed into the pharynx, and entry into the esophagus is aided by having the patient swallow. The position of the gastroesophageal junction is best identified during this initial introduction and with the use of minimal air insufflation. A sliding hiatal hernia may be reduced by passage of the endoscope and thus go undetected on subsequent withdrawal. Most endoscopists then aim toward the pylorus and duodenum, position the scope well into the second part of the duodenum, and systematically inspect the interior of the duodenum and stomach and esophagus as the scope is withdrawn. When the antrum has been visualized, the incisura angularis appears as a constant ridge on the lesser curve. Turning the lens of the scope 180 degrees (retroflexion) allows inspection of the fundus and cardia. Attention is paid to the "frenulum" of the esophagogastric junction, which corresponds to the angle of His, and to the closeness with which the cardia grips the scope. A grading system to classify this aspect of hiatal function has been devised by L.D. Hill and appears to correlate with esophageal acid exposure. The instrument is then straightened and withdrawal through the cardia and esophagus continued. Three landmarks are measured: the level of the crura (observed as a slitlike narrowing that closes when the patient is asked to sniff), the level of the anatomic gastroesophageal junction (identified as the position where the more dilated stomach with vertically running rugal folds becomes the tubular esophagus with smooth mucosa), and the level of the squamo-columnar junction. A hiatal hernia is present when the gastroesophageal junction is more than 2 cm above the crura and Barrett's esophagus when the squamocolumnar junction is more than 2 cm above the gastroesophageal junction. The diagnosis of Barrett's esophagus should be confirmed by demonstrating specialized (intestinal type) columnar epithelium on biopsy. Barrett's esophagus may be diagnosed if specialized epithelium is identified above the gastroesophageal junction, regardless of the measured length of the columnar segment.

The advantages of endoscopy as the initial investigation for foregut symptoms are that a wide range of disease processes can be detected, suspicious lesions can be biopsied, and lesions such as strictures can be treated at the same sitting. The disadvantages are that it is an invasive procedure with small but measurable risks of oversedation, aspiration, and instrumental perforation and some areas, especially in the region of the upper esophageal sphincter, are difficult to visualize. Mucosal disease such as peptic ulceration can be thoroughly examined, and complications of gastroesophageal reflux disease (e.g., esophagitis, stricture, or Barrett's esophagus) may be detected. Even if a purely functional disease such as achalasia is suspected, endoscopic visualization of the cardia is vital to exclude an infiltrating tumor as a cause of the symptoms.

Barium upper gastrointestinal studies complement endoscopy in providing important structural information and some functional information, especially when the entire examination is recorded on video rather than as a series of still films. The pharynx and upper esophageal sphincter are evaluated in the upright position, and both anteroposterior and lateral views are required. Movement of the hyoid and larynx, epiglottis, soft palate, and tongue are easily identified and their relationship to cricopharyngeal opening and compliance of the cervical esophagus determined. Aspiration, if observed, can be timed and residual barium remaining after a swallow identified. Esophageal body peristalsis is studied in the recumbent and upright positions. A swallowed bolus normally generates a stripping wave (primary peristalsis), which clears the bolus completely. Residual material rarely stimulates a secondary peristaltic wave. Usually a second pharyngeal swallow is required. Motility disorders characterized by disorganized activity with simultaneous contractions give rise to "tertiary waves," often with a segmented appearance of the barium column, sometimes described as a “beading” or “corkscrew” appearance. A hiatal hernia, best seen in the recumbent position, may be reducible in the upright position. Barium studies are of little value in detecting reflux: not only are they insensitive, but motility disorders causing retrograde transport of barium may be mistaken for gastroesophageal reflux.

ESOPHAGEAL FUNCTION STUDIES

STATIONARY ESOPHAGEAL MANOMETRY

Esophageal pressures are measured by transducers that are either connected to or are an integral part of a catheter that is passed transnasally into the esophagus. The transducers are spaced at 5 cm intervals. Pressures may be measured by external transducers connected to a water-perfused multilumen catheter having side holes cut in each channel at the point where the measurement of pressure is to be recorded.[2,3] These are still the most common systems in routine use and are durable and relatively inexpensive. Increasingly, solid-state miniature transducers mounted directly on the catheter itself are being used.[4] They are fragile and expensive, but they have the advantage of a faster response rate, of causing no additional stimulation in the pharynx from perfusate, and of recording pressure independent of body position. They are essential for ambulatory studies. Typical catheters are illustrated in Fig. 4-1.

Indications

Nonobstructive Dysphagia. Most patients with dysphagia or odynophagia are candidates for manometry when barium studies or endoscopy have failed to show a physical obstruction but a motility disorder is suspected. This can be confirmed only by manometry.

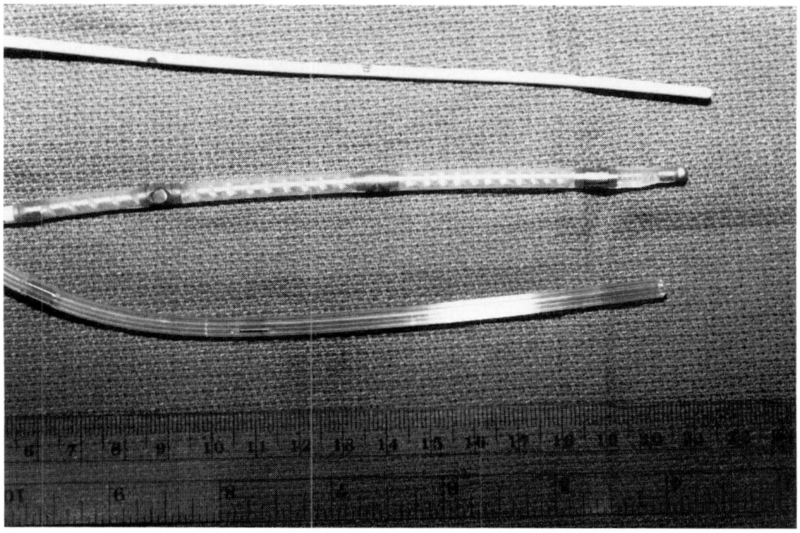

Fig. 4-1. Three different types of motility catheters in common use. The lower catheter is used with the water-perfused system (Arndorfer, Greendale, Wisc.). The upper two catheters have solid-state sensors (top, Sentron, Irving Tex.; middle, Konigsberg, Pasadena, Calif.).

Noncardiac Chest Pain. Central chest pain resembling angina pectoris in location, character, and pattern of radiation (e.g., to the neck, jaw, or arms) may arise from the esophagus. An esophageal cause is generally not considered until extensive cardiac investigation has excluded obvious coronary artery disease. Of the estimated 600,000 new cardiac catheterizations carried out annually in the United States, in 30% of patients no abnormality will be found.[5] Of these, 50% can be demonstrated to have an abnormality in the esophagus, the most common of which is increased esophageal acid exposure. The scope of this problem is therefore significant, especially since simply excluding cardiac disease gives little reassurance to patients, who continue to seek consultation for their symptoms. In contrast, patients in whom a definite esophageal etiology can be demonstrated respond positively to this news.[6,7] Such patients are often younger than 40 years old and have pain bearing little relationship to exercise. Patients with primarily exertional chest pain constitute about 25% of referrals to the motility laboratory for the evaluation of angina-like chest pain. Another group of patients are those with known coronary artery disease who respond poorly to medical therapy and in whom a concomitant esophageal cause is being sought.

Gastroesophageal Reflux Disease. This disease may affect the lower esophageal sphincter, the esophageal body, or the upper esophageal sphincter. Although many gastroenterologists do not perform manometry on patients with gastroesophageal reflux disease routinely, there are many reasons why it is helpful. First, in the assessment of gastroesophageal reflux disease it is important to know the reason for the increased esophageal acid exposure. A defective sphincter is found in more than 50% of patients with increased esophageal acid exposure.[8] Patients with gastroesophageal reflux disease caused by a defective sphincter respond well to antireflux surgery. In contrast, the finding of a normal lower esophageal sphincter in a patient with gastroesophageal reflux disease should prompt a more thorough search for other underlying causes.[9] The most common nonsphincteric causes are to be found in the stomach and include acid hypersecretion,[10] delayed gastric emptying,[11] or gastric dilatation due to aerophagia.

Second, the status of esophageal body peristalsis is critical in planning antireflux operations. Preoperative manometry helps identify defective peristalsis and allows the surgeon to substitute an operation with a lesser risk of obstruction, such as a partial fundoplication, of which the Belsey procedure is the most common.[12] In addition, if the esophageal body is manometrically short (i.e., the distance between the upper border of the lower esophageal sphincter and the lower border of the upper esophageal sphincter is below the normal range), this may interfere with the ability of the surgeon to place the wrap in the abdomen without tension, or it increases the risk of inadvertently placing the wrap around the upper stomach. In this situation a thoracic approach is used to allow maximum mobilization of the esophagus and permit the performance of a gastroplasty to ensure a tension-free repair with proper abdominal placement of the wrap. These considerations are highly relevant to the decision to offer a laparoscopic antireflux procedure. In a patient with uncomplicated reflux who has no esophageal shortening or in whom a hiatal hernia, if present, is reducible and esophageal body peristalsis is adequate, a transabdominal Nissen fundoplication can be expected to produce good results.[9] These are the patients most suited to laparoscopic treatment.[13]

Manometry may also reveal an underlying motility disorder as the primary diagnosis, perhaps rendering surgery unnecessary. Dilation should be performed in patients with benign esophageal strictures and the symptomatic response assessed before manometry is carried out. The motility of the body can be altered depending on the degree of stenosis.[14] A more meaningful assessment of esophageal body function can be made after dilatation. Thus it can be seen that accurate information on the functional status of the esophageal body is essential in assessing patients with gastroesophageal reflux disease.

Third, manometry is known to be the most accurate way of locating the lower esophageal sphincter prior to placement of a pH electrode for 24-hour monitoring in patients suspected of having gastroesophageal reflux disease.[15] Finally, postoperative manometry objectively assesses if the goal of the operation has been attained and encourages the surgeon to modify his technique in the light of the results.

Patient Preparation

Manometric studies are carried out after an overnight fast. All drugs known to influence motility and acid exposure are stopped 48 hours prior to the study. The nostril is anesthetized topically with a 4% cocaine solution. Passage of the catheter is accomplished by having the patient sit upright while the catheter is advanced along the floor of the nostril. After entry into the nasopharynx is established, the catheter is advanced until it lies just above the cricopharyngeus. At this point the patient takes a bolus of water through a straw, holds it in the mouth, and at the moment of swallowing the catheter is advanced through the open cricopharyngeus. Alternatively, the catheter can be passed with the patient in the supine position. When the catheter is just above the cricopharyngeus, the patient's head is bent forward until the chin touches the chest. The patient is asked to swallow in this position and the catheter is simultaneously passed into the esophagus. Further passage of the catheter is continued until all the side holes are in the stomach. The patient then lies supine on the bed and is encouraged to relax (Fig. 4-2). The patient should be allowed time to become accustomed to the presence of the tube in the nasopharynx. Proceeding with the study

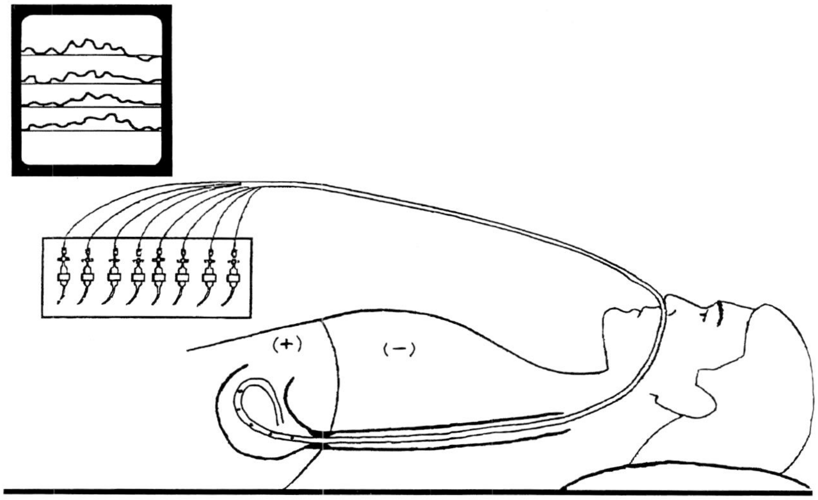

Fig. 4-2. Patient in supine position with water-perfused motility catheter passed into the stomach prior to stationary pull-through of the lower esophageal sphincter. The pressure transducers are connected to a polygraph that produces a hard copy of the tracing for subsequent analysis.

too soon often leads to artifact as the patient is unable to refrain from repeated swallowing.

Technique

A manometric study consists of three components: assessment of the lower esophageal sphincter characteristics, esophageal body contractility and waveforms, and assessment of the upper esophageal sphincter characteristics.

Assessment of the Lower Esophageal Sphincter. At the start of the test the catheter is passed into the stomach. As the catheter is slowly withdrawn in 1 cm increments, the high-pressure zone of the lower esophageal sphincter is reached by the uppermost transducer. The lower (distal) border of the lower esophageal sphincter is the point where the resting pressure leaves the gastric baseline and the upper border the point where it reaches the esophageal baseline. Between these two points is the respiratory inversion point; here the positive deflections with inspiration change to negative deflections. This represents the point where the transmission of abdominal pressure converts to intrathoracic pressure and is thought to represent the attachment of the phrenoesophageal membrane. Three components of the lower esophageal sphincter are measured: the *resting pressure* is the pressure in midrespiration measured at the respiratory inversion point, the *overall length of the sphincter* is the distance from the distal border to the proximal border, and the *abdominal length* is the distance from the distal border of the lower esophageal sphincter to the respiratory inversion point. All these features are illustrated in the tracing in Fig. 4-3. The values for each of these components from each transducer are expressed as an average. If any one component is below the 5th percentile of normal, the sphincter is mechanically defective. These values are a resting pressure of <6 mm Hg, an overall length of <2 cm, or an abdominal length of <1 cm.[8] The pressures in the high-pressure zone are a combination of the intrinsic pressure of the lower esophageal sphincter, intra-abdominal pressure, and compression by the crura of the diaphragm. In hiatal herniation the diaphragmatic and intrinsic components are sometimes separated rather than superimposed, resulting in a very long high-pressure zone described as a "double hump."

If manometry is carried out using a catheter with four transducers radially oriented at the same level, the pressures around the circumference can be integrated into a three-dimensional image (Fig. 4-4), the volume of which (sphincter pressure vector volume) is a quantitative measure of lower esophageal sphincter resistance. A volume below the 5th percentile of normal is a more sensitive measure of mechanical deficiency of the lower esophageal sphincter than the parameters described above. The prevalence of a defective lower esophageal sphincter increases with increasing severity of gastroesophageal reflux disease, being lowest in patients without evidence of endoscopic injury and highest in patients with stricture or Barrett's esophagus.[16]

The chief source of confusion during the station pull-through is the artifact introduced when the patient swallows. If the patient swallows as the catheter is moved to another station, the pressure falls because of lower esophageal sphincter relaxation and then rises during the postrelaxation phase. Estimation of the pressure at each station may be difficult unless a sufficient time interval elapses to permit

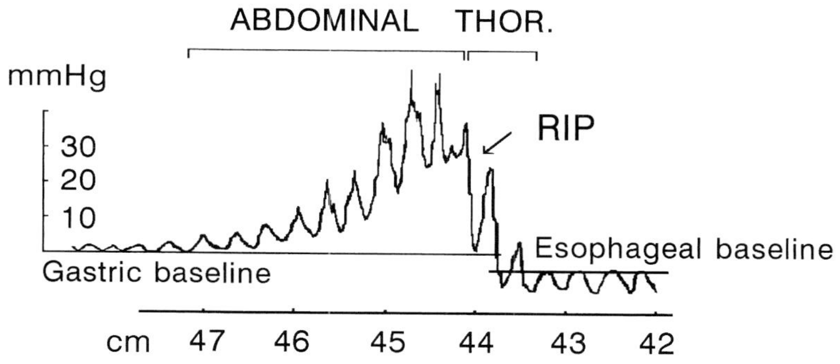

Fig. 4-3. Characteristic manometric features of the lower esophageal sphincter. Abdominal plus thoracic length equals overall length.

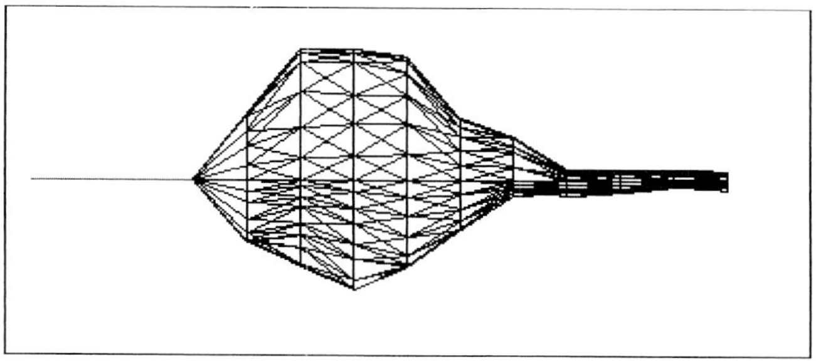

Fig. 4-4. Three-dimensional sphincter pressure image in a normal volunteer.

stabilization of the reading to occur after a swallow. The long performance time and the need for a cooperative patient have prompted workers to examine alternatives to the station pull-through technique. One alternative is the rapid pull-through method in which the catheter is drawn through the lower esophageal sphincter at a steady rate of 1 cm/sec while the patient holds his breath. Although this test is still performed by some laboratories, it suffers from lack of reproducibility and has consequently fallen out of favor.[17] A more physiologic method that also avoids swallow-induced artifact is the slow motorized pull-through technique.[18] This method, in which the catheter is pulled at a slow constant speed of 1 mm/sec, causes no pharyngeal stimulation to swallow and allows the patient to breathe normally. It can be conducted in about one third of the time taken for stepwise station pull-through. High-quality artifact-free tracings are easy to obtain, and since the respiratory inversion point can be identified, the contributions of the intra-abdominal and intrathoracic portions of the lower esophageal sphincter can be measured (Fig. 4-5). Current indications suggest that it may become the preferred method to examine the lower esophageal sphincter.

Measurement of Lower Esophageal Sphincter Relaxation. The lower esophageal sphincter pressure normally drops to gastric baseline immediately after the swallow and before the oncoming peristaltic wave reaches the lower esophagus (Fig. 4-6).

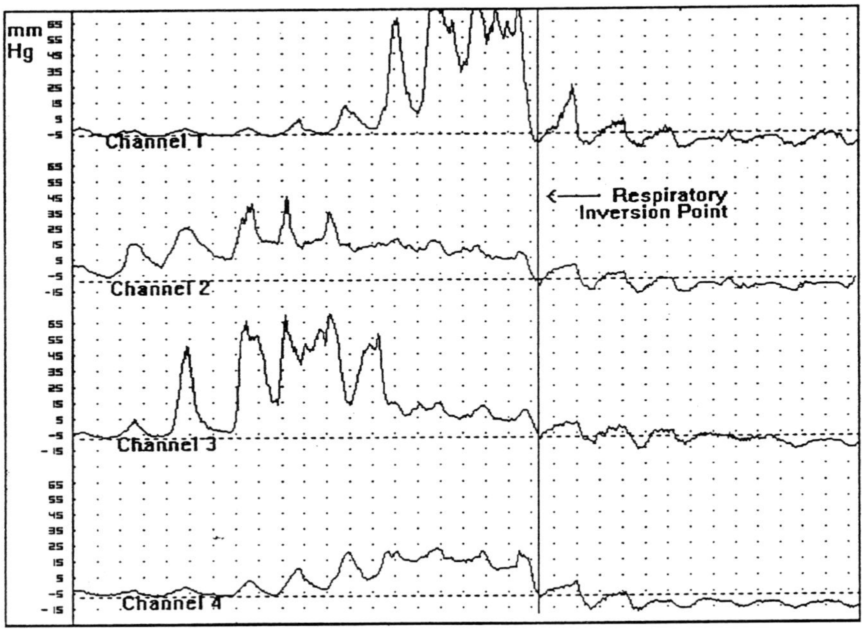

Fig. 4-5. Evaluation of the characteristics of the lower esophageal sphincter in a normal subject obtained by the slow motorized pull-through technique. The four tracings are obtained from four circumferentially arranged pressure sensors, all located at the same level but at 90-degree angles to one another.

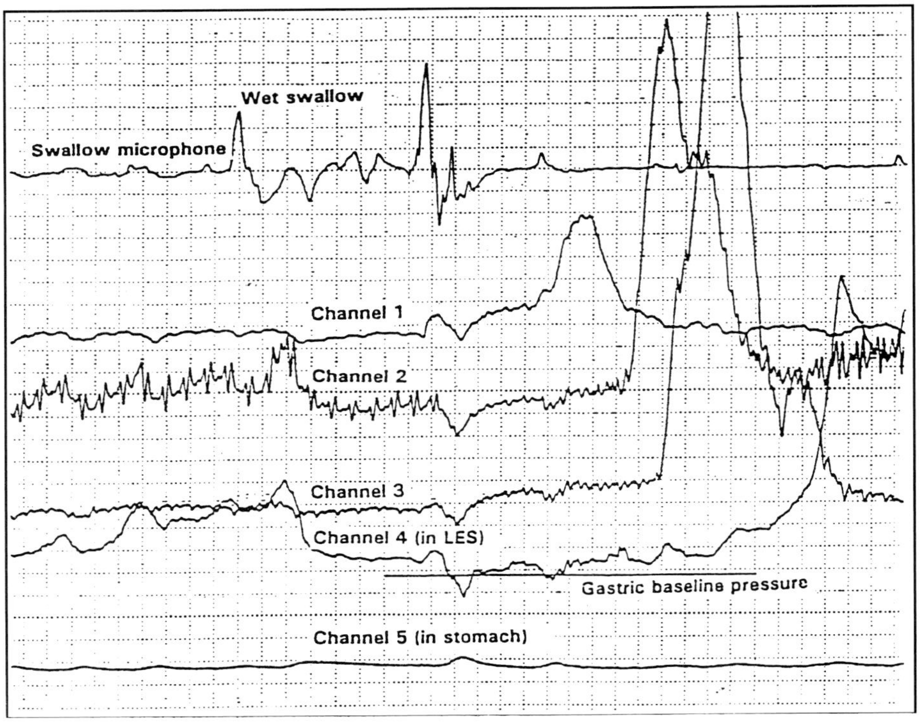

Fig. 4-6. Normal lower esophageal sphincter relaxation. Channels 1, 2, and 3 are in the esophageal body and show a peristaltic contraction wave in response to a 5 ml bolus swallow. Channel 4 is within the lower esophageal sphincter and relaxes to gastric baseline in response to the swallow.

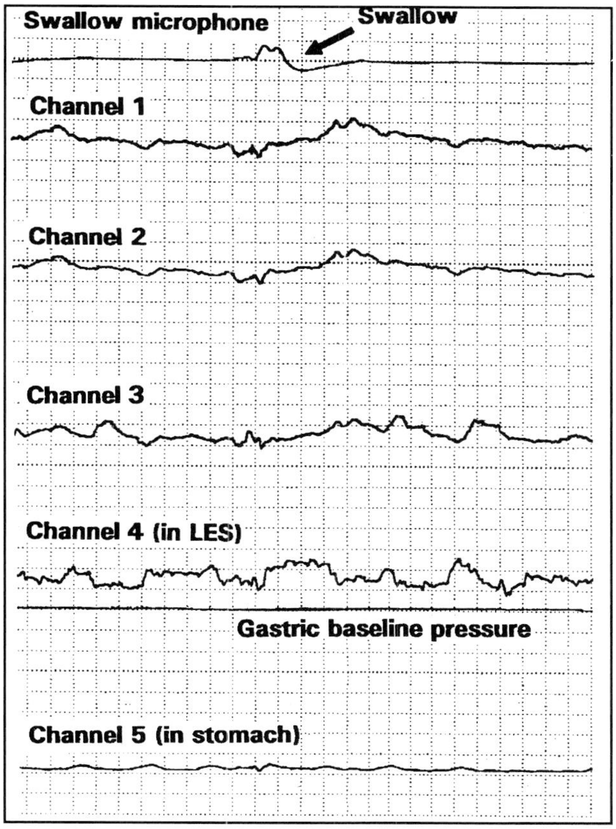

Fig. 4-7. A patient with achalasia. Channel 4 is within the lower esophageal sphincter. Note that in response to a 5 ml bolus swallow there are low-amplitude simultaneous waves in channels 1 to 3, whereas no relaxation is seen in channel 4.

Relaxation of the lower esophageal sphincter is classically absent or incomplete in patients with achalasia (Fig. 4-7), but it may be incomplete in other diseases such as diffuse esophageal spasm and malignant infiltration.[19] It also occurs after a fundoplication that is too tight or incorrectly situated around the upper stomach. A catheter is positioned in the lower esophageal sphincter to assess relaxation and a series of swallows obtained by giving boluses of 5 ml water.

Relaxation of the lower esophageal sphincter can be a difficult feature to examine manometrically. After a swallow (in addition to lower esophageal sphincter relaxation) the lower esophageal sphincter moves craniad, causing the transducer to return momentarily to the upper stomach.[20] Thus apparent relaxation may reflect longitudinal movement of the transducer off the lower esophageal sphincter. This is avoided by positioning the transducer near the upper part of the lower esophageal sphincter or by using several closely spaced transducers to straddle the lower esophageal sphincter.

Esophageal Body Manometry. Following assessment of the lower esophageal sphincter the catheter is positioned so that the transducers span the length of the

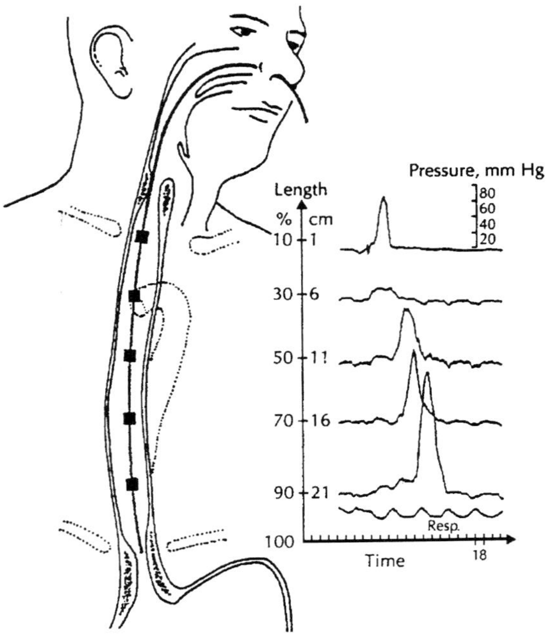

Fig. 4-8. Positioning of the five pressure sensors for analysis of esophageal body motility during stationary manometry. The upper sensor is located 1 cm below the lower border of the cricopharyngeus muscle. The remaining sensors trail the length of the esophagus at 5 cm intervals. An example of the tracing obtained from a single swallow is shown on the right. (From Stein HJ, DeMeester TR, Hinder RA. Outpatient physiological testing and surgical management of foregut motility disorders. Curr Probl Surg 24:418-555, 1992.)

esophageal body (Fig. 4-8). The peristaltic response to 10 swallows of 5 ml water is measured. The features of individual contractions are the amplitude, duration, slope (dP/dT), and morphology (i.e., whether single, double, or triple peaked) (Fig. 4-9). The amplitude is affected by the diameter of the catheter and by the size and the temperature of the bolus. We recommend performing wet swallows with a 5 ml bolus of water at room temperature. Transmission of a contraction from one level to the next forms a wave and is assessed by the speed of wave propagation and by noting any interruption of the wave. In practice any wave traveling faster than 20 cm/sec is described as simultaneous. Such waves do not contribute to propulsion. Most commercially available manometric systems automatically measure these features of contractions and their progression down the esophagus as waves and relate the results to those of normal subjects.

Assessment of the Upper Esophageal Sphincter. The position, length, and resting pressure of the upper esophageal sphincter and its relaxation on swallowing are assessed with a technique similar to that used for the lower esophageal sphincter. Since pressure changes at the upper esophageal sphincter are much faster than those in the lower esophageal sphincter, a high paper speed (25 mm/sec) is necessary to evaluate the timing of events, and the responsiveness of the system must be sufficient

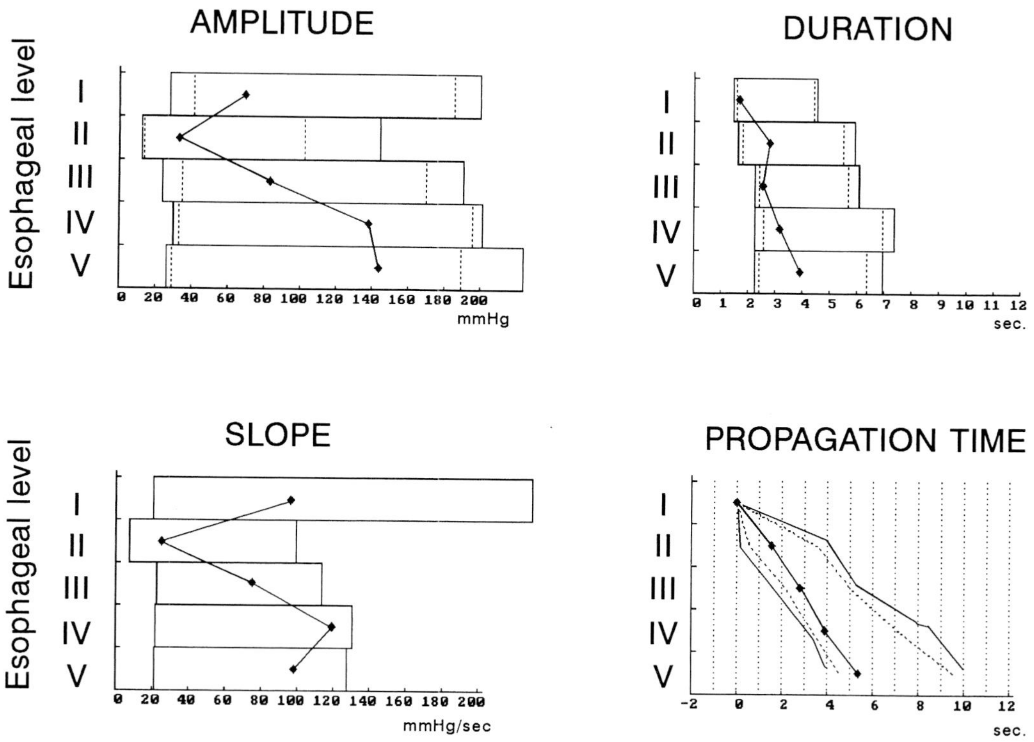

Fig. 4-9. Esophageal body motility results obtained during stationary manometry in a normal subject. Analysis is based on the median values obtained from 10 sequential swallows of 5 ml of water. The level of the pressure sensor is shown on the y-axis. I corresponds to the catheter 1 cm below the cricopharyngeus, II is 6 cm below the cricopharyngeus, etc. (see Fig. 4-8). Results for amplitude, duration, slope, and propagation of the esophageal waves are shown. The lines represent the patient's values. The boxes show the normal ranges obtained in a study of 50 volunteers, with the dotted line representing the 10th and 90th percentiles and the outer limit of the boxes the 5th and 95th percentiles. This subject is within the normal range for all parameters. Abnormalities are diagnosed when any value lies outside the normal ranges.

to reflect the rapid changes in pressure without damping. Solid-state transducers have excellent responsiveness but cannot be placed at close intervals along the catheter as this would make them too rigid and impossible to swallow.

Interpretation

The features identified by manometric studies have been validated by relating the manometric features to simultaneous video fluoroscopic examination. Studies by Kahrilas et al.[21] have shown that the amplitude of contraction increases as the wave travels down the esophagus. An ineffective contraction was described as one that allowed "barium escape," and the amplitude necessary to prevent barium escape was greater in the distal esophagus than the proximal. Thresholds above which peristaltic clearance of barium was complete were 18 mm Hg in the cervical esophagus, 25 mm Hg at the aortic arch, 30 mm Hg at the retrocardiac level, and 43 mm Hg in the ampulla. In the distal esophagus, barium escape was very likely if the contraction amplitude was <30 mm Hg. Similar studies by Hewson et al.[22] have shown that a wave traveling faster than 6.25 cm/sec is associated with abnormal bolus transit.

The pattern of manometric abnormalities is the basis for classification of motility disorders. The best known is *achalasia*, a disorder characterized by incomplete or absent relaxation of the lower esophageal sphincter and absent esophageal body peristalsis. The resting lower esophageal sphincter pressure may or may not be elevated.[23] The typical response to a swallow in the esophageal body is a low-pressure elevation in all the esophageal channels simultaneously, indicating that the entire esophagus behaves like a common cavity filled with fluid. The resting esophageal baseline pressure is often positive with respect to the gastric baseline, indicating outflow resistance. A subgroup of patients with achalasia is characterized by simultaneous high-pressure esophageal body contractions, often associated with retrosternal chest pain. Surgery for this variant, sometimes known as vigorous achalasia, generally requires a long myotomy of the esophageal body in addition to myotomy of the lower esophageal sphincter. The extent of the simultaneous waves on manometry is used as a guide to gauge the proximal extent of the myotomy. *Diffuse esophageal spasm* is a condition characterized by intermittent peristalsis alternating with simultaneous contractions in the esophageal body.[24,25] These patients typically complain of both chest pain and dysphagia. *Nutcracker esophagus*, the commonest primary esophageal motility disorder, is characterized by peristaltic waves of increased amplitude (median >180 mm Hg) or duration.[26,27] It is often associated with central chest pain. *Hypertensive lower esophageal sphincter* is a disorder in which the resting pressure of the lower esophageal sphincter is above normal, but it relaxes with swallowing. Some of these patients ultimately develop classic achalasia or diffuse esophageal spasm on follow-up.

In *secondary motility disorders* the disordered peristalsis is secondary to identifiable esophageal pathology. The most common cause is the reduction of peristaltic amplitude associated with severe reflux disease. Once the amplitude of esophageal contractions has dropped below the lower limit of normal, neither surgical nor medical treatment is likely to improve it.[12,28,29] Treatment should be directed toward abolishing reflux before irreversible damage to the esophageal body has occurred. The other relatively common secondary motility disorder is scleroderma, a connective tissue disorder that causes infiltration of fibrous tissue into the lower esophageal sphincter and esophageal body, leading to profound lower esophageal sphincter hypotonia and absence of esophageal body peristalsis.

MEASUREMENT OF ESOPHAGEAL ACID EXPOSURE: 24-HOUR pH MONITORING

Indications

Twenty-four–hour esophageal pH monitoring is the principal method of diagnosing gastroesophageal reflux and has effectively replaced all other "dipstick" methods of measuring esophageal acid exposure.[30,31] It is indicated in any patient with symptoms suggestive of gastroesophageal reflux disease unless the symptoms are trivial or are abolished by a 12-week course of acid suppression therapy with H_2 blockers or omeprazole. If symptoms persist or recur on cessation of therapy, the diagnosis should be confirmed objectively by 24-hour pH monitoring. This is especially important in patients who are being considered for antireflux repair. Atypical presentations of gastroesophageal reflux disease are also common. They include noncardiac chest pain (following a negative cardiac evaluation), respiratory symptoms of adult-onset asthma, aspiration and nocturnal wheezing, chronic laryngitis, and in the pediatric patient persistent neonatal vomiting, apnea, and failure to thrive. Twenty-four–hour pH monitoring in such patients allows the opportunity to confirm or refute the diagnosis of gastroesophageal reflux disease and to relate the patient's symptoms during the monitored period to episodes of reflux.

Technique

Esophageal pH monitoring is performed following manometric localization of the upper border of the lower esophageal sphincter. Inferring the position from endoscopic measurements or noting the abrupt transition from acidic to neutral pH is not sufficiently accurate for reliable probe positioning.[15] The patient is advised to fast for at least 6 hours prior to passage of the pH probe to minimize the risk of vomiting during probe positioning. Patients should stop all medications that interfere with gastric motility and secretion 48 hours prior to the procedure. We have found that patients taking omeprazole should discontinue this medication 2 weeks before testing since prolonged acid suppression can produce a false negative result. We find glass electrodes with an in-built reference electrode (Ingold probes, Mui Scientific, Toronto, Ontario) are more accurate and stable at the extremes of the pH range than antimony electrodes. Antimony probes are widely used and are an acceptable alternative, but they do require the use of an external reference lead and do not reliably measure pH in the "alkaline" range (pH 6 to 8).[32] The pH probes are calibrated before and after the test in buffer solutions at pH 1 and 7, and the drift in pH must be within 0.2 unit of the standard for accurate interpretation of the results.

The pH probe is passed through the anesthetized nostril into the stomach, a fact easily determined by recording a pH of 1 to 2. Withdrawal of the probe into the esophagus ensures that it has not curled and that the measured distance is 5 cm above the manometrically defined upper border of the lower esophageal sphincter. The probe is taped to the nostril and looped behind the ear to maintain a stable position with minimal patient discomfort. The pH recordings are stored on a portable data recorder strapped to the patient's side.

The patients are instructed to carry out their normal daily activities on return home but to avoid strenuous exertion. During the day they are asked to remain in the upright position and are given a diet sheet listing foods with a pH in the range of 5 to 7. They are provided with a diary and asked to note the times of meals, retiring for sleep, and rising the following morning and to record the presence and duration of each of their symptoms. Many commercially available data logging devices have buttons to indicate mealtimes, position (whether upright or supine), and symptoms. Experience has shown that patients may not remember to press the correct button at the correct moment, and the information is not reliable unless supplemented by a diary, which is reviewed with the patient by the laboratory personnel the next day. Smoking and alcohol are prohibited during the recording period. The patients return to the laboratory the following day, and the data logging device is downloaded onto an IBM personal computer for subsequent analysis.

Interpretation

In healthy individuals the esophageal pH is between 4 and 7 over 94% of the time (Fig. 4-10).[33] Short episodes can be observed when the esophageal pH drops below 4, but these usually are only seen during the daytime, often postprandially, and are rapidly cleared by primary peristaltic waves reaching the distal esophagus and by the neutralizing effect of swallowed saliva.[34] These events can be termed "physiologic reflux." Abnormal esophageal acid exposure can be defined as that exceeding the 95th percentile of healthy normal subjects.

The single measurements of the percent time the pH is below a certain threshold, although concise, does not reflect how the exposure occurred (a few long episodes or frequent short episodes). Previous data indicated that patients with reflux episodes of long duration and those who reflux during the recumbent period ("supine refluxers") have more severe disease than those who have frequent short reflux episodes occurring predominantly during the daytime ("upright refluxers").[35] Upright reflux represents an exacerbation of physiologic reflux and is often associated with aerophagia. Many such patients have a normal lower esophageal sphincter. In contrast, supine reflux is associated with clearance defects and often occurs in patients who have either a profound esophageal body motility disorder (e.g., scleroderma or after long esophageal myotomy) or impairment of peristalsis secondary to severe reflux. The worst disease is found in patients with excessive reflux both during the day and during the night ("combined refluxers") (Fig. 4-11). A composite scoring system has been derived that integrates several different features of the pH record into a single measurement of esophageal acid exposure. The score is calculated from the six parameters shown in the Table 4-1. Each of these parameters is not uniformly sensitive when applied to a population of patients with gastroesophageal reflux disease. The percent time pH is <4 in the supine period is the most sensitive and the total number of reflux episodes is the least. The score is derived for each of the six parameters by dividing the patient's actual value for that parameter by the standard deviation found in normal volunteers for that parameter. The individual scores are summed and values >14.8 are above the 95th percentile of normal. Further details of how the score is derived are explained elsewhere,[33] but a commercially available computer software package is available (Gastrosoft, Inc., Irving, Tex.). Esophageal pH monitoring is the most

Table 4-1. Values of 24-hour esophageal monitoring when pH is <4 in 50 healthy volunteers

	Mean	SD	Median	Min.	Max.	95th Percentile
Total time pH <4 (%)	1.5	1.4	1.2	0	6.0	4.5
Upright time pH <4 (%)	2.2	2.3	1.6	0	9.3	8.4
Supine time pH <4 (%)	0.6	1.0	0.1	0	4.0	3.5
No. of episodes	19.0	12.8	16.0	2.0	56.0	46.9
No. of episodes ≥5 min	0.8	1.2	0	0	5.0	3.5
Longest episode (min)	6.7	7.9	4.0	0	46.0	19.8
Composite score	6.0	4.4	5.0	0.4	18.0	14.7

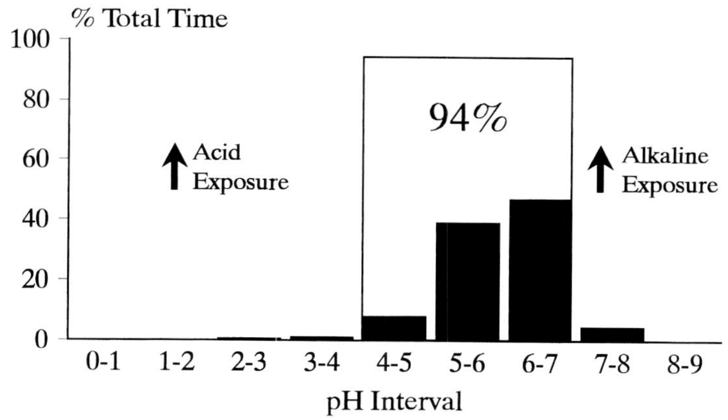

Fig. 4-10. Normal range for esophageal pH expressed as the median percentage of the total time spent at each pH interval in 50 normal volunteers. Note that 94% of the time is spent within a pH range of 4 to 7. (From DeMeester TR, Stein HJ. Ambulatory 24-hour pH monitoring—what is abnormal? In Richter JE, ed. Ambulatory Esophageal pH Monitoring. New York: Igaku-Shoin, 1991, pp 81-92.)

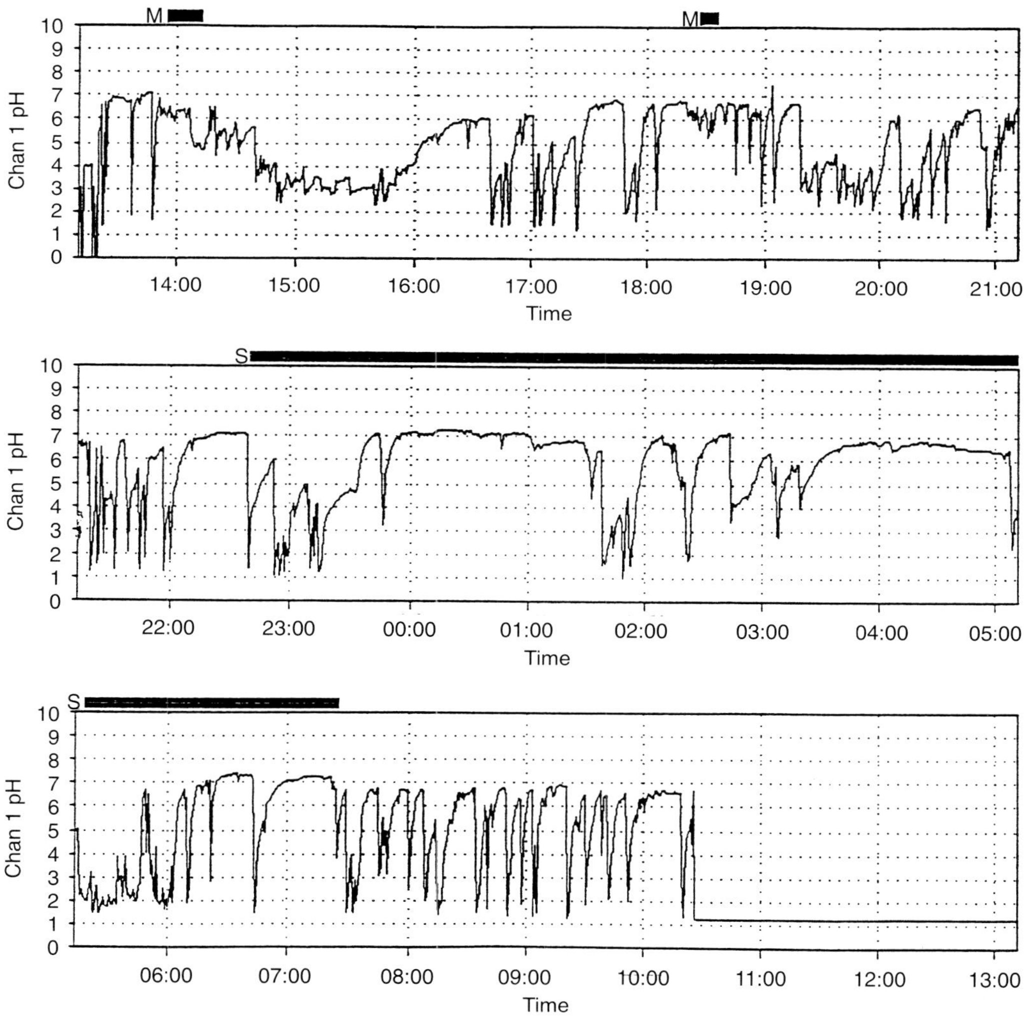

Fig. 4-11. The 24-hour esophageal pH recording from a patient with reflux in the upright and supine positions. Each of the three tracings indicates an 8-hour time period. The pH is shown on the y-axis. M = meal period; S = supine period. Note the frequent and often prolonged drops in esophageal pH to below 4. The record was interrupted at 10:30 A.M.

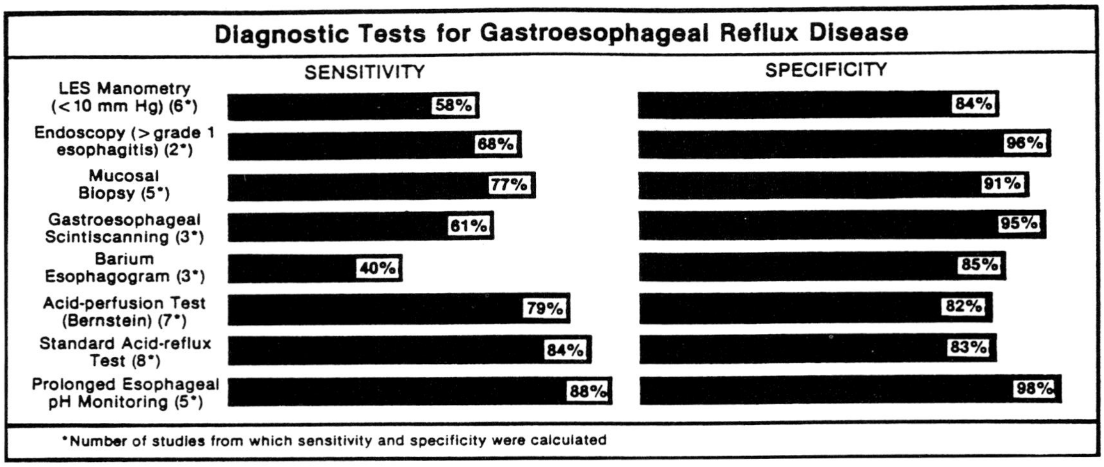

Fig. 4-12. Sensitivity and specificity of diagnostic tests for gastroesophageal reflux disease in the recent literature. (From Bonavina L, DeMeester TR. Prolonged esophageal pH monitoring. In Sigel B, ed. Diagnostic Patient Studies in Surgery. Philadelphia: Lea & Febiger, 1986, p 358.)

sensitive and most specific diagnostic test for the detection of gastroesophageal reflux disease (Fig. 4-12).

When measured in this way esophageal acid exposure in normal subjects is independent of nationality or dietary habits, and when the composite score is used, it is also independent of sex.[32] The test quantitates the actual time the esophageal mucosa is exposed to gastric acid, measures the ability of the esophagus to clear refluxed acid, and correlates esophageal acid exposure to the patient's symptoms.

In addition to the measurement of acid exposure, pH monitoring can also be used to detect excessive alkaline exposure (pH >7) in the esophagus. Normal alkaline exposure in the esophagus is related to saliva secretion. Salivary pH can be elevated in the presence of bacterial overgrowth associated with dental decay or pooling of saliva caused by a stricture or certain motility disorders. If these factors are excluded, increased alkaline exposure in the esophagus may be caused by gastroesophageal reflux of alkaline gastric juice, implying contamination of the gastric juice with duodenal juice containing bile and pancreatic enzymes.[36] This is especially important in complicated forms of gastroesophageal reflux disease such as Barrett's esophagus.[37-39] If duodenogastric reflux is suspected, 24-hour monitoring of the stomach with a pH probe placed 5 cm below the lower border of the lower esophageal sphincter may confirm this finding (see below).

ADDITIONAL TESTS

Dual Esophageal pH Monitoring

Investigation of patients who have respiratory symptoms such as nocturnal cough, wheeze, asthma, or recurrent aspiration pneumonia may include pH monitoring of both the proximal and distal esophagus.[40] We use two pH electrodes positioned in the esophagus, one 5 cm above the upper border of the lower esophageal sphincter and one 1 cm below the lower border of the upper esophageal sphincter. The ideal location of the two probes is determined by prior stationary manometry. The probes are marked and tied together with fine silk ligatures. The two probes can be passed through the nostril simultaneously, and the ligatures prevent displacement of the proximal pH probe during swallowing. Reflux of gastric acid up to the region of the cricopharyngeus is very rare in healthy subjects, particularly during the supine period.[41] In addition, the pH recordings can be examined following the study to identify whether reflux episodes are propagated from the lower esophagus to the upper esophagus. A key feature of this test is the correlation between drops in pH in the esophagus and the symptoms experienced by the patient during the monitored period. If a clear relation can be established, abolition of reflux should be followed by good symptomatic relief provided there is no motility disorder.

Provocative Testing

In the standard acid reflux test the stomach is loaded with hydrochloric acid and reflux in response to various straining maneuvers is detected by a pH probe.[42] This test is still useful in patients with hypochlorhydria and a history suggestive of gastroesophageal reflux disease. Such patients may have symptoms from alkaline reflux or may have prolonged suppression of gastric acid from omeprazole consumption. Other measures such as the acid clearance test and the pH withdrawal gradient are of historical interest only.

The Bernstein test, in which hydrochloric acid is dripped into the esophagus via a nasogastric tube, is sometimes used to determine if a patient's symptoms are reproduced by acid exposure, with the assumption that a positive test implies reflux disease.[43] It is basically a measure of esophageal mucosal sensitivity and has recently been used to demonstrate that patients with Barrett's esophagus have a less sensitive mucosa than patients with esophagitis. It has been largely superseded by the use of 24-hour pH monitoring, which in effect is an "endogenous" Bernstein test.

The edrophonium test is occasionally performed in a patient with central chest pain of suspected esophageal origin.[44] Although edrophonium often causes marked increases in peristaltic amplitude, the end point of the test is reproduction of the patient's typical symptoms rather than the generation of a specific motility abnormality.

Ambulatory (24-Hour) Esophageal Manometry

Ambulatory esophageal manometry is a recently developed technique for assessing the characteristics of esophageal body peristalsis over a 24-hour period. It is performed with a solid-state catheter connected to a portable microdigitrapper that is capable of recording and storing the large amount of data obtained when recording esophageal activity over a full circadian cycle. The catheter assembly we use consists of a 7 F probe that has four pressure transducers and is positioned in the lower esophagus 5 cm proximal to the upper border of the lower esophageal sphincter. The pressure transducers accurately measure pressure changes of up to 400 mm Hg and show a drift of less than 15% over a 24-hour period. The sensors are located 5, 10, 15, and 25 cm proximal to the upper border of the lower esophageal sphincter (Fig. 4-13). Analysis of esophageal body motility is performed using the distal three channels, whereas the most proximal sensor is situated in the pharynx and is used to flag swallows.[45] At the end of the 24-hour study the data are unloaded from the microdigitrapper onto an

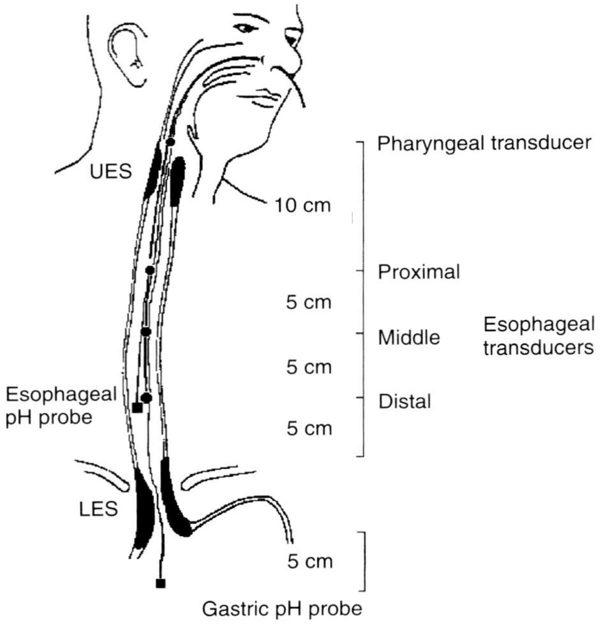

Fig. 4-13. Positioning of the ambulatory manometry catheter. The solid-state sensors are identified by the black circles. The upper sensor is positioned in the pharynx, whereas the three distal sensors are located in the esophageal body. Note that this catheter can be passed along with two pH probes (black squares). One is positioned in the esophagus 5 cm above the upper border of the lower esophageal sphincter to monitor esophageal acid exposure and the other in the stomach 5 cm below the lower border of the lower esophageal sphincter to monitor gastric pH.

IBM-compatible computer. Fully automated analysis is performed with a commercially available software package (Multigram, Gastrosoft, Inc.).[46]

The great advantage of ambulatory motility is that it demonstrates esophageal dysfunction during the patient's normal daily activities, especially during meals.[47] It provides a much more comprehensive picture of esophageal function than is possible by examining the response to 10 swallows of 5 ml of water while lying supine in the esophageal laboratory. Analysis of the data is more complex than for stationary motility. Most analytical software programs divide the 24-hour study into three periods, the meal period, the upright period, and the supine period. The same basic parameters as in stationary manometry are analyzed, including the number of swallowing sequences and the morphology and amplitudes of contraction at each level in the esophagus. Waves can be divided into those which are completely peristaltic (progressive waves at all three levels), incompletely peristaltic (simultaneous between any two adjacent levels), or simultaneous (all three levels simultaneous). Peristaltic waves are described as effective if the amplitude is above the required threshold at each level. Lower amplitudes in peristaltic waves are described as possibly effective and very low amplitudes or nonperistaltic waves as ineffective. The range of normal for each class of wave during mealtimes, the supine period, and the upright period has been determined, and the software program relates an individual patient's values to the range of normal (Fig. 4-14).

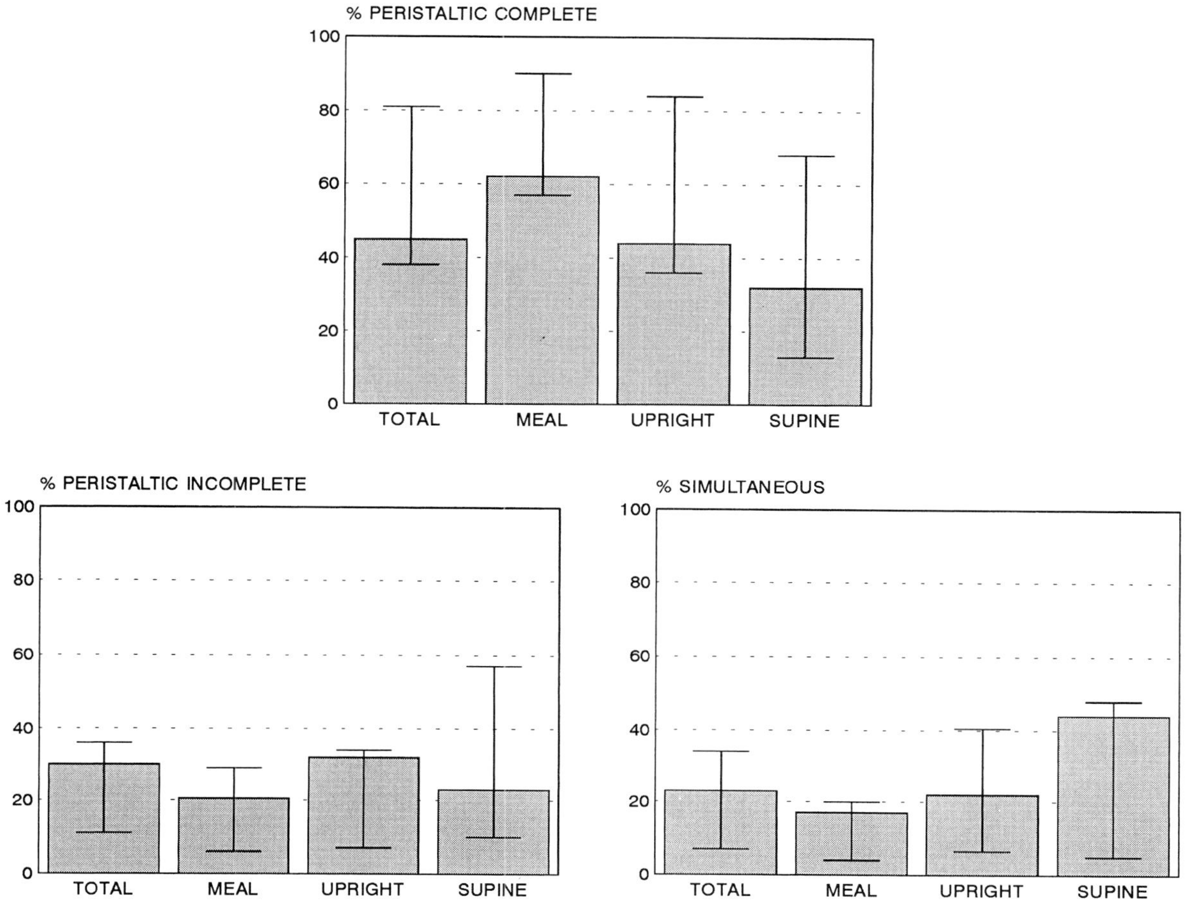

Fig. 4-14. Graphic analysis of 24-hour ambulatory manometry in a normal subject. The x-axis shows the time period. The y-axis shows the percent of waves. Normal ranges established in 25 healthy volunteers are shown by the line bars (5th and 95th percentiles). The upper graph indicates the percent of waves that were completely peristaltic. The middle graph shows the percent of waves in which peristalsis was incomplete because of either an interrupted or dropped wave. The lower graph indicates the percent of waves that were simultaneous between two or all three sensors. Note that the subject lies within the normal ranges for all parameters. Also, note that the normal ranges indicate that the esophageal motility becomes progressively better organized (percent of waves completely peristaltic) from the supine to the upright to the meal period.

In healthy persons the esophagus becomes progressively more organized from the supine to the upright to the meal period, a feature reflected in both the increased frequency of esophageal contractions and a higher prevalence of complete peristaltic waves that are effective.[48] Loss of this improved organization of esophageal activity during mealtimes is a subtle sign of motility disorder, and when fewer than 50% of waves during the meal period are effective and peristaltic, there is a significant correlation with the onset of dysphagia.

Other advantages of ambulatory esophageal motility monitoring are that the chance of the patient experiencing symptoms that can be correlated with esophageal motility events is greatly increased when the study is performed over 24 hours. Compared with stationary motility, much more data can be recorded (about 100 times as many events and in a variety of physiologic situations). It is more likely to pick up distal esophageal motor disorders, which are common in patients with long-standing gastroesophageal reflux disease (Fig. 4-15). The technique is also useful in classifying nonobstructive esophageal motor disorders, particularly nutcracker

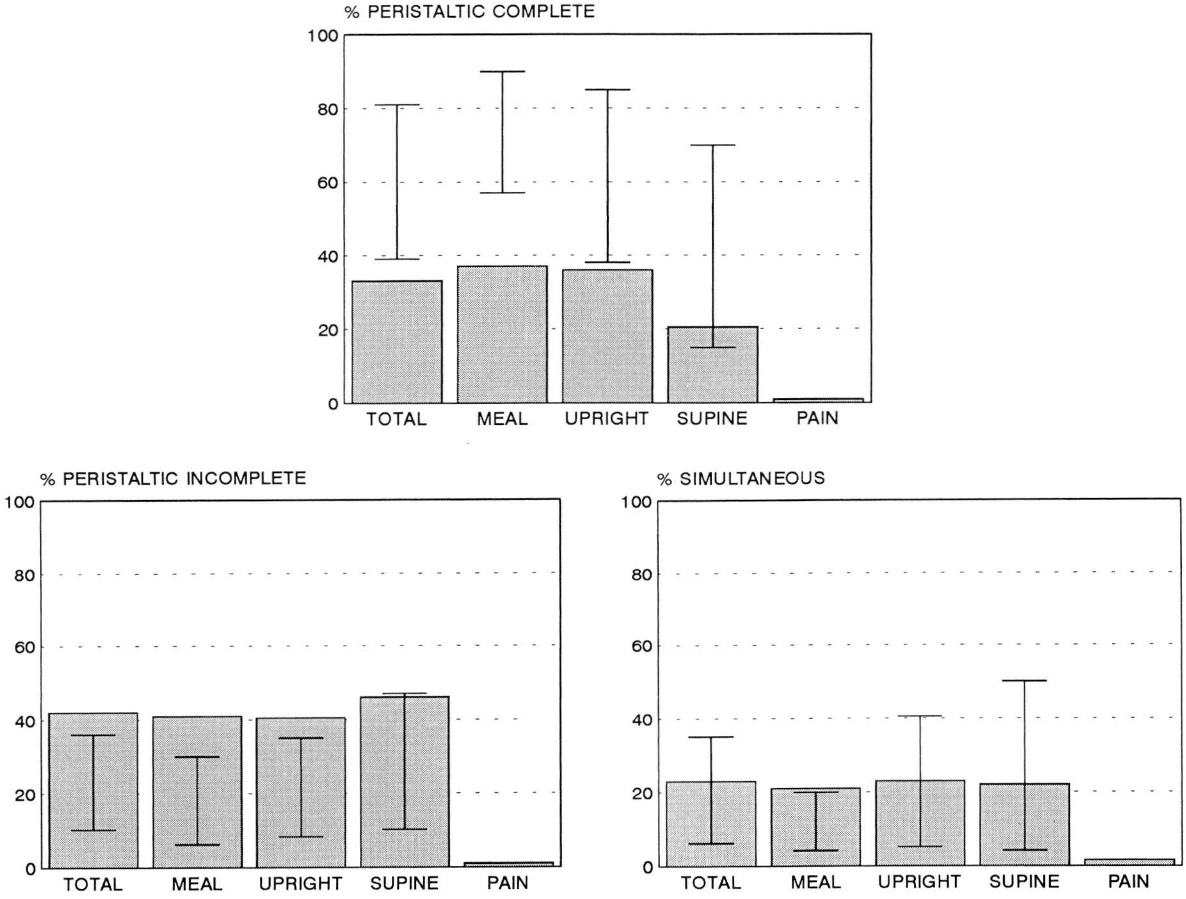

Fig. 4-15. Graphic analysis of 24-hour ambulatory manometry in a patient with gastroesophageal reflux disease and mild dysphagia for which no mechanical obstruction was identified. The x-axis shows the time period. The y-axis shows the percent of waves. Normal ranges established in 25 healthy volunteers are shown by the line bars (5th and 95th percentiles). The upper graph indicates the percent of waves that were completely peristaltic. The middle graph shows the percent of waves in which peristalsis was incomplete because of either an interrupted or dropped wave. The lower graph indicates the percent of waves that were simultaneous between two or all three sensors. Note that the patient falls well below the normal range for percent of peristaltic complete waves, especially during mealtimes, because of an abnormally high percent of incomplete waves (interrupted and dropped) during meal and upright periods. The patient has a defect in esophageal body motility as a result of reflux disease and was treated by a partial wrap rather than the traditional Nissen fundoplication to prevent postoperative dysphagia.

esophagus and diffuse esophageal spasm. The percent of effective contractions during mealtimes appears to be especially helpful in patients with nonobstructive dysphagia, and there is a good correlation between the presence of dysphagia and the finding of <50% effective waves during mealtimes (Fig. 4-16). The clarification of esophageal motility disorders obtained by the use of ambulatory manometry has reduced the need to perform provocative testing such as the edrophonium test.

Esophageal Bile Probe

Another recently developed technique for investigating the composition of the material that refluxes into the lower esophagus is a portable spectrophotometric device capable of continuously measuring the concentration of bile in the ambulatory setting.[49] A fiberoptic cable is connected to a light source and data logger and is worn on the patient's side (Bilitec 2000, Fig. 4-17). The light source emits light at 470 nm, which is close to the wavelength of maximum absorbance of bilirubin. The light is transmitted across a 2 mm space to a white Teflon reflector that reflects the light back to the probe (Fig. 4-18). In the absence of bilirubin all the light emitted is reflected back, whereas in the presence of bilirubin the absorbance of light is directly related to the concentration of bilirubin and the amount of light reflected back to the probe is proportionally reduced. Validation studies have indicated that the sensor is accurate in detecting bilirubin in both an acid and alkaline pH environment.[50] The cable is passed into the esophagus and positioned 5 cm above the upper border of the lower esophageal sphincter. The bile probe is usually passed in conjunction with an esophageal pH probe to correlate pH changes with changes in bilirubin concentration. One potential pitfall is that the yellow colorings in foodstuffs (e.g., butter) may interfere with the absorption of bilirubin, leading to artifi-

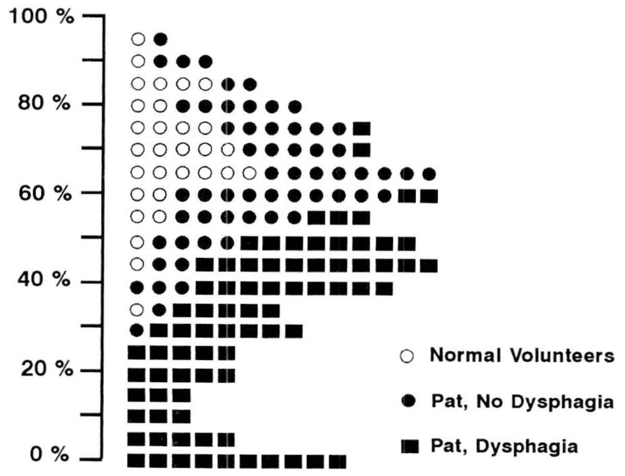

Fig. 4-16. Percent of effective contractions during meals in a series of patients who were investigated for foregut disease with 24-hour ambulatory manometry because of suspected esophageal body motor disorders. pH testing showed all patients were free of reflux disease. Note that in those patients with dysphagia, over 90% had less than 50% effective contractions during meals.

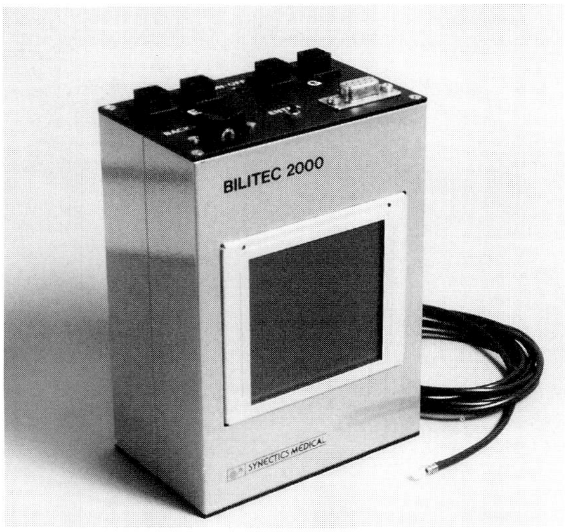

Fig. 4-17. Bilitec 2000 system. The data logger gives a continual graphic display of bilirubin absorbance. The data are also stored for subsequent downloading and analysis onto a personal computer.

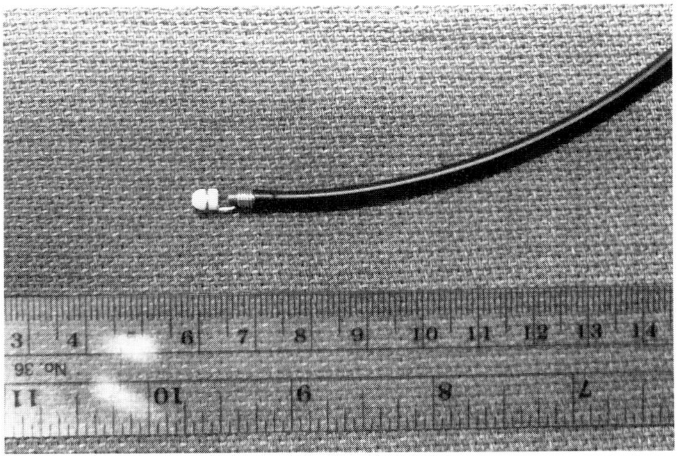

Fig. 4-18. Distal end of the Bilitec fiberoptic cable. The light is emitted from the probe and passes across a 2 mm space to a Teflon reflector that reflects the nonabsorbed light back to the probe.

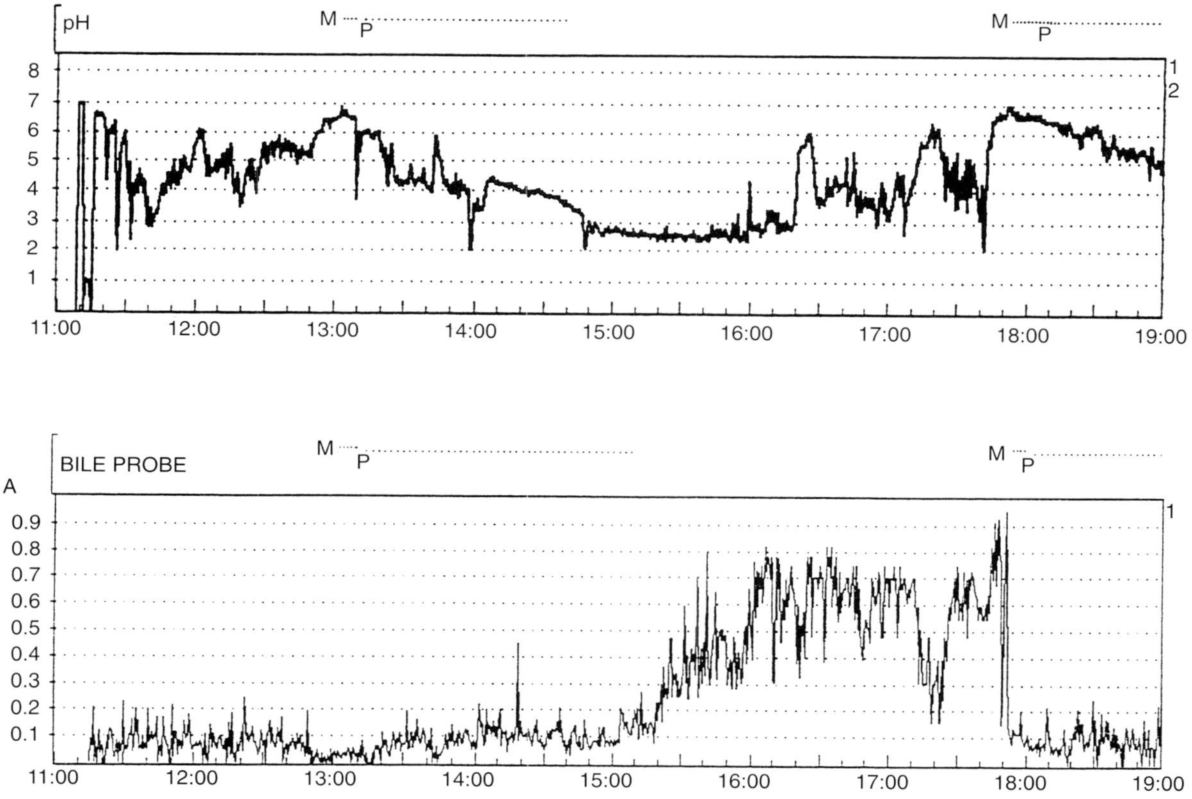

Fig. 4-19. Combined esophageal pH monitoring (upper trace) and esophageal bilirubin monitoring (lower trace) in a patient with Barrett's esophagus. Each trace represents the same 8-hour period (11:00 to 19:00 hours). In addition to the frequent and prolonged falls in esophageal pH to a level <4, note the high esophageal exposure to bilirubin (absorption >0.14) between 15:00 and 18:00 hours). High bilirubin recordings are observed at both low and normal esophageal pH levels.

cially high values. We restrict the patient's diet to narrow selection of plain foods or a liquid diet for this test and use an absorbance threshold of above 0.14 to indicate the presence of bilirubin in the esophageal lumen.[49]

Using the Bilitec probe to investigate healthy volunteers and patients with gastroesophageal reflux disease we have observed that bilirubin rarely refluxes into the esophagus of control subjects (upper limit of normal <3% total time of monitoring with absorbance >0.14). In patients with complicated reflux disease (e.g., Barrett's esophagus), bilirubin is detected within the esophageal lumen for 15% to 20% of the total time and may be present for >30% of the supine period (Fig. 4-19). These data support the view that patients with Barrett's esophagus reflux a complex mixture of both acid and duodenal juice into the esophagus.[51] Additionally, the presence of bilirubin in the esophagus of Barrett's patients occurs both at pH values <4 and at pH values >4, indicating that pH monitoring may not detect the full extent of the reflux disease in these patients.

GASTRIC FUNCTION STUDIES

MEASUREMENT OF GASTRIC EMPTYING

The stomach is divided functionally into two parts that complement each other in function. The proximal stomach serves as a reservoir for solid foodstuff and is capable of receptive and adaptive relaxation after meals. In addition, the fundus exerts a continuous tonic contraction that is responsible for the emptying of liquids. It is electrically inert and appears to be under direct vagal control. The motor activity of the gastric body and antrum are regulated by the gastric pacemaker, which is located one third the distance down the greater curvature.[52] The pacemaker discharges with a regular rhythm of about three per minute and sweeps across the stomach from the greater curvature toward the lesser curvature and in an aborad direction.

The pacesetter potential or basal electrical rhythm of the stomach controls the rate of action potentials, the electric counterpart of muscle contractions. Action potentials do not follow each pacesetter potential but follow the pattern of the migrating myoelectric complex, which is composed of interdigestive cycles of steadily increasing motor activity to a brief crescendo, the activity front, lasting for 2 to 3 minutes and occurring every 70 to 150 minutes.[53] After the patient feeds, each pacesetter potential is followed by a weaker action potential that is associated with regular muscle contractions.

Gastric emptying is affected by the composition and consistency of the ingested meal.[54] Liquids empty most rapidly, semisolids more slowly, and solids the slowest. The emptying of liquids and semisolids follows an exponential decline, whereas when solids are ingested there is an initial plateau phase without any obvious emptying followed by a linear emptying of the foodstuff. Foods with a high protein content tend to empty most rapidly, whereas high fat and calorie composition in a meal tend to slow the rate of gastric emptying. These factors are of importance when comparing rates of gastric emptying in different patients and controls.

Measurement of gastric emptying is best performed with isotopically labeled meals. Following ingestion of the meal, anterior and posterior images of the area of interest are obtained by a gamma camera collimator for a period of 60 seconds every 15 minutes. Studies are best performed with patients in the upright position. The counts are corrected for decay and the geometric mean values are determined from both the anterior and posterior images. Fig. 4-20 shows the normal median values and the 5th and 95th percentiles that were established in 20 healthy volunteers for solid (^{99m}Tc-labeled chicken liver and beef stew), semisolid (^{99m}Tc-labeled oatmeal), and liquid (^{111}InDTPA-labeled water) emptying. Abnormalities in gastric emptying may be identified when the $t_{1/2}$ is outside the normal range (above or below the 5th and 95th percentiles). A better assessment of gastric emptying abnormalities is made by plotting the patient's emptying curve against the normal values to see if and when the patient falls outside the normal range.

Abnormalities of gastric emptying may be categorized as rapid or prolonged. *Rapid gastric emptying* is associated with symptoms of dumping and diarrhea. It is uncommon in the unoperated stomach. It typically occurs in patients following vagotomy who have increased tone in the fundus of the stomach with rapid emptying of liquids into the duodenum and upper small bowel. Additionally, gastric fundoplication without vagotomy will speed the gastric emptying rate for both solids and liquids. Rapid gastric emptying may also accompany partial gastric resections.

Delayed gastric emptying is common in patients complaining of foregut symptoms. Patients complain of early satiety, bloating, epigastric pain, and flatulence, which may lead to regurgitation and heartburn symptoms. If the condition is untreated, it may progress to repeated vomiting with dehydration and electrolyte imbalance. The causes of delayed gastric emptying are outlined below.

- Infective
  - Septicemia
  - Viremia
- Inflammatory
  - Gastritis
    - Bile reflux
    - Bacterial *(Helicobacter pylori)*
    - Chemical (alcohol)
  - Peptic ulcer
    - Pyloric stenosis
  - Pancreatitis
- Metabolic
  - Diabetes mellitus
  - Hypothyroidism
- Systemic
  - Scleroderma
- Iatrogenic
  - Drug abuse (opiate narcotics)
- Traumatic
  - Multiple trauma
  - Head injuries
  - Burns
  - Spinal injury
- Mitotic
  - Carcinoma
    - Distal stomach
    - Pancreatic head
    - Peritoneal metastasis
    - Retroperitoneal tumors
- Postoperative
  - Ileus
  - Adhesions
  - Vagotomy
  - Roux stasis syndrome

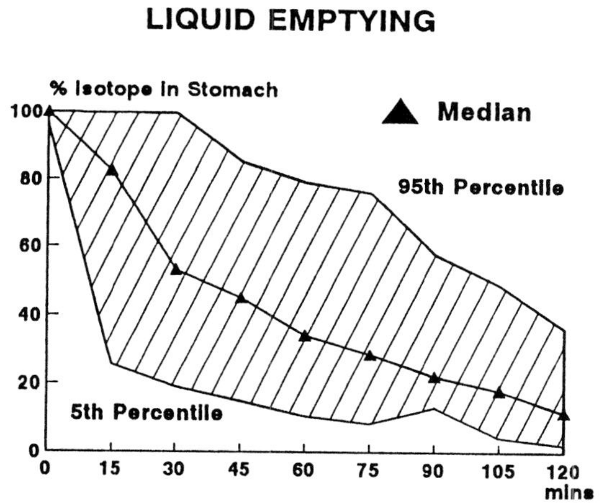

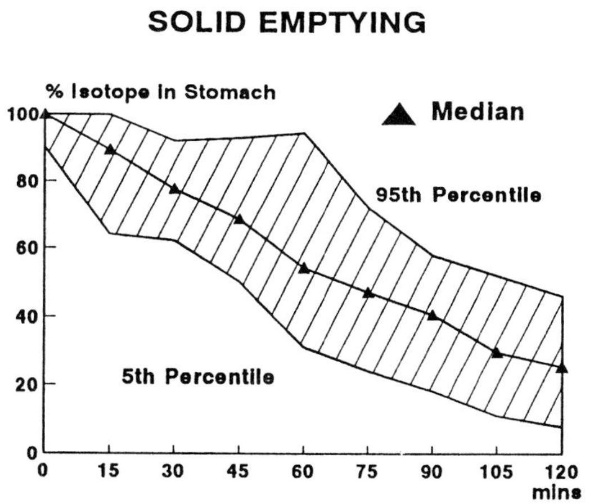

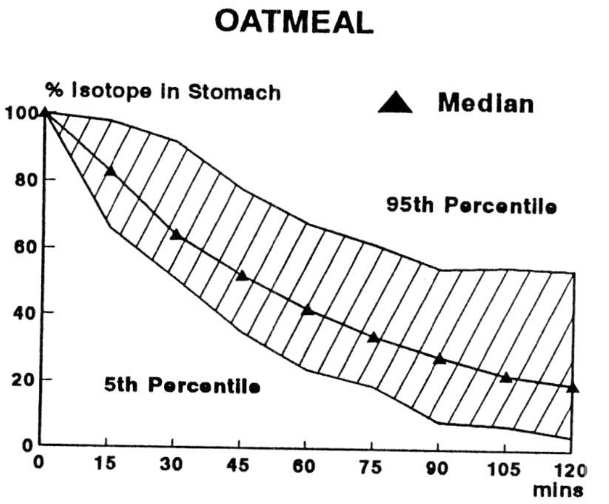

Fig. 4-20. Median, 5th, and 95th percentile ranges for gastric emptying of liquid, solid, and oatmeal established in 20 healthy volunteers. (From Clark GWB, Jamieson JR, Hinder RA, et al. The relationship of gastric pH and the emptying of solid, semisolid and liquid meals. J Gastrointest Motil 5:273-279, 1993.)

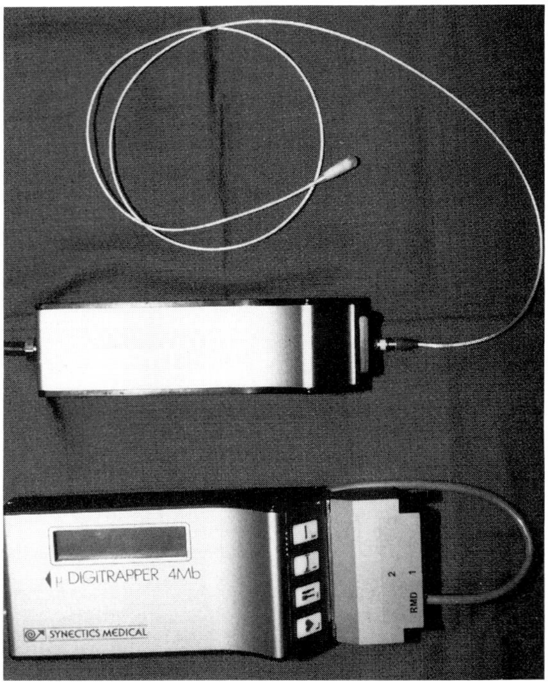

Fig. 4-21. Hardware for monitoring of ambulatory gastric emptying. The Geiger counter probe is passed transnasally into the patient's stomach before ingestion of the labeled meal. The probe is connected to a preamplifier attached to a portable microdigitrapper.

A recently developed technique to evaluate gastric emptying in an ambulatory setting is now available (Synectics Medical, Irving, Tex.).[55] A portable Geiger counter is connected to a preamplifier and a portable microdigitrapper, which can collect counts over a 24-hour circadian cycle (Fig. 4-21). The probe is passed transnasally and positioned in the proximal stomach 5 cm distal to the lower border of the lower esophageal sphincter. The patient then ingests up to three isotopically labeled meals over the ensuing 24 hours, and at the end of the study the data are unloaded onto a personal computer for analysis. In addition, the gastric emptying probe can be combined with gastric pH monitoring or antroduodenal manometry. Fig. 4-22 shows a typical normal gastric emptying trace obtained with this technique.

AMBULATORY 24-HOUR GASTRIC pH MONITORING

Gastric pH monitoring is used in the evalaution of the gastric secretory state and provides information to the surgeon regarding the basal gastric pH, the effect of medications on the gastric pH,[56,57] and the presence of duodenogastric reflux based on patterns of gastric alkalinization[58,59] and suggests the diagnosis of gastric hypersecretion and delayed gastric emptying.

The studies are best performed with glass electrodes, which are more accurate than antimony in the gastric environment. The probe is passed transnasally and positioned in the fundus 5 cm below the lower border of the lower esophageal sphincter and connected to a microdigitrapper. Gastric pH analysis is performed

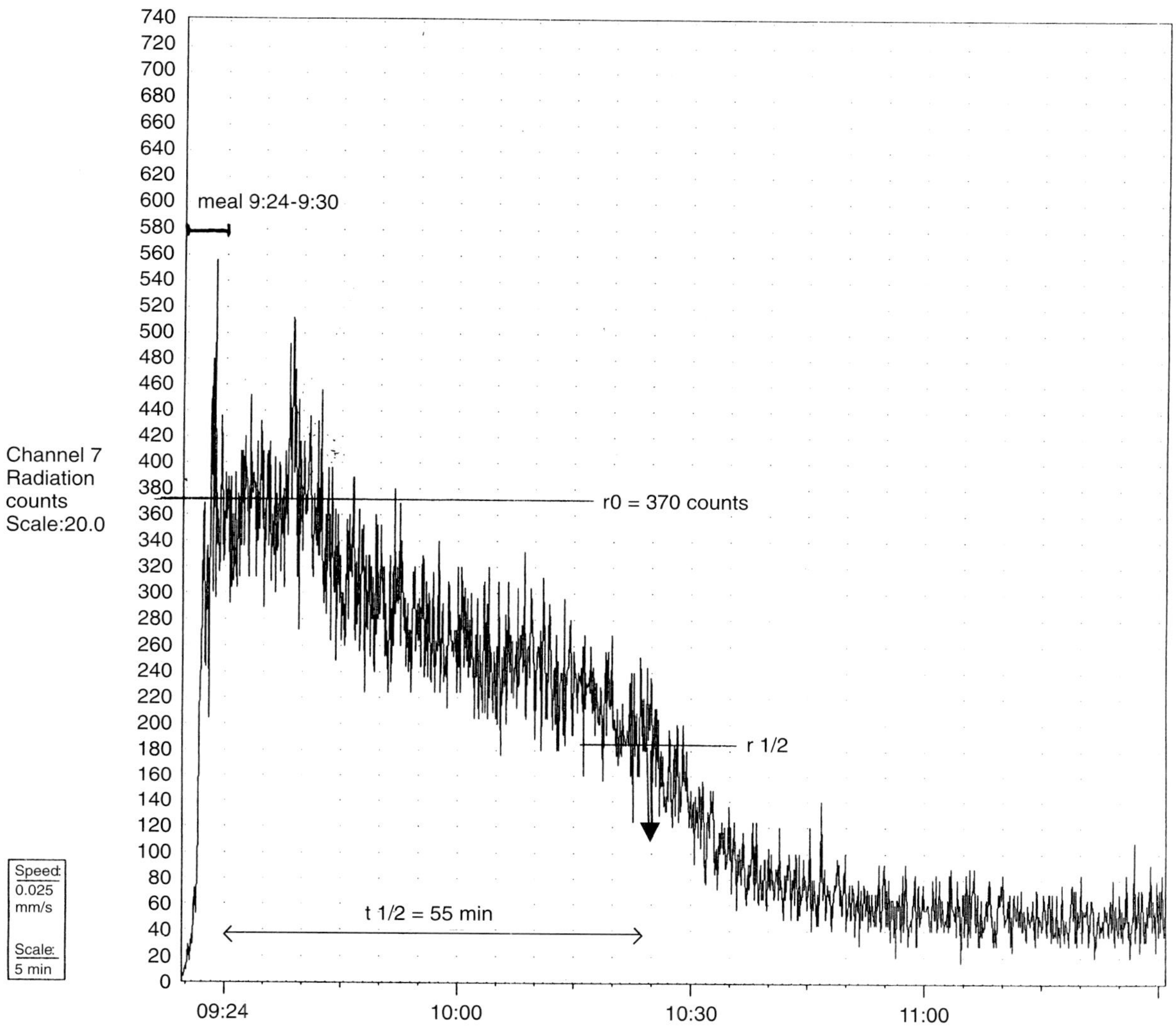

Fig. 4-22. Typical ambulatory gastric emptying tracing. Radioactivity counts are displayed along the y-axis and time is displayed along the x-axis. The ^{99m}Tc-labeled egg sandwich was ingested between 9:24 and 9:30 A.M. The median plateau count was estimated to be 370 counts and the $t_{1/2}$ (time for the counts to drop by 50%) was 55 minutes.

over a 24-hour circadian cycle with the patient off all medications for at least 48 hours (and omeprazole for 2 weeks). A diary is kept of mealtimes, upright and supine periods, and symptoms experienced during the study. At the end of the study the data are unloaded onto a personal computer for subsequent analysis.

Analysis is performed with commercially available computer software that measures a set of parameters describing the circadian gastric pH pattern based on the percent time spent at a pH band, that is, between whole-number pH thresholds during the upright, supine, meal, and postprandial period; the number of times the pH moved from lower band into a higher band; the most common pH below 2 or the baseline pH; the most common pH of the meal plateau; and the pattern of pH decline from the plateau.[60,61]

To quantitate alkaline duodenogastric reflux the gastric pH record is divided into the upright period, the supine period, the prandial pH plateau period, and the postprandial pH decline period. For each of these periods the following parameters are calculated:

1. The pH frequency distribution (the percentage time the gastric pH was at the pH interval 0 to 1, 1 to 2, 2 to 3, 3 to 4, 4 to 5, 5 to 6, 6 to 7, and >7)
2. The frequency of pH changes (the incidence of pH movements from a lower into a higher pH interval)
3. The duration of pH exposure expressed as the longest time the pH remained at a pH interval during the monitoring period
4. The duration-frequency of pH exposure expressed as the number of times the pH remained at a pH interval for >5 minutes

Discriminate analysis has shown that a scoring system based on 16 variables of these parameters can differentiate the gastric pH profile of normal volunteers from patients with classic duodenogastric reflux disease. When applied prospectively, this scoring system was superior to *o*-diisopropyl iminodiacetic acid (DISIDA) scanning with cholecystokinin stimulation in the diagnosis of excessive duodenogastric reflux and detected the disease with a sensitivity of 90% and a specificity of 100%.[62,63]

Gastric hypersecretion can also be evaluated by gastric pH monitoring. The percent time spent in each of the pH bands 0 to 1, 1 to 2, 2 to 3, etc. can be plotted graphically and compared to the normal ranges established in healthy volunteers. The supine gastric pH recording is especially helpful in the diagnosis of gastric hypersecretion. Fig. 4-23 shows an example of a patient who is outside the normal range for percent time the gastric pH was between the band 0 to 1 during the supine period. Acid hypersecretion can also be diagnosed when the patient's cumulative frequency distribution graph of gastric pH falls to the left of the normal range. This "left shift" in gastric pH correlates well with the presence of duodenal ulcer disease, whereas a "right shift" in gastric pH consequent to an increased time above pH 3 correlates well with the presence of antral gastritis.[64]

ADDITIONAL TESTS

Gastric Acid Analysis

Gastric acid analysis is the traditional method for diagnosing gastric acid hypersecretion.[65] It is indicated in patients with peptic ulcer disease, particularly those patients resistant to conventional treatment and those with recurrent ulcer following vagotomy, in whom the test can be used to evaluate the completeness of the vagotomy (insulin stress test), and gastroesophageal reflux disease mainly in the presence of a competent lower esophageal sphincter.

The procedure is performed after an overnight fast in patients who have been off all antisecretory medications for 48 hours (and omeprazole for 2 weeks). The stomach is intubated with a 16 F Salem Sump nasogastric tube. By means of intermittent manual suction, basal acid secretion is determined by collecting gastric secretions for two 15-minute periods. The volume of secretion is recorded and the hydrogen ion concentration determined by titration with 0.2 N sodium hydroxide to pH 7. The maximal acid output is determined by collecting 15-minute aliquots of gastric secretion over a 1-hour period following stimulation of the gastric secretory state with intravenous pentagastrin in doses of 6 μg/kg. The peak acid output is determined by selecting the two consecutive highest stimulated periods. The values obtained are usually expressed in milliequivalents per hour. The upper limit of normal for these

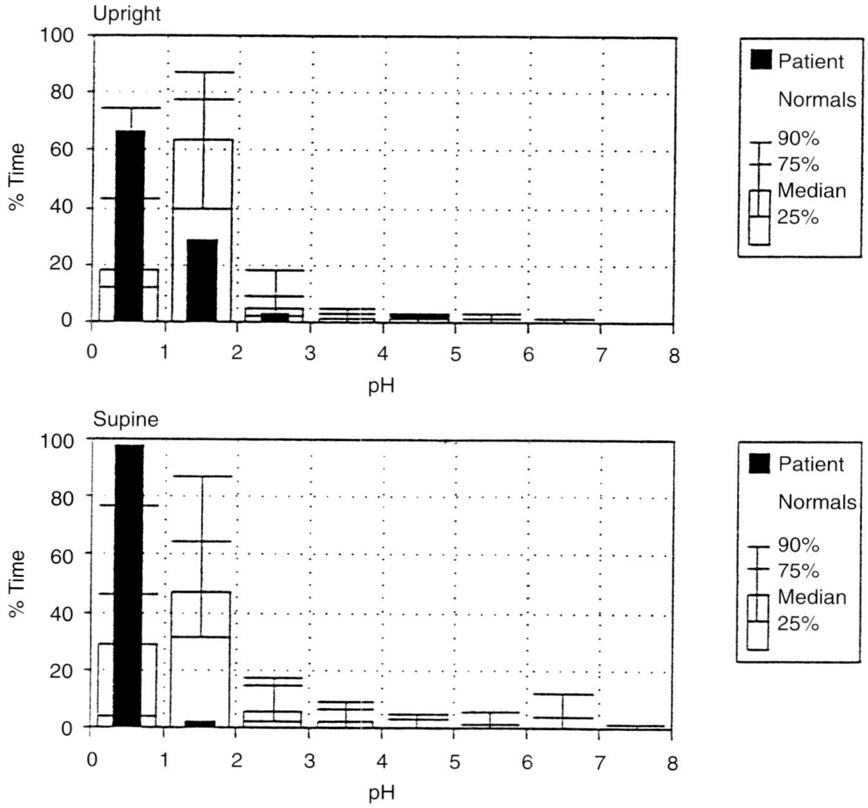

Fig. 4-23. Distribution of gastric pH by percent time spent at bands 0 to 1, 1 to 2, 2 to 3, etc. during the upright (upper) and supine (lower) periods. The patient's value is shown by the dark bars with normal ranges shown in the key boxes. During the supine time the patient spent an abnormally long percent of time at the pH interval 0 to 1, suggesting gastric acid hypersecretion. This suspicion was confirmed by subsequent gastric acid analysis.

values is a basal acid output <5 mEq/hr, maximal acid output <20 mEq/hr, and peak acid output <35 mEq/hr. An estimation of the fasting serum gastrin level is performed when collecting the basal acid output. Normally the fasting serum gastrin is <100 picomoles/L.

Patients with gastroesophageal reflux disease are usually suspected of being hypersecretors when reflux is found in the presence of a mechanically competent lower esophageal sphincter or when there is a past history or coexisting duodenal ulcer disease. When hypersecretion is identified and the patient has a concomitant duodenal ulcer or a documented history of an ulcer, consideration must be given to performing a highly selective vagotomy at the time of Nissen fundoplication; however, it should be noted that we do not advocate adding a vagotomy to an antireflux procedure as a routine measure.

Gastric Bile Probe

The Bilitec 2000 system with its fiberoptic cable can be positioned in the stomach rather that the distal esophagus. The probe is positioned 5 cm below the lower border of the lower esophageal sphincter and gastric exposure to bilirubin measured for up to 24 hours. The technique was described previously in the section on esophageal function studies. Early studies in our laboratory have indicated that gastric exposure to bilirubin (absorption >0.14) occurs up to 15% of the time in normal subjects. The use of this technique in the stomach and its role in the investigation of patients are currently under investigation.

Cholescintigraphy

Scintigraphic imaging of bile reflux into the stomach can be performed after intravenous injection of 5 μCi of ^{99m}Tc-labeled iminodiacetic acid derivatives such as disofenin (DISIDA). The isotope is concentrated in the gallbladder, and the flow of bile can be followed by gamma camera imaging of the upper abdomen, gallbladder, and stomach. The first series of images are performed at 5-minute intervals for 60 minutes. Emptying of the gallbladder is encouraged by intravenous injection of 20 mg/kg of a synthetic analogue of cholecystokinin and flow of bile into the stomach can be imaged. The diagnosis of duodenogastric reflux is based on the observation of positive counts from the stomach within the first 30 minutes following the injection of cholecystokinin. The test has a low specificity and consequently has limited use in the diagnosis of pathologic duodenogastric reflux.

REFERENCES

1. Costantini M, Crookes PF, Bremner RM, et al. Value of physiological assessment of foregut symptoms in a surgical practice. Surgery 114:780-787, 1993.
2. Pope CE. Effect of infusion on force of closure measurements in the human esophagus. Gastroenterology 58:779-786, 1970.
3. Arndorfer RC, Stef JJ, Dodds WJ, et al. Improved infusion system for intraluminal esophageal manometry. Gastroenterology 73:23-27, 1977.
4. Humphries TJ, Castell DO. Pressure profile of esophageal peristalsis in normal humans as measured by direct intraesophageal transducers. Dig Dis 22:641-645, 1977.
5. Richter JE, Bradley LA, Castell DO. Esophageal chest pain: Current controversies in pathogenesis, diagnosis and therapy. Ann Intern Med 110:67-78, 1989.
6. Weilgosz ET, Fletcher RH, McCants CB, et al. Unimproved chest pain in patients with minimal or no coronary disease: A behavioral phenomenon. Am Heart J 108:67-72, 1984.
7. Ward BW, Wu WC, Richter JE, et al. Long-term follow-up of symptomatic status of patients with noncardiac chest pain: Is diagnosis of esophageal etiology helpful? Am J Gastroenterol 82:215-218, 1987.
8. Zaninotto G, DeMeester TR, Schwizer W, et al. The lower esophageal sphincter in health and disease. Am J Surg 155:104-111, 1988.
9. DeMeester TR, Bonavina L, Albertucci M. Nissen fundoplication for gastroesophageal reflux disease—evaluation of primary repair in 100 consecutive patients. Ann Surg 204:9-20, 1986.
10. Barlow AP, DeMeester TR, Ball CS, et al. The significance of the gastric secretory state in gastroesophageal reflux disease. Arch Surg 124:937-941, 1989.
11. Schwizer W, Hinder RA, DeMeester TR. Does delayed gastric emptying contribute to gastroesophageal reflux disease? Am J Surg 157:74-81, 1985.
12. Stein HJ, Bremner RM, Jamieson J, et al. Effect of Nissen fundoplication on esophageal motor function. Arch Surg 127:788-791, 1992.
13. Weerts JM, Dellemagne G, Hamoir E, et al. Laparoscopic Nissen fundoplication: Detailed analysis of 132 patients. Surg Laparosc Endosc 3:359-364, 1993.
14. Zaninotto G, DeMeester TR, Bremner CG, et al. Esophageal function in patients with reflux-induced strictures and its relevance to surgical treatment. Ann Thorac Surg 47:362-370, 1989.

15. Mattox HE. The placement of the pH electrode. In Richter JE, ed. Ambulatory Esophageal pH Monitoring. New York: Igaku-Shoin, 1991, pp 41-49.
16. Stein HJ, DeMeester TR, Naspetti R, et al. Three dimensional imaging of the lower esophageal sphincter in gastroesophageal reflux disease. Ann Surg 214:374-384, 1991.
17. Welch RW, Drake ST. Normal lower esophageal sphincter pressure: A comparison of rapid vs. slow pull-through. Gastroenterology 78:1446-1451, 1980.
18. Costantini M, Bremner RM, Hoeft SF, et al. The slow motorized pull-through: An improved technique to evaluate the lower esophageal sphincter. Gastroenterology 103:A1407, 1992.
19. Tucker HJ, Snape WJ, Cohen S. Achalasia secondary to carcinoma: Manometric and clinical features. Ann Intern Med 89:315-318, 1978.
20. Dodds WJ, Stewart ET, Hogan WJ, et al. Effect of esophageal movement in intraluminal esophageal pressure recording. Gastroenterology 67:592-600, 1974.
21. Kahrilas PJ, Dodds WJ, Hogan WJ. Effect of peristaltic dysfunction on esophageal volume clearance. Gastroenterology 94:73-80, 1988.
22. Hewson EG, Ott DJ, Dalton CB, et al. Manometry and radiology. Complementary studies in the assessment of esophageal motility disorders. Gastroenterology 98:626-632, 1990.
23. Katz PO. Achalasia. In Castell DO, Richter JE, Dalton CB, ed. Esophageal Motility Testing. New York: Elsevier, 1987, pp 107-117.
24. Vantrappen G, Janssens J, Hellmans J, et al. Achalasia, diffuse esophageal spasm and related motility disorders. Gastroenterology 76:450-457, 1979.
25. Richter JE. Diffuse esophageal spasm. In Castell DO, Richter JE, Dalton CB, eds. Esophageal Motility Testing. New York: Elsevier, 1987, pp 118-129.
26. Benjamin SB, Gerhardt DC, Castell DO. High-amplitude, peristaltic esophageal contractions associated with chest pain and/or dysphagia. Gastroenterology 77:478-483, 1979.
27. DeMeester TR, O'Sullivan GC, Bermudez G, et al. Esophageal function in patients with angina-type chest pain and normal coronary angiograms. Ann Surg 196:488-498, 1982.
28. Stein HJ, Bremner RM, Jamieson JR, et al. Effect of Nissen fundoplication on esophageal motor function. Arch Surg 127:788-791, 1992.
29. Singh P, Adamopoulos A, Taylor RH, et al. Oesophageal motor function before and after healing of oesophagitis. Gut 33:1590-1596, 1992.
30. Richter JE, Castell DO. Gastroesophageal reflux: Pathogenesis, diagnosis and therapy. Ann Intern Med 97:93-99, 1982.
31. DeMeester TR, Wang CI, Wernly JA, et al. Technique, indications and clinical use of 24-hr esophageal pH monitoring. J Thorac Cardiovasc Surg 799:656-667, 1980.
32. Wu W. Ambulatory esophageal pH monitoring: The equipment and probes. In Richter JE, ed. Ambulatory Esophageal pH Monitoring. New York: Igaku-Shoin, 1992, pp 13-22.
33. Jamieson JR, Stein HJ, DeMeester TR, et al. Ambulatory 24-hr esophageal pH monitoring: Normal values, optimal thresholds, sensitivity, specificity and reproducibility. Am J Gastroenterol 87:1102-1111, 1992.
34. Helm JF, Dodds WJ, Hogan WJ, et al. Acid neutralizing capacity of human saliva. Gastroenterology 83:69-74, 1982.
35. DeMeester TR, Johnson LF, Joseph GJ, et al. Patterns of gastroesophageal reflux in health and disease. Ann Surg 184:459-470, 1976.
36. Lin KM, Ueda RK, Hinder RA, et al. Etiology and importance of alkaline esophageal reflux. Am J Surg 162:553-557, 1991.
37. Attwood SEA, DeMeester TR, Bremner, CG, et al. Alkaline gastroesophageal reflux: Implications in the development of complications in Barrett's columnar-lined lower esophagus. Surgery 106:764-770, 1989.
38. Gillen P, Keeling P, Byrne PJ, et al. Implications of duodenogastric reflux in the pathogenesis of Barrett's oesophagus. Br J Surg 75:540-543, 1988.
39. Iftikhar SY, Ledingham S, Steele RJC, et al. Bile reflux in columnar-lined Barrett's oesophagus. Ann R Coll Surg Eng 75:411-416, 1993.
40. Jacob P, Kahrilas PJ, Herzon G. Proximal esophageal pH-metry in patients with "reflux laryngitis." Gastroenterology 100:305-310, 1991.
41. Singh S, Richter JE. Twenty-four-hour esophageal pH measurement. Prob Gen Surg 9:104-123, 1992.

42. Skinner DB, Booth DJ. Assessment of distal esophageal function in patients with hiatal hernia and/or gastroesophageal reflux. Ann Surg 172:627-637, 1970.
43. Bernstein LM, Baker CA. A clinical test for esophagitis. Gastroenterology 34:760-781, 1958.
44. deCaestecker JS, Pryde A, Heading RC. Comparison of intravenous edrophonium and oesophageal acid perfusion during oesophageal manometry in patients with non-cardiac chest pain. Gut 29:1029-1034, 1988.
45. Bremner RM, Hoeft SF, Costantini M, et al. Pharyngeal swallowing. The major factor in clearance of esophageal reflux episodes. Ann Surg 218:364-370, 1993.
46. Bremner RM, Costantini M, Hoeft SF, et al. Manual verification of computer analysis of 24-hour esophageal motility. Biomed Instrum Technol 27:49-55, 1993.
47. Eypasch EP, Stein HJ, DeMeester TR, et al. A new technique to define and clarify esophageal motor disorders. Am J Surg 159:144-152, 1990.
48. Stein HJ, DeMeester TR. Indications, technique, and clinical use of ambulatory 24-hour esophageal motility monitoring in a surgical practice. Ann Surg 217:128-137, 1993.
49. Bechi P, Pucciani F, Baldini F, et al. Long-term ambulatory enterogastric reflux monitoring. Validation of a new fiberoptic technique. Dig Dis Sci 38:1297-1306, 1993.
50. Burdiles P, Hoeft SF, Clark GWB, et al. Evaluation of a fibre-optic sensor for bilirubin. Gastroenterology 104:A485, 1993.
51. Champion G, Singh S, Bechi P, Richter JE. Duodenogastric reflux—relationship to esophageal pH and response to omeprazole. Gastroenterology 104:A51, 1993.
52. Hinder RA, Kelly KA. Human gastric pacesetter potential. Site of origin, spread and response to gastric transection and proximal vagotomy. Am J Surg 133:29-33, 1977.
53. Hermon-Taylor J, Code CF. Localization of the duodenal pacemaker and its role in the organization of duodenal myoelectric activity. Gut 12:40-47, 1971.
54. Clark GWB, Jamieson JR, Hinder RA, et al. The relationship of gastric pH and the emptying of solid, semisolid and liquid meals. J Gastrointest Motil 5:273-279, 1993.
55. Hoeft SF, DeMeester TR, Peters JH, et al. Ambulatory monitoring of gastric emptying. Gastroenterology 104:A521, 1993.
56. Etienne A, Fimmel CJ, Bron BJ, et al. Evaluations of pirenzepine on gastric acidity in healthy volunteers using ambulatory 24 hour intragastric pH-monitoring. Gut 26:241-245, 1985.
57. Fimmel CJ, Etienne A, Cilluffo T, et al. Long-term ambulatory gastric pH monitoring: Validation of a new method and effect of H_2 antagonists. Gastroenterology 88:42-51, 1985.
58. Fuchs KH, DeMeester TR, Albertucci M, et al. Quantification of the duodenogastric reflux in gastroesophageal reflux disease. In Siewart JH, Holscher AH, eds. Diseases of the Esophagus. 1988, pp 831-835.
59. Hinder RA, Fuchs KH, Barlow AP, et al. Prolonged measurement of intragastric pH. In Read NW, ed. Gastrointestinal Motility: Which Test? Petersfield, England: Wrightson Biomedical Publishing, 1989, pp 121-127.
60. Barlow AP, Hinder RA, DeMeester TR. Principles of 24 hour pH monitoring and its clinical applications. Gastroenterology 98:A27, 1989.
61. Fuchs KH, DeMeester TR, Hinder RA, et al. Computerized identification of pathological duodenogastric reflux using 24-hour gastric pH monitoring. Ann Surg 213:13-20, 1991.
62. Stein HJ, Hinder RA, DeMeester TR, et al. Clinical use of 24-hour gastric pH monitoring vs. *o*-diisopropyl iminodiacetic acid (DISIDA) scanning in the diagnosis of pathological duodenogastric reflux. Arch Surg 125:966-971, 1990.
63. Stein HJ, Smyrck TC, DeMeester TR, et al. Clinical value of endoscopy and histology in the diagnosis of duodenogastric reflux disease. Surgery 112:796-804, 1992.
64. Stein HJ, DeMeester TR, Peters JH, et al. Technique, indications, and clinical use of ambulatory 24-hour gastric pH monitoring in a surgical practice. Surgery (in press).
65. Jenkins JX, Lanspa SJ. Acid secretory tests in the diagnosis of foregut surgical disease. Probl Gen Surg 9:104-123, 1992.

Part

II

Esophageal Motor Disorders

Chapter

5

Endoscopic Approach to Hypopharyngeal Diverticulum

Jean-Marie Collard, M.D.

Transoral management of hypopharyngeal pouches has received wide acceptance since the beginning of the twentieth century. Inverting the diverticular sac into the digestive lumen and encircling it with a ligature for a few days until the sac necrosed was a popular procedure 60 years ago.[1] The ligature and the sac could be removed with gentle traction. The final result was a superficially ulcerated area at the level of the mouth of the esophagus.

Even more popular was the technique described by Mosher[2] in 1917. The common wall between the esophageal lumen and the diverticular sac was divided with punch forceps to create a common cavity. Rather than being retained in the diverticular sac after swallowing, food was pushed into the common cavity and the lower cervical esophagus by pharyngeal contraction. Mosher noted that "a small crescentic rim was to be left at the bottom of the pouch to wall off the mediastinum" to prevent perforation and that "should symptoms return it should be an easy matter to cut the common wall still more." Mosher discontinued the procedure when one of his patients developed mediastinitis and died.

The concept of creating a common cavity endoscopically was restored to favor by Dohlman and Mattsson[3] and later by others.[4-6] They introduced diathermy for coagulating the common wall prior to cutting. This endoscopic procedure, however, was not widely used by esophageal surgeons during the following decades because some patients complained of persistent dysphagia after the operation[7] and required division of the wall at the second and even the third stage.[8] Moreover, perforation and mediastinitis occurred as a result of failure to identify the bottom of the diverticulum during division of the distal part of the wall. More recently, Dutch ENT surgeons such as Van Overbeek and Hoeksema[9] published their experience with this endoscopic procedure. Their series is the largest reported to date. The innovative feature was the use of the CO_2 laser beam to coagulate and cut the common wall.[10,11] More than 500 patients have been treated with few postoperative complications and a very high short-term success rate.[12]

Recent developments in minimal access surgery and instrumentation have led to improved methods for coagulation and division of the esophageal wall as well as the use of endoscopic stapling devices to suture the opposing walls of the sac and the esophagus at the same time they are divided[13] (Fig. 5-1).

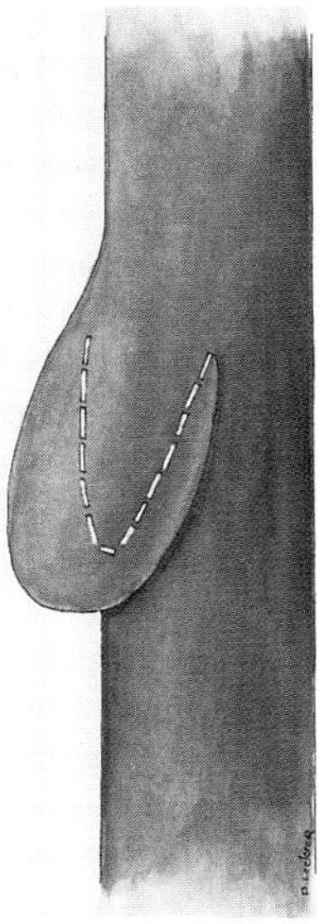

Fig. 5-1. Principle of creating a common cavity with the esophageal lumen and the hypopharyngeal diverticulum.

ANATOMIC CONSIDERATIONS AND INDICATIONS

The recent studies of Cook and associates on the biomechanics of the upper esophageal sphincter,[14] cricopharyngeal bar,[15] and Zenker's diverticulum[16] have clearly shown that in the two latter situations there is a resistance to flow through the upper esophageal sphincter as a result of incomplete sphincter opening. This necessitates an increase in hypopharyngeal intrabolus pressure to preserve a normal transsphincteric flow. The same group observed that unlike cricomyotomy without resection of the pouch, resection of the diverticulum without cricomyotomy failed to normalize sphincter opening and intrabolus pressure. This emphasizes the critical role played by the upper esophageal sphincter in the genesis of hypopharyngeal diverticulum, which is not a disease in itself but only the consequence of a motility disorder. Any treatment of hypopharyngeal diverticulum should include abolishment of stasis in the pouch as well as enlargement of the mouth of the esophagus to correct the underlying motility disorder. The endoscopic division of the common wall between the lumen of the cervical esophagus and that of the diverticulum fulfills both of these criteria. Indeed, the anatomic structures that form the upper esophageal sphincter are included in the common wall and they are severed when it is divided. Lateral retraction of the divided cricopharyngeus muscle and the muscular layers of the cervical esophagus creates a V-shaped defect between the two lumina, resulting in a common cavity.

At present we see that these principles should not be applied to small hypopharyngeal diverticula. A major reason for this is that the common wall needs to be long enough so that the esophageal wall can be cut over a distance of 3 cm or more, achieving an adequate myotomy (placement of one cartridge of staples and preferably more than one on the common wall). Although the upper esophageal sphincter has been shown to correspond to the cricopharyngeus muscle,[14] division of the muscular layers of the cervical esophagus distal to the cricopharyngeus is necessary to achieve a myotomy capable of opening the esophageal mouth adequately. This is supported by manometric studies on patients with cricopharyngeal dysfunction[17] and by the

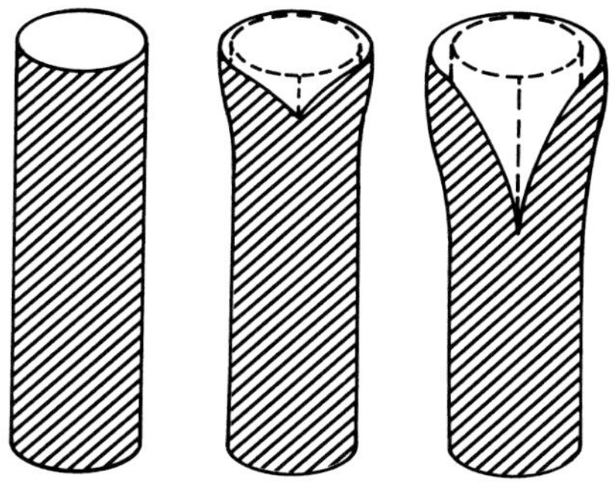

Fig. 5-2. The longer the cut in the wall, the greater the enlargement of the tip of any soft tubular structures.

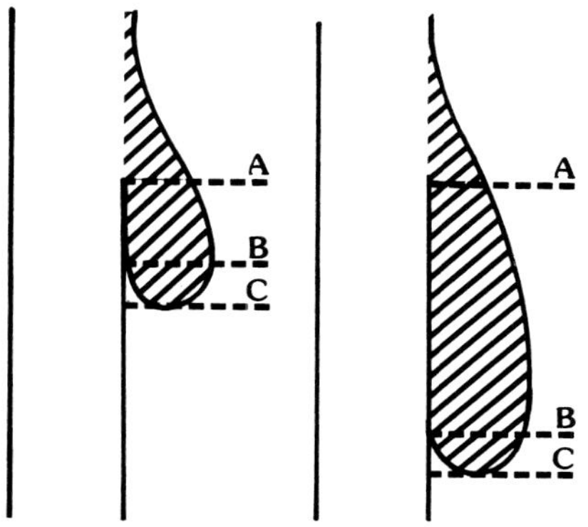

Fig. 5-3. A small (left) and a large (right) diverticulum. A = proximal border of the common wall before division; B = proximal edge of the residual spur; C = bottom of the diverticulum. The length of the spur is relatively long in a small diverticulum (AB/BC = 2), whereas it is relatively short in a large one (AB/BC = 7).

experience with open surgery. A general principle for widening the diameter of any tubular structure is that the longer the longitudinal section of the wall, the greater the gain in diameter (Fig. 5-2). The length of the common wall is best evaluated endoscopically at operation. Indeed, a preoperative estimation of the size of the common wall on side-view roentgenograms depends on correction factors for magnification and/or reduction. Superimposition of the bottom of the diverticulum and the clavicle, which is sometimes observed on roentgenograms, also makes evaluation difficult. The common wall can be readily observed at operation when the striated muscles of the neck, the pharynx, and the proximal esophagus are relaxed by anesthesia. The stapling procedure permits the bottom of the diverticulum to be pushed downward and the common wall to be stretched, providing a cut length somewhat greater than that which had been estimated preoperatively.

A second reason for not approaching a small diverticulum endoscopically is that the ratio of the length of the residual spur at the bottom of the diverticulum to the section length would be much greater than that achieved after sectioning of the common wall of a larger diverticulum (Fig. 5-3). This would render the maneuver ineffective. Clinical experience with two patients who had only incomplete symptomatic relief after endoscopic management of a small diverticulum supports this concept, whereas five patients in whom one or more than one cartridge of staples could be applied to the common wall had a more satisfactory outcome.

The third reason is that endoscopic identification of the opening of a very small diverticulum into the esophageal lumen may be difficult because the two lips of the diverticuloscope can collapse this opening into a simple slit by stretching the oropharyngeal wall. This can lead to catching of the lower lip of the diverticuloscope in the slit and perforation of a small diverticulum.

In view of these anatomic considerations the following surgical strategy may be proposed:

1. Diverticula of 1 cm or less should be treated exclusively by open transcervical myotomy of the cricopharyngeus muscle and the muscular wall of the proximal esophagus. The mucosa of the diverticulum usually realigns itself with that of the cervical esophagus.
2. Diverticula of 1 to 2 cm are best treated by transcervical myotomy and diverticulopexy.[18,19]
3. Medium-sized diverticula of 3 to 4 cm can be treated either by transcervical myotomy and diverticulopexy or by endoscopic division of the common wall. However, further experience and long-term follow-up of endoscopic techniques are required prior to widespread use. At present we reserve the endoscopic procedure for elderly patients, especially those admitted to the hospital with aspiration-related pneumonia or those with a history of multiple respiratory infections. Patients undergoing reoperation after failure of a transcervical operation on the diverticulum or patients with a history of thyroid lobectomy may also be candidates since the left recurrent nerve must be protected.
4. A diverticulum of 6 cm or more creates a mass effect and cannot be placed behind the pharynx. Diverticula of this size are best treated by resection and myotomy.[19]

Advantages of the Endoscopic Approach

In general the merits of the endoscopic procedure are as follows:

1. The procedure takes 5 minutes or less.
2. Only a short-acting, light general anesthetic is required.
3. The excellent magnified view of the diverticular wall permits detection of any mucosal irregularity, which can be readily biopsied to exclude any neoplastic change.
4. The anatomic structures that form the upper esophageal sphincter, that is, the cricopharyngeus muscle and the muscular fibers of the proximal esophagus, are included in the common wall and divided at the same time, which results in a true myotomy.
5. The procedure allows early oral feeding after operation.
6. The hospital stay is short.
7. There is no residual neck scar.

The particular benefits of stapling include the following:

1. Stapling of the two edges of the V-shaped opening results in excellent hemostasis and no contamination of the cervical spaces by the digestive contents.
2. Perforation of the bottom of the common cavity is unlikely since the incision ends a few millimeters proximal to the distal tip of the anvil, even with the sawed-off version. The lower risk of perforation compared with the coagulating methods should give the surgeon a feeling of security and reduce the potential for a second-stage division later.
3. The diverticulum can be tapered by pushing the bottom downward with the tip of the anvil, elongating the common wall and reducing the length of the residual spur.

4. Expensive instruments such as a laser source, which has minimal application in a general surgery practice, are unnecessary.

ENDOSCOPIC STAPLING TECHNIQUE

Preoperative Management

Patients are admitted to the hospital the day before the operation. They are restricted to water, coffee, or tea until the operation and are given topical antibiotics for decontamination of the oropharynx. Those patients admitted on an emergency basis for acute pneumonitis due to aspiration of the diverticular contents are first given intravenous antibiotics and intensive respiratory physiotherapy for a few days before surgery.

Patient Positioning and Anesthesia

The patient is placed in the recumbent position on the operating table with the head hyperextended. A short-acting, light general anesthetic such as propofol or alfentanil is given in a low dose. A small-diameter endotracheal tube is introduced transnasally.

Instrumentation

A double-lipped diverticuloscope, a 30 mm endoscopic linear stapler, a light source, a light conductor, a 5 mm diameter telescope, a microcamera similar to that used for laparoscopy or thoracoscopy, and a television screen are necessary to perform this procedure. The endoscope we initially used was the Weerda diverticuloscope (Karl Storz, Tuttlingen, Germany), the two lips of which can be angulated and approximated to fit each patient's unique oropharyngeal anatomy. However, it soon became evident that the original Weerda diverticuloscope was too large for patients with prominent incisors and those with a narrow oropharyngeal channel. Therefore, together with Karl Storz, we designed a new diverticuloscope (Fig. 5-4) that is narrower and permits the introduction of the linear stapler alongside the light conductor and telescope. The latter was angulated to permit connection to the side of the microcamera so that it would not interfere with the stapler.

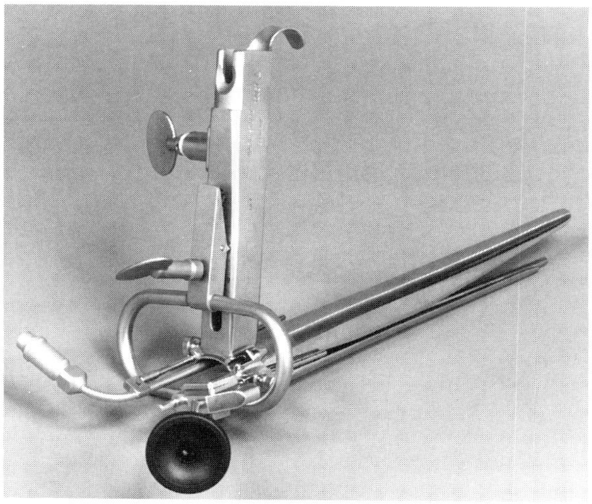

Fig. 5-4. The modified Weerda endoscope. The two lips can be moved away from each other and angulated. Two lateral channels accommodate a 5 mm diameter telescope and a light conductor.

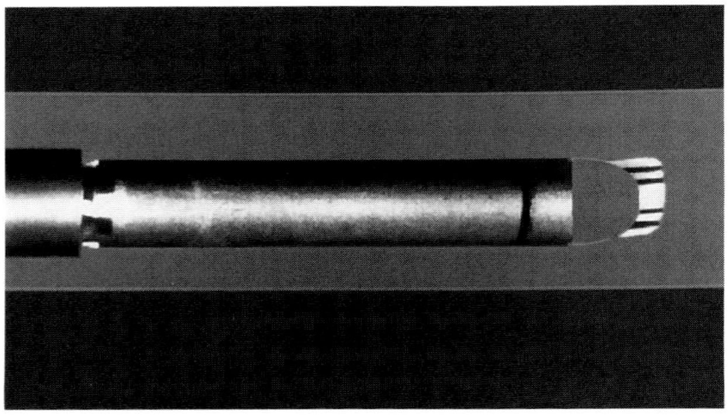

Fig. 5-5. Distal end of the original anvil of the 30 mm endoscopic linear stapler. The segment located beyond the distal end of the staple receptacles (green area) was sawed off to minimize the size of the spur at the bottom of the common cavity.

We also modified the original 30 mm linear stapler (Fig. 5-5). The part of the anvil distal to the staple receptacles was sawed off to reduce the length of the spur at the bottom of the common cavity following endoscopic division of the common wall. This modification does not change the basic characteristics of the stapler. It still has a section length of 2.7 cm and a stapling length of 3 cm.

Procedure

The modified double-lipped diverticuloscope is introduced into the mouth and the pharynx under direct vision, the larynx is lifted forward, and the diverticular opening is identified. The lower lip is inserted into the diverticular sac and the upper lip into the cervical esophageal lumen. The two lips are moved away from each other to expose the wall between the two lumina. The saliva retained in the diverticular sac is suctioned and the mucosa is carefully inspected. The modified linear stapler is introduced into the pharynx through the diverticuloscope (Fig. 5-6). The two forks of the stapler are placed across the common wall, that is, the anvil into the diverticular sac and the cartridge of staples into the cervical esophageal lumen (Fig. 5-7). After midline approximation of the two forks, the trigger of the gun is squeezed to permit forward displacement of the knife and delivery of three rows of staples on each side. After the two forks are separated, the stapler is removed as the cricopharyngeus muscle forces the two stapled wound edges to retract laterally. The muscle, which is located within the common wall, has also been divided. The medial slit thus becomes a V-shaped opening between the two lumina (Fig. 5-8). A second cartridge is applied along the distal segment of the common wall to complete its division. When hemostasis of the two wound edges is ensured, the diverticuloscope is removed and the patient is aroused.

Postoperative Course

The patient is allowed to drink the evening following the operation. A soft diet is begun on the first postoperative day, and the patient is discharged from the hospital

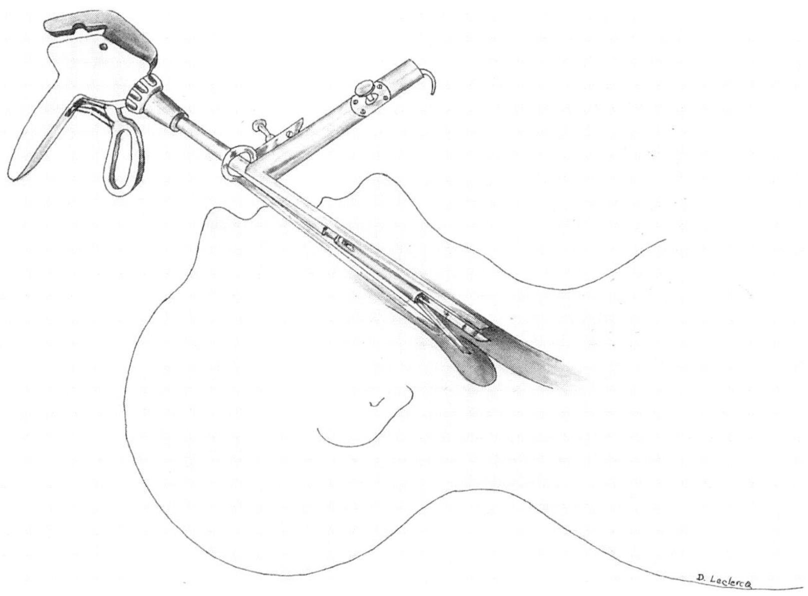

Fig. 5-6. Introduction of the endoscopic linear stapler through the modified Weerda diverticuloscope.

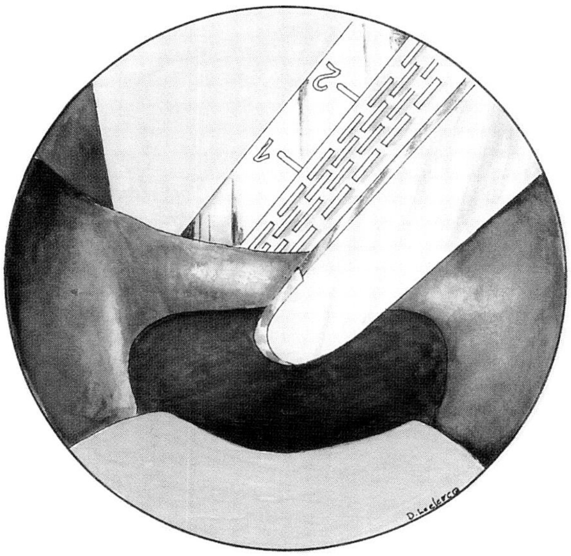

Fig. 5-7. The endoscopic linear stapler is placed across the common wall, the anvil into the diverticulum, and the cartridge of staples into the cervical esophageal lumen.

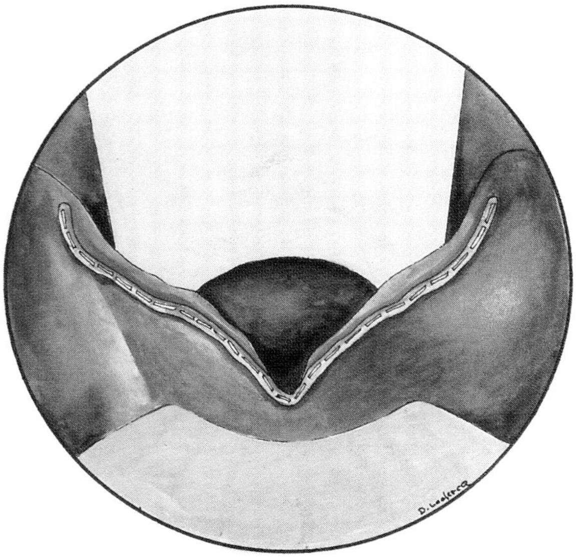

Fig. 5-8. The divided cricopharyngeal muscle allows the two wound edges to move away from each other. A triple line of staples ensures hemostasis of the two wound edges and prevents any contamination of the adjacent cervical spaces by the digestive contents.

at the end of the day. Before leaving the hospital, the patient is instructed on dietary restrictions during the first postoperative week. A barium swallow study is performed as an outpatient procedure 1 week after surgery. An esophageal motility study is performed at follow-up in patients who agree to submit to further investigation.

Clinical Experience

From November 1991 to July 1993, 17 patients were operated on for hypopharyngeal diverticulum at the Louvain Medical School Hospital in Brussels. A transcervical myotomy of the cricopharyngeus muscle and the muscular layers of the cervical esophagus was performed in one patient with a small diverticulum. A transcervical myotomy plus diverticulectomy was carried out in three patients, two of whom had a large diverticulum that extended to the thoracic inlet and the mediastinum and one in whom the diverticulum was perforated during diagnostic esophagoscopy. A transcervical myotomy plus diverticulopexy was performed in six patients; three had a small diverticulum and three had a medium-sized diverticulum and either a narrow oropharyngeal channel or severe arthrosis of the cervical spine that precluded accurate positioning of the original Weerda diverticuloscope.

Seven patients were treated by endoscopic division of the common wall; five of them were over 75 years of age. Of these seven patients, two had been admitted to the hospital emergently with acute pneumonitis due to aspiration of the diverticular contents. Five underwent elective repair. Symptomatology included cervical dysphagia (n = 6), respiratory infection (n = 4), and regurgitation (n = 7). A laparoscopic Nissen fundoplication for gastroesophageal reflux was performed during the same operation in two patients. One patient had a history of recent neck surgery (the

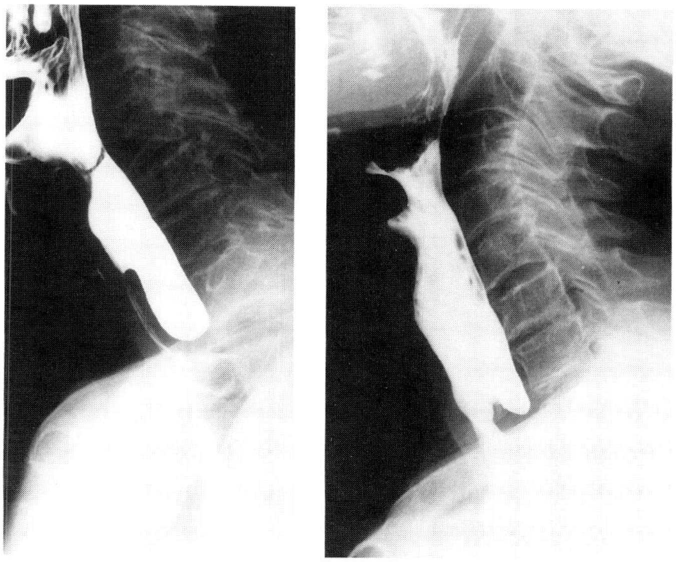

A B

Fig. 5-9. Barium swallow study before **(A)** and immediately after **(B)** endoscopic division of the common wall in an 80-year-old patient with a history of previous neck surgery. Although the length of the common wall was estimated not to exceed 25 mm on preoperative roentgenograms, one cartridge of staples and the distal end of a second cartridge could be applied to the common wall by pushing the bottom of the diverticulum downward with the distal tip of the anvil at operation. Note the spur at the bottom of the common cavity.

surgeon did not find the hypopharyngeal diverticulum at cervicotomy). In another patient a gastroenterologist had attempted without success to cut the proximal segment of the common wall using a flexible esophagoscope.

Postoperative body temperature never exceeded 37° C in the five patients who underwent the transoral procedure alone. The first four patients were discharged from the hospital a few days after the operation and the last three patients the day after surgery.

Symptomatic relief was achieved in five patients at follow-up of 1 to 20 months. A 45-year-old truck driver who had a diverticulum 2 cm in length complained of slight dysphagia when he ate bread without drinking water while driving his truck. The seventh patient, a 75-year-old man operated on following unsuccessful management of a 2 cm diverticulum using a flexible endoscope, remained nervous about eating coarse meat. The five patients with a good result had a diverticulum in which the common wall with the esophagus was found to be 3 cm or more at endoscopic evaluation under general anesthesia. The two patients who underwent laparoscopic Nissen fundoplication at the same operation had no residual symptoms of reflux.

Postoperative barium swallow studies showed the presence of a spur at the bottom of the common cavity in six patients (Fig. 5-9). Shrinkage of a small diverticulum was observed in one patient who nevertheless experienced residual dysphagia when eating bread. Only two patients agreed to undergo follow-up esophageal motility studies. Upper esophageal sphincter pressure was reduced by 40% and 58%, respectively, compared with the preoperative value.

CONCLUSION

We now have at our disposal several surgical modalities to treat benign esophageal disorders such as hypopharyngeal diverticulum. A good surgeon should be skilled in using all the available options, allowing him to individualize treatment. Endoscopic division of the common wall between the esophagus and the diverticulum is not an "all-purpose" technique. This lack of selectivity most likely explains why the results published by some esophageal surgeons have been far from optimal. Although the stapling method affords simplicity, reliability, and security, further experience is needed to provide long-term data. Particular attention should be directed toward evaluating the outcome of the residual spur and the diverticular remnant left behind and to learning how to manage failures.

REFERENCES

1. Imperatori CJ. Endoscopic treatment of pulsion diverticulum. Ann Otol Rhinol Laryngol 36:1175-1180, 1927.
2. Mosher HP. Webs and pouches of the esophagus, their diagnosis and treatment. Surg Gynecol Obstet 25:175-187, 1917.
3. Dohlman G, Mattsson O. The endoscopic operation for hypopharyngeal diverticula. Arch Otolaryngol 71:744-752, 1960.
4. Hollinger PH, Schild JA. The Zenker's (hypopharyngeal) diverticulum. Ann Otol Rhinol Laryngol 78:679-688, 1969.
5. MacKay IS. The treatment of pharyngeal pouch. J Laryngol Otol 98:183-190, 1976.
6. Trible WM. The surgical treatment of Zenker's diverticulum: Endoscopic vs. external operation. South Med J 68:1260-1262, 1975.
7. Hollinger PH, Johnston KC. Endoscopic surgery of Zenker's diverticula: Experience with the Dohlman technique. Ann Otol Rhinol Laryngol 70:1117-1123, 1961.
8. Todd GB. The treatment of pharyngeal pouch. J Laryngol Otol 88:307-315, 1974.
9. Van Overbeek JJ, Hoeksema PE. Endoscopic treatment of the hypopharyngeal diverticulum: 211 cases. Laryngoscope 92:88-91, 1982.
10. Van Overbeek JJ, Hoeksema PE, Edens ET. Microendoscopic surgery of the hypopharyngeal diverticulum using electro-coagulation of carbon dioxide laser. Ann Otol Rhinol Laryngol 93:34-36, 1984.
11. Knegt PP, de Jong PC, Van der Schrans EJ. Endoscopic treatment of the hypopharyngeal diverticulum with the CO_2 laser. Endoscopy 17:205-206, 1985.
12. Van Overbeek JJ, Wouters B. Surgical techniques for functional dysphagia. In Inouye T, Fukuda H, Sato T, Hinohara T, eds. Recent Advances in Bronchoesophagology. Amsterdam: Elsevier, 1990, pp 131-134.
13. Collard JM, Otte JB, Kestens PJ. Endoscopic stapling technique of esophagodiverticulostomy for Zenker's diverticulum. Ann Thorac Surg 56:573-576, 1993.
14. Cook IJ, Dodds WJ, Dantas RO, Massey B, Kern MK, Lang IM, Brasseur JG, Hogan WJ. Opening mechanisms of the human upper esophageal sphincter. Am J Physiol 20:748-759, 1989.
15. Dantas RO, Cook IJ, Dodds WJ, Kern MK, Lang IM, Brasseur JG. Biomechanics of cricopharyngeal bars. Gastroenterology 99:1269-1274, 1990.
16. Cook IJ, Gabb M, Panagopoulos V, Jamieson GG, Dodds WJ, Dent J, Shearman DJ. Pharyngeal (Zenker's) diverticulum is a disorder of upper esophageal sphincter opening. Gastroenterology 103:1229-1235, 1992.
17. Orringer MB. Extended cervical esophagomyotomy for cricopharyngeal dysfunction. J Thorac Cardiovasc Surg 80:669-678, 1980.
18. Lerut T, Vandekerkhof J, Leman G, Guelinckx PJ, Dom R, Gruwez JA. Cricopharyngeal myotomy for pharyngo-esophageal diverticula. In DeMeester TR, Matthews HR, eds. Benign Esophageal Disease. St. Louis: CV Mosby, 1987, pp 351-363.
19. Hauters P, Segol P, Leroux Y, Gignoux M. Place de la myotomie du cricopharyngien associée à une diverticulopexie dans le traitement du diverticule de Zenker (quinze années d'expérience). Ann Chir 42:726-730, 1988.

Chapter

6

Thoracoscopic Myotomy of the Lower Esophageal Sphincter and Esophageal Body

Jeffrey H. Peters, M.D. • *Tom R. DeMeester, M.D.*

Dysphagia is the primary symptom of esophageal motor disorders. Its perception by the patient is a balance between the severity of the underlying abnormality causing the dysphagia and the adjustment made by the patient in altering his eating habits. Consequently, any complaint of dysphagia must include an assessment of the patient's dietary history. Does the patient experience pain, choking, or vomiting when eating; does he require liquids with the meal; is he the last to finish or have interrupted a social meal because of difficulty in swallowing; or has he been admitted to the hospital for food impaction? These assessments, in addition to the patient's nutritional status, help to quantitate the severity of dysphagia and are important in determining the indications for surgical therapy.

The extent of surgical myotomy designed to improve the patient's swallowing ability will depend on the underlying cause of nonobstructive dysphagia. In principle we are making a defect to correct a defect. The results can profoundly improve the patient's ability to ingest food but rarely restores the function of the esophageal body to normal.

A clear understanding of the physiologic mechanism of swallowing and a precise determination of the motility abnormality giving rise to the dysphagia are essential for choosing the best therapeutic approach. This usually entails a complete esophageal motility evaluation. Endoscopy is necessary only to exclude the presence of tumor or inflammatory changes as the cause of dysphagia.

Disorders of the esophageal phase of swallowing result from abnormalities in the propulsive pump action of the esophageal body or the relaxation of the lower esophageal sphincter (Fig. 6-1). These disorders result either from primary esophageal abnormalities or from generalized neural, muscular, or collagen vascular disease. With the introduction of standard esophageal manometry, specific primary esophageal motility disorders can be distinquished from a host of nonspecific motility abnormalities. These include achalasia, diffuse esophageal spasm, so-called nutcracker esophagus, and a hypertensive lower esophageal sphincter.[1,2] The manometric characteristics of these disorders are listed on p. 85. The boundaries between the primary esophageal motor disorders are, however, vague and intermediate types exist.[3] This, in part, is attributable to the analysis of 10 wet swallows performed in a

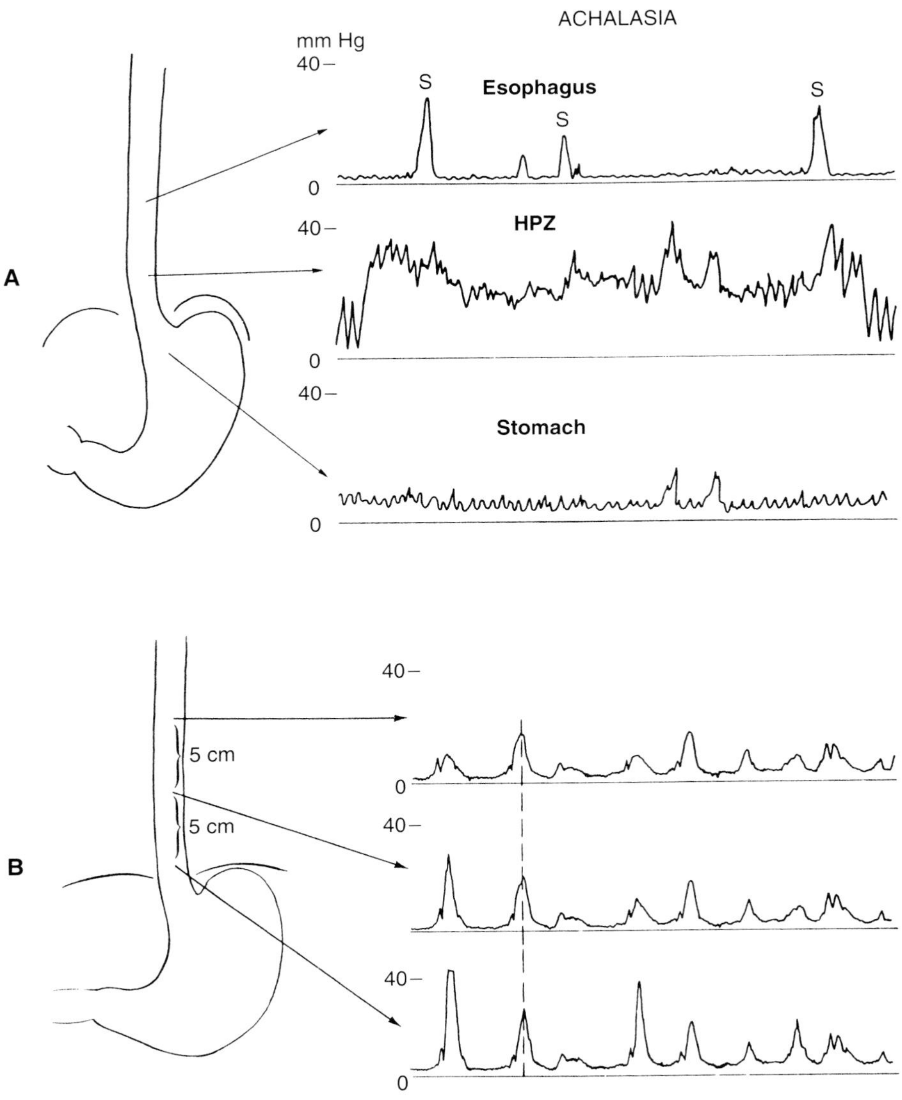

Fig. 6-1. Motility record demonstrating **(A)** hypertension of the distal esophageal sphincter and failure of the sphincter to relax on swallowing and **(B)** elevation of intraluminal esophageal pressure and aperistalsis in the body of the esophagus. Swallows are followed only by tertiary contractions, as illustrated by the dotted line. S = swallows; HPZ = lower esophageal high-pressure zone synonymous with lower esophageal sphincter. (From Waters PF, DeMeester TR. Foregut motor disorders and their surgical management. Med Clin North Am 65:1235, 1981.)

Current Classification of Esophageal Motility Disorders

Primary Esophageal Motility Disorders

Achalasia, "vigorous" achalasia
Diffuse and segmental esophageal spasm
Nutcracker esophagus
Hypertensive lower esophageal sphincter
Nonspecific esophageal motility disorders

Secondary Esophageal Motility Disorders

Collagen vascular diseases: Progressive systemic sclerosis, polymyositis and dermatomyositis, mixed connective tissue disease, systemic lupus erythematosus, etc.
Chronic idiopathic intestinal pseudo-obstruction
Neuromuscular diseases
Endocrine and metastatic disorders

Manometric Characteristics of Primary Esophageal Motility Disorders

Achalasia

Incomplete lower esophageal sphincter (LES) relaxation (<75% relaxation)
Aperistalsis in the esophageal body
Elevated LES pressure >26 mm Hg
Increased intraesophageal baseline pressures relative to gastric baseline

Diffuse esophageal spasm

Simultaneous (nonperistaltic contractions) (>20% of wet swallows)
Repetitive and multipeaked contractions
Spontaneous contractions
Intermittent normal peristalsis
Contractions may be of increased amplitude and duration

Nutcracker esophagus

Mean peristaltic amplitude in the distal esophagus >180 mm Hg
Normal peristaltic sequence

Hypertensive LES

Elevated LES pressure (>26 mm Hg)
Normal LES relaxation
Normal peristalsis in esophageal body

Nonspecific esophageal motility disorders

Decreased or absent amplitude of esophageal peristalsis
Increased number of nontransmitted contractions
Abnormal waveforms
Normal mean LES pressure and relaxation

laboratory setting, which has hampered accurate diagnosis. The recently introduced technique of ambulatory 24-hour monitoring of esophageal motor activity permits classification of esophageal motor disorders based on more than 1000 contractions recorded during different physiologic states (i.e., normal daily activity, eating, and sleeping) and improves the diagnostic accuracy of foregut motility testing.[4]

ACHALASIA

The best-known and understood primary motility disorder of the esophagus is achalasia, which occurs with a prevalence of 6/100,000 population per year.[5] Although complete absence of peristalsis in the esophageal body has been proposed as the major abnormality, present evidence indicates achalasia is a primary disorder of the lower esophageal sphincter. This is based on 24-hour outpatient esophageal motility monitoring showing up to 5% of contractions can be peristaltic even in advanced disease.[6-8] Abnormal esophageal peristalsis develops as a result of the increased resistance provided by the nonrelaxing lower esophageal sphincter. This is supported by experimental studies in which a loosely placed Gore-Tex band around the gastroesophageal junction in cats did not change sphincter pressures but resulted in impaired relaxation of the lower esophageal sphincter and led to a markedly increased frequency of simultaneous contractions and a decrease of contraction amplitude in the esophageal body.[9] This was associated with dilatation of the esophagus on x-ray films and was reversible after removal of the band. Clinical observations in patients with pseudoachalasia due to tumor infiltration, a tight stricture in the distal esophagus, or an antireflux procedure that is too tight also indicate that dysfunction of the esophageal body can be caused by the increased outflow obstruction of a nonrelaxing lower esophageal sphincter. The observation that esophageal peristalsis can return in patients with classic achalasia following dilatation or myotomy further supports that this is a primary disease of the lower esophageal sphincter.[10,11]

The pathogenesis of achalasia is presumed to be a neurogenic degeneration that is either idiopathic or due to infection. In experimental animals the disease has been reproduced by destruction of the nucleus ambiguus and the dorsal motor nucleus of the vagus nerve. In patients with the disease, degenerative changes have been shown in the vagus nerve and in the ganglia in the Auerbach plexus of the esophagus itself.[12] This degeneration results in hypertension of the lower esophageal sphincter, failure of the sphincter to relax on deglutition, elevation of intraluminal esophageal pressure, and subsequent loss of progressive peristalsis in the body of the esophagus. The combination of a nonrelaxing sphincter, which causes a functional retention of ingested material in the esophagus, and elevation of intraluminal pressure from repetitive pharyngeal air swallowing results in dilatation of the esophageal body. With time, the functional disorder results in anatomic alterations seen on roentgenographic studies as a dilated esophagus with a tapering, beaklike narrowing of the distal end (Fig. 6-2). There is usually an air-fluid level in the esophagus that reflects the degree of resistance imposed by the nonrelaxing sphincter. As the disease progresses, the esophagus becomes massively dilated and tortuous.

A subgroup of patients with otherwise typical features of classic achalasia have simultaneous contractions of the esophageal body that can be of high amplitude. This manometric pattern has been termed vigorous achalasia and chest pain episodes are a common finding in these patients.[13] Differentiation of vigorous achalasia from diffuse esophageal spasm can be difficult. In both diseases a video roentgenographic examination can show a corkscrew deformity of the esophagus and diverticulum formation (Fig. 6-3).

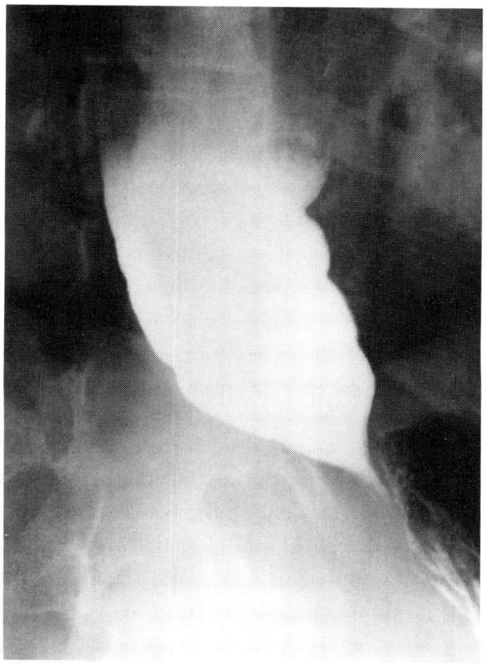

Fig. 6-2. Barium esophagogram showing a markedly dilated esophagus and characteristic "bird's beak" in achalasia. (From Waters PF, DeMeester TR. Foregut motor disorders and their surgical management. Med Clin North Am 65:1235, 1981.)

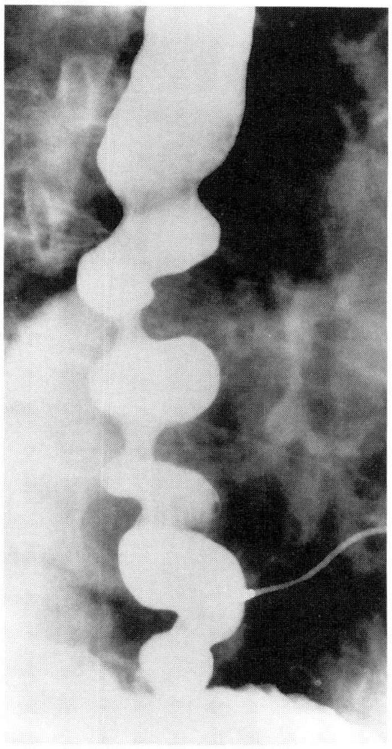

Fig. 6-3. Barium esophagogram of patient with diffuse esophageal spasm showing the "cork-screw" deformity.

Table 6-1. Follow-up results after myotomy or balloon dilation in patients with achalasia

Reference	No. of Patients	Mortality	Follow-Up (yr)	Good to Excellent Response (%)
Surgical myotomy				
Black et al. (1976)[16]	108	0	4	65
Menzies et al. (1978)[17]	102	0	8	98
Okike and Payne (1979)[18]	456	1	1-17	85
Ellis et al. (1984)[19]	113	0	3.5	91
Csendes et al. (1988)[11]	100	0	6.8	92
Balloon dilatation				
Sanderson et al. (1970)[20]	408			81
Okike and Payne (1979)[18]	431	2	1-18	65
Vantrappen and Janssens (1983)[15]	403	17	7.8	76

Treatment Options

It is impossible to relieve the functional obstruction of a nonrelaxing sphincter effectively with drugs. Many have been tried, but they have been found to be of limited clinical value. This can only be achieved by an uncontrolled instrumental rupture of the sphincter muscle or by surgical myotomy.[14,15] Complete destruction of the sphincter is to be avoided, as it results in free gastroesophageal reflux, esophagitis, and stricture secondary to reflux disease. Pneumatic dilation has been suggested as adequate treatment but only relieves dysphagia and pharyngeal regurgitation in 70% of patients. When questioned carefully, it becomes clear that patients tend to overemphasize the benefits of pneumatic dilation and are slow to accept that the procedure was a failure. Consequently, surgical myotomy is delayed, leading to progressive esophageal dilatation and the resulting tortuosity. Whether a patient with newly diagnosed esophageal achalasia is best treated by forceful dilation or by operative cardiomyotomy remains controversial. Both large retrospective reviews and prospective randomized studies comparing the two modes of therapy indicate that surgical myotomy is associated with low morbidity and gives better long-term results (Table 6-1). Consequently, the data support surgical myotomy as the procedure of choice; however, in practice most patients are treated by dilation. An inherent risk of pneumatic dilation is rupture of the esophagus. This is reported to occur in 2% of patients, but in carefully monitored studies the incidence can be as high as 15%. Although it has been reported that a myotomy after previous balloon dilation is more difficult, this has not been a universal experience unless the cardia has been ruptured. In this situation, operative intervention either immediately or after healing has occurred can be difficult.

MYOTOMY OF THE LOWER ESOPHAGEAL SPHINCTER

In performing a surgical myotomy of the lower esophageal sphincter there are four important principles: (1) minimal dissection of the cardia, (2) adequate distal myoto-

Table 6-2. Gastroesophageal reflux following esophageal myotomy for achalasia

Reference	No. of Patients	Postoperative Reflux
Without antireflux procedure		
Ferguson and Burford (1960)[21]	44	4
Belsey (1966)[22]	64	10
Jara et al. (1979)[23]	121	63
Okike and Payne (1979)[18]	456	14
Bjorck et al. (1982)[24]	41	8
Pai et al. (1984)[25]	16	0
Ellis et al. (1984)[19]	113	4
	855	103 (12%)
With antireflux procedure		
Belsey (1966)[22]	62	0
Peyton et al. (1974)[26]	8	2
Okike and Payne (1979)[18]	16	1
Bjorck et al. (1982)[24]	11	0
Pai et al. (1984)[25]	17	2
	114	5 (4%)

my to reduce outflow resistance, (3) prevention of postoperative reflux, and (4) prevention of rehealing of the myotomy site. The development of a reflux-induced stricture as a result of the loss of sphincter competency after a myotomy is a serious problem that usually necessitates esophagectomy.

If simultaneous esophageal contractions are associated with the sphincter abnormality, so-called vigorous achalasia, then the myotomy should extend over the distance of the motility abnormality as mapped by the preoperative motility study. Failure to do so will result in continuing dysphagia and a dissatisfied patient. The use of a fundoplication after a myotomy to prevent reflux has been debated (Table 6-2). Recent studies have shown that when an antireflux procedure is added to the myotomy it should be a partial fundoplication. A 360-degree fundoplication is associated with progressive retention of swallowed food, regurgitation, and aspiration to a degree that exceeds the patient's preoperative symptoms.

Whether to add an antireflux procedure to the surgical myotomy is a difficult choice. A balance must be struck between relieving the outflow resistance responsible for achalasia and allowing free reflux through an incompetent sphincter. Some authors have chosen to perform a meticulous myotomy without an antireflux procedure, carefully limiting the extent of the dissection and distal myotomy in an effort to minimize postoperative reflux, whereas others have combined the myotomy with a partial or complete fundoplication. Our initial experience with minimally invasive esophageal myotomy is based on the following principles:

1. Use of a thoracoscopic rather than a laparoscopic approach
2. Minimal dissection of the esophagus and esophageal hiatus to preserve the normal anatomic antireflux mechanisms

3. Precise control of the distal extent of the myotomy, limiting it to the anatomic gastroesophageal junction
4. Definition of the gastroesophageal junction via an intraluminal flexible endoscope
5. No antireflux procedure

Technique

The procedure is performed with the patient in the left lateral decubitus position. A double-lumen endotracheal tube is used to allow selective ventilation of the right lung (Fig. 6-4, *A*).

Port Placement. A four-port technique is employed in addition to a small (1-inch) incision along the left costal margin for placement of retracting instruments (Fig. 6-4, *B*). A 10 mm port placed posterior to the scapula in the fourth intercostal space is used for the camera. Meticulous hemostasis when creating the trocar holes is important. Bleeding from the trocar site is common and very troublesome during the procedure, particularly in the camera port. Air is allowed to enter the thorax and the left lung is slowly deflated with some assistance from the shaft of the telescope. A second 10 mm port is placed high and anterior in the second or third intercostal space at the anterior axillary line. A Babcock clamp placed through this port is used as a lung retractor following incision of the inferior pulmonary ligament. The right-handed surgeon's port is placed at the midaxillary line in the sixth or seventh intercostal space. The position should be such that the electrocautery hook placed through the right-handed trocar is directly above the esophagus, not approaching it from an angle. Placing this trocar too high can cause difficulty in performing the myotomy near the gastroesophageal junction. The left-handed surgeon's trocar is placed low, inferior and posterior, above the diaphragm in the ninth or tenth intercostal space. Finally a 1-inch incision is made along the left costal margin directly above the esophagus for placement of three instruments: a fan retractor to displace the diaphragm inferiorly, a long vein retractor to retract the crura superiorly, and a suction irrigation device. With selective ventilation of the right lung it is not necessary to insufflate the left hemithorax. One of the advantages of thoracoscopy is that airtight ports are not necessary, allowing small incisions and the placement of standard instruments. We have found that angled viewing laparoscopes/thoracoscopes are preferable to zero-degree scopes.

Retraction. Proper retraction and exposure of the esophageal hiatus is critical to the dissection and requires some attention at the outset. The diaphragm should be forcefully displaced inferiorly via the large fan retractor, completely exposing the esophageal hiatus. Identification and dissection of the esophagus are aided by the concomitant use of an endoscope within the esophageal lumen, allowing displacement of the esophagus to the left (Fig. 6-5). In patients with achalasia the esophagus is often dilated and easily seen. The mediastinal pleura overlying the terminal esophagus is divided sharply with scissors, and the inferior pulmonary ligament is divided for 2 to 3 cm (Fig. 6-6). A Babcock clamp placed through the high anterior port is used to retract the left lower lobe and left lung toward the superior thorax.

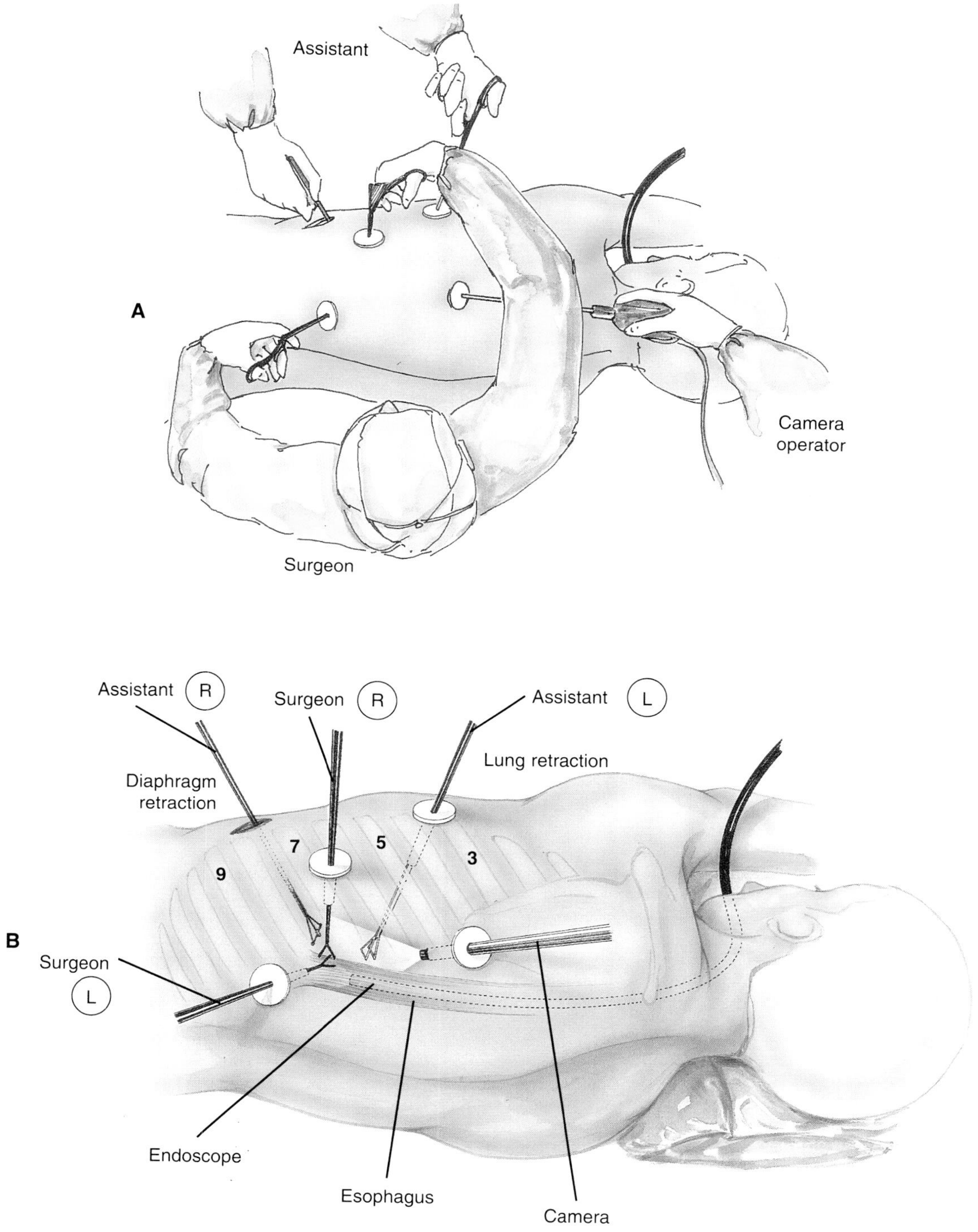

Fig. 6-4. A, Patient and surgeon positioning for thoracoscopic esophageal myotomy. **B,** Trocar placement. Four 10 mm Thoracoports and a single 2- to 3- inch incision are used here.

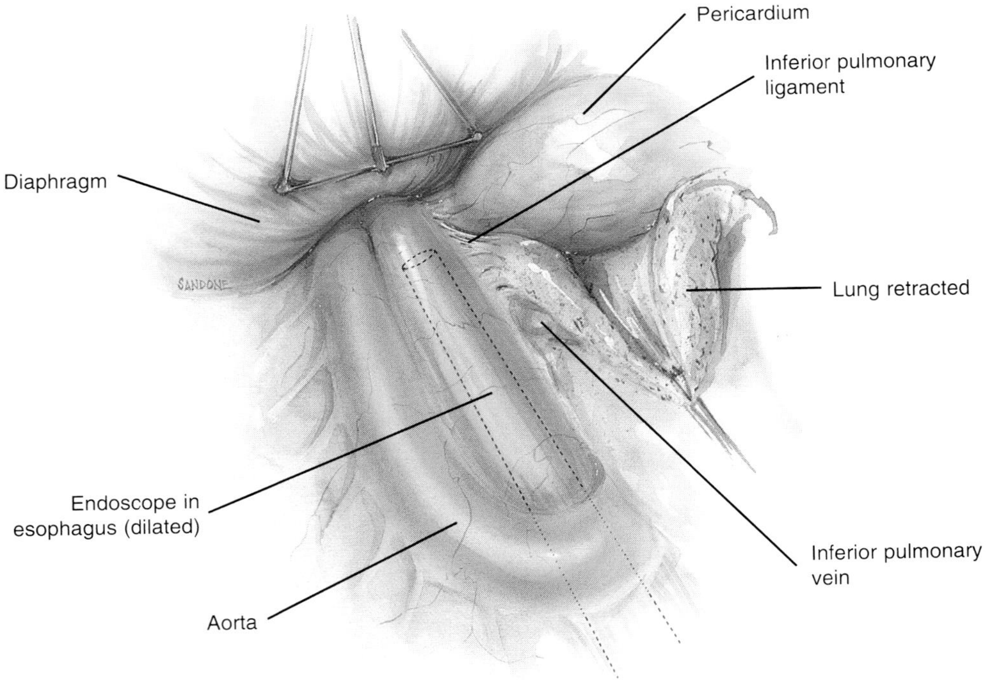

Fig. 6-5. Thoracoscopic esophageal myotomy illustrating the exposure obtained with video-assisted technology, permitting the traditional myotomy of the esophageal lower sphincter or body to be performed without a thoracotomy. The diaphragm is forcefully retracted toward the patient's abdomen with a fan-shaped retractor inserted through a small incision along the left costal border. The left lower lung is retracted superiorly and anteriorly with a Babcock clamp placed in a high anterior port.

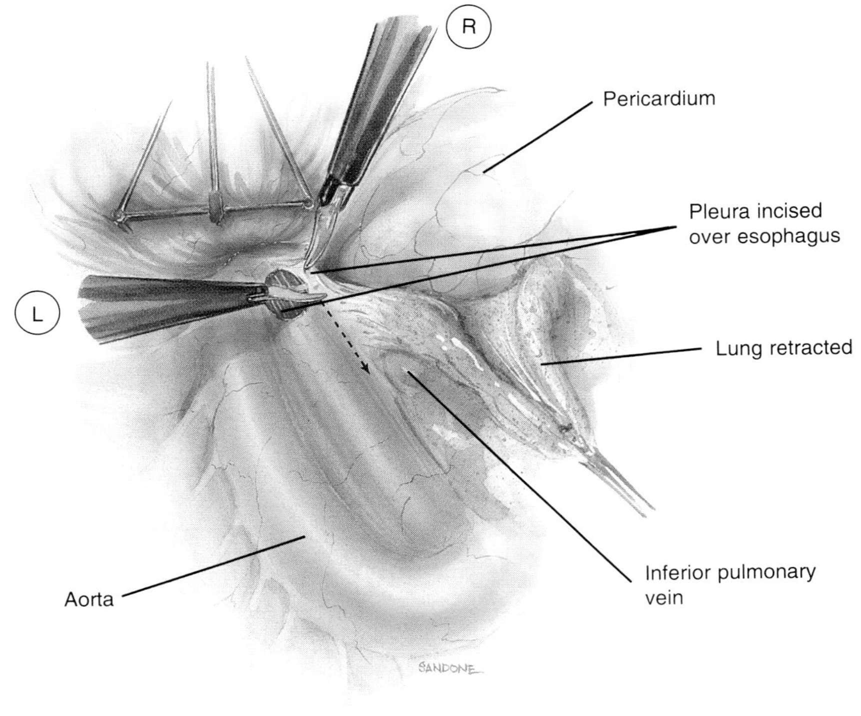

Fig. 6-6. Videoscopic view of the initial dissection for myotomy of the lower esophageal sphincter. The pleura overlying the lower esophagus is being incised.

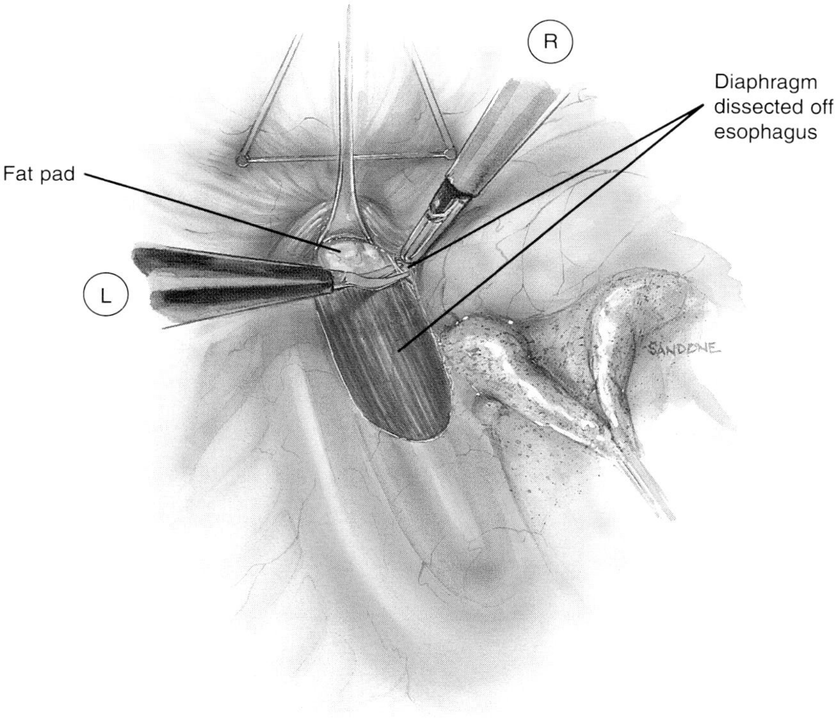

Fig. 6-7. The initial dissection is continued by dissecting the crura of the diaphragm at the gastroesophageal junction.

Initial Dissection. The dissection is consciously kept to a minimum, preserving normal hiatal structures. The crural arch is dissected just as the esophagus passes beneath, allowing placement of a long vein retractor underneath the arch and retraction of the crura away from the esophagus. The gastric serosa usually becomes evident and is recognized by its more distinct white color. No attempt is made to mobilize any portion of the stomach, only to visualize the gastroesophageal junction (Fig. 6-7).

The Myotomy. The myotomy is begun 2 to 3 cm above the gastroesophageal junction and performed with an L-hook electrocautery probe (Fig. 6-8). The magnification of the telescope usually allows clear visualization of the longitudinal and circular muscle fibers. Insufflation via the intraluminal endoscope will allow the mucosa to pouch out between the cut ends of the muscle, clearly outlining the myotomized segment. In addition, the endoscope within the lumen of the esophagus can be used to help prevent mucosal injury by applying suction to collapse the mucosa prior to using the electrocautery. Once the esophageal mucosa is clearly identified, the myotomy is carried distally with an electrocautery probe or scissors. The inferior extent of the myotomy is carefully inspected through the endoscope. The myotomy is completed when it has reached the endoscopic gastroesophageal junction and the spasm of the valve commonly associated with achalasia is alleviated.

Closure. At the completion of the procedure the dependent portion of the left chest is filled with water and air is insufflated via the endoscope to check for esoph-

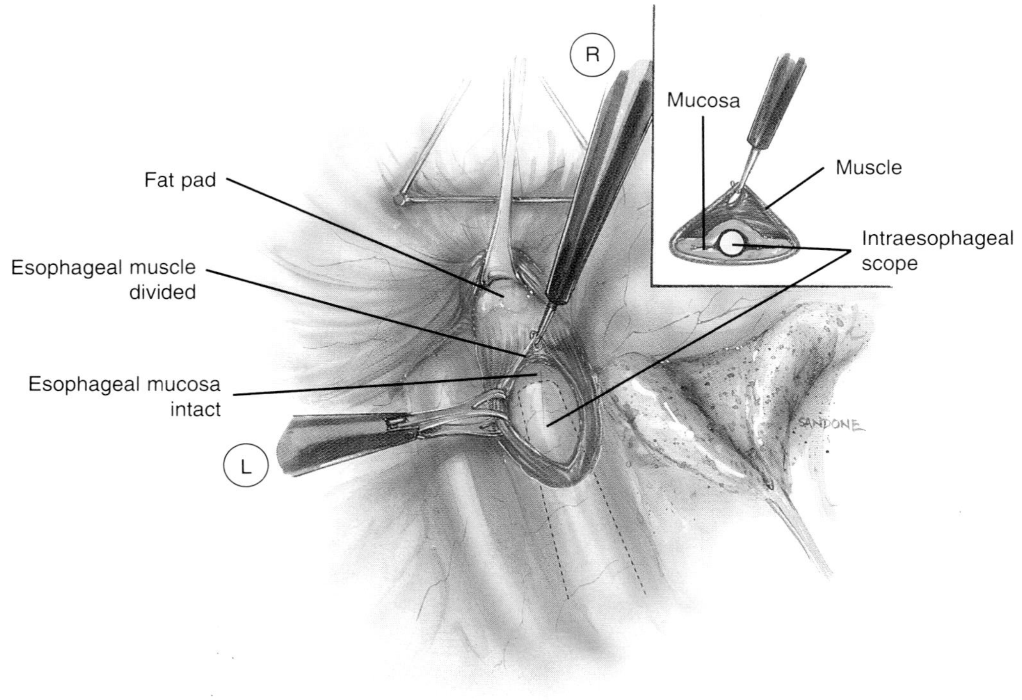

Fig. 6-8. The myotomy is begun 2 to 3 cm above the gastroesophageal junction and carried out with an L-hook electrocautery instrument. Note the intraluminal endoscope is an aid in defining the gastroesophageal junction. The inset demonstrates collapse of the mucosa as suction is applied via the endoscope just prior to the application of electrocautery.

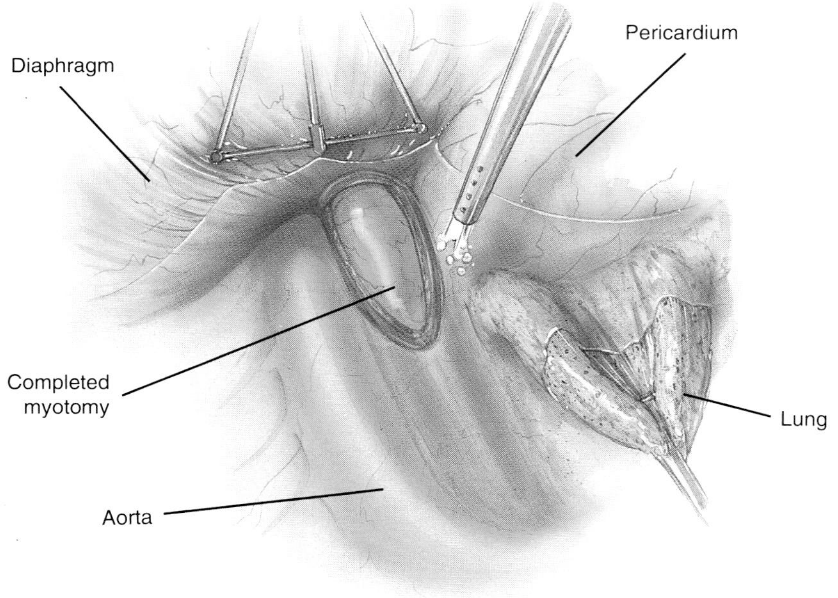

Fig. 6-9. Following completion of the myotomy the lower chest and esophagus are irrigated with water. The integrity of the esophageal mucosa is checked by insufflating air via the intraluminal endoscope.

ageal mucosal integrity. A small-caliber chest tube is placed and the left lung reinflated under direct vision. All trocars are removed and the wounds closed in a two-layer fashion (Fig. 6-9).

Postoperative Care

A nasogastric tube is not necessary; its placement may be potentially hazardous following myotomy. A video contrast esophogram is obtained the day following surgery and the patient allowed liquids. Hospital stay in the absence of comorbid disease is generally 2 to 3 days.

Results

Critical analysis of the results of therapy for motor disorders of the esophagus requires objective measurement. The use of symptoms alone as an end point to evaluate therapy may be misleading. The propensity of patients to unconsciously modify their diet to avoid difficulty swallowing is underestimated, making an assessment of results based on symptoms unreliable. Furthermore, insufficient reduction in outflow resistance may allow progressive dysphagia and esophageal dilatation to develop slowly over the course of years. Objective measurements of the decrease in outflow resistance should therefore be included in any careful evaluation of treatment results.

A variety of objective measurements may be used, including improvements in lower esophageal sphincter pressure, esophageal baseline pressure, and scintigraphic assessment of esophageal emptying time. Esophageal baseline pressure, usually negative relative to gastric pressure, is increased in patients with achalasia because of accumulation of air and food in the esophagus. Given that the goal of therapy is to eliminate the outflow resistance of a nonrelaxing sphincter, measurement of improvements in esophageal baseline pressure and scintigraphic transit time may be better indicators of success, but they are rarely reported.

Eckardt et al.[27] recently investigated whether the effect of pneumatic dilation in patients with achalasia could be predicted on the basis of objective measurements. Lower esophageal sphincter pressure was the most valuable measurement for predicting long-term clinical response. A postdilation sphincter pressure <10 mm Hg predicted a good response. Fifty percent of the patients studied had postdilation sphincter pressures between 10 and 20 mm Hg and a 2-year remission rate of 71%. Importantly, 16 of 46 patients were left with a postdilation sphincter pressure of >20 mm Hg and had an unacceptable outcome.

Open Surgery. Csendes et al.[11] reported the long-term follow-up of 81 patients randomized into groups undergoing forceful dilation and surgical myotomy. They showed that myotomy was associated with a significant increase in the diameter at the gastroesophageal junction and a decrease in the middle third of the esophagus on follow-up roentgenographic studies. There was also a greater reduction in sphincter pressure and improvement in the amplitude of esophageal contractions following myotomy. Of interest, 13% of patients regained some peristalsis after dilation compared with 28% after surgery. These findings were shown to persist over 5 years of follow-up, at which time 95% of those treated with surgical myotomy were doing well. Of those who had dilation, only 54% were doing well, 16% required redilation, and 22% eventually required surgical myotomy to obtain relief.

Bonavina et al.[10] report good to excellent results with transabdominal myotomy and Dor fundoplication in 94% of patients after a mean follow-up of 5.4 years. Eighty-one of 193 patients underwent postoperative 24-hour esophageal pH study, and only 8.6% of these demonstrated abnormal esophageal acid exposure. Similar to the study of Csendes et al.,[11] they report recovery of peristalsis in the esophageal body in several of their patients who volunteered for follow-up manometry. This would suggest that the deterioration of esophageal body function in patients with achalasia is secondary to the outflow obstruction of the hypertensive, nonrelaxing lower esophageal sphincter and is reversible if the obstruction is completely resolved without an inordinate delay. Stipa et al.[28] also reported good to excellent long-term results after myotomy in 85% of 101 patients with achalasia after a median follow-up of approximately 10 years. No operative mortality occurred in either of these series, attesting to the safety of the procedure.

Thoracoscopic Myotomy. Early experience with endosurgical esophageal myotomy is encouraging. Pellegrini et al.[29] have reported a series of 17 patients. Fifteen underwent thoracoscopic surgery and two laparoscopic surgery. All patients had dysphagia as well as a dilated esophagus with a bird-beak deformity demonstrated on upper gastrointestinal series. Manometry revealed a mean lower esophageal sphincter pressure of 32 mm Hg, incomplete sphincter relaxation on swallowing, and no primary esophageal peristalsis. Postoperatively, the mean lower esophageal sphincter pressure was 10 mm Hg. Most patients were fed on postoperative day 2. The average hospital stay was 3 days. There were no deaths or major complications. The relief of dysphagia was graded as excellent in 12 patients, good in two patients, fair in two patients, and poor in one patient.

Our experience with thoracoscopic myotomy of the lower esophageal sphincter includes 12 patients. Two patients required conversion to open surgery, in the first to inspect the dissection and in the second because of a small perforation at the gastroesophageal junction just after the completion of the myotomy. This was recognized immediately and repaired following thoracotomy. The patient did well. The median age of these patients was 65 years (range 30 to 83 years). The average length of thoracoscopic surgery was 223 minutes and the average length of hospitalization was 4 days.

Physiologic studies revealed a significant reduction in mean lower esophageal sphincter pressure (Fig. 6-10) with little change in sphincter length characteristics (Fig. 6-11). Excellent to good results were achieved in the majority of patients (Fig. 6-12).

Diffuse and Segmental Esophageal Spasm

Diffuse esophageal spasm is characterized clinically by substernal chest pain and/or dysphagia. This esophageal motor disorder differs from classic achalasia in that it is primarily a disease of the esophageal body, produces a lesser degree of dysphagia, causes more chest pain, and has less effect on the patient's general condition. True symptomatic diffuse esophageal spasm is a rare condition, occurring about five times less frequently than achalasia.

The etiology and neuromuscular pathophysiology of diffuse esophageal spasm are unclear. The basic motor abnormality is rapid progression of contractions down the esophagus secondary to an abnormality in the latency gradient. Hypertrophy of

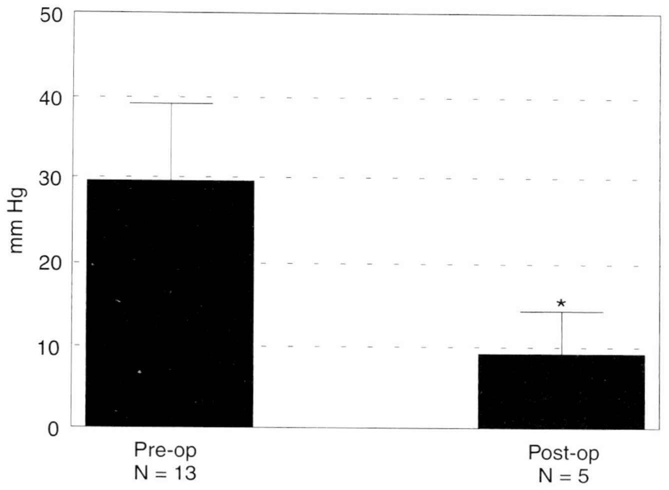

Fig. 6-10. Mean lower esophageal sphincter pressures before and after thoracoscopic esophageal myotomy. * = $p < 0.05$ vs. preoperatively.

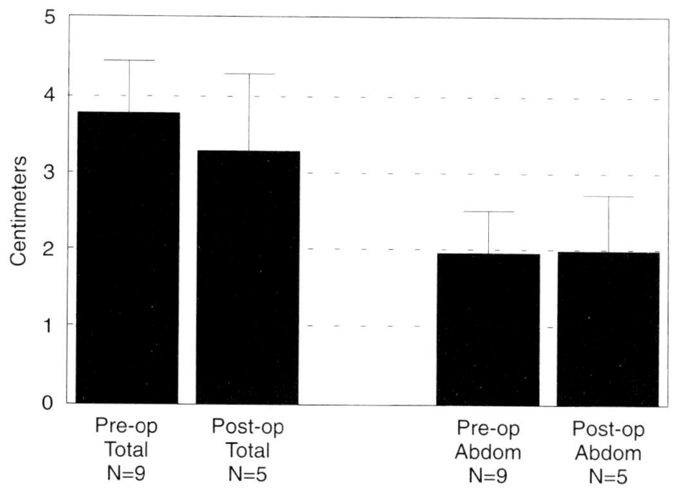

Fig. 6-11. Mean lower esophageal sphincter total and abdominal lengths before and after thoracoscopic esophageal myotomy.

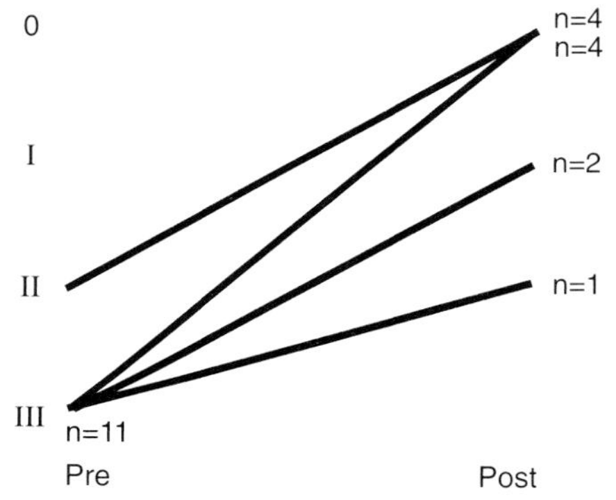

Fig. 6-12. Mean values for the clinical stage of patients before and after thoracoscopic esophageal myotomy.

the muscular layer of the esophageal wall and degeneration of the esophageal branches of the vagus nerve have been observed in this disease, although this is not a constant finding.[30,31] Manometric abnormalities in diffuse esophageal spasm may be present over the total length of the esophageal body but are usually confined to the distal two thirds. In segmental esophageal spasm the manometric abnormalities are confined to a short segment of the esophagus.

The classic manometric finding in these patients is characterized by the frequent occurrence of simultaneous and repetitive esophageal contractions that may be of abnormally high amplitude or long duration. Key to the diagnosis of diffuse esophageal spasm is that the esophagus retains a degree of peristaltic performance in excess of that seen in achalasia. A criterion of 20% or more simultaneous contractions in 10 wet swallows has been used to diagnose diffuse esophageal spasm.[32] This figure is, however, arbitrary and often debated. Recently a different approach has been proposed to diagnose diffuse esophageal spasm. Discriminate analysis has identified a series of abnormalities on the ambulatory motility record of patients with classic diffuse esophageal spasm. A composite score based on these parameters of the ambulatory motility record has allowed diagnoses of the disease with a sensitivity of 90% and a specificity of 100%. When applied prospectively, this scoring system identified severely deteriorated esophageal motor function in symptomatic patients despite the absence of the classic motility abnormalities of diffuse spasm on standard manometry.

The lower esophageal sphincter in patients with the disease usually shows normal resting pressure and relaxation on deglutition. A hypertensive sphincter with poor relaxation may also be present. In patients with advanced disease the radiographic appearance of tertiary contractions appears helical and has been termed corkscrew esophagus or pseudodiverticulosis. Patients with segmental or diffuse esophageal spasm can compartmentalize the esophagus and develop an epiphrenic or midesophageal diverticulum.

A long esophageal myotomy is indicated for dysphagia caused by any motor disorder characterized by segmental or generalized simultaneous contractions in a patient whose symptoms are not relieved by medical therapy. Such disorders include diffuse and segmental esophageal spasm, vigorous achalasia, and nonspecific motility disorders associated with a mid- or epiphrenic esophageal diverticulum. The recent introduction of 24-hour ambulatory motility studies has greatly aided in the identification of patients with symptoms of dysphagia and chest pain who might benefit from surgical myotomy.

The decision to operate depends on the patient's symptoms, diet, life-style adjustments, and nutritional status. The symptom of chest pain alone is not an indication for a surgical procedure.

In patients selected for myotomy of the esophageal body, preoperative manometry is essential to determine the proximal extent. Most surgeons extend the myotomy distally across the lower esophageal sphincter to reduce outflow resistance.

MYOTOMY OF THE ESOPHAGEAL BODY

Technique

The technique of long esophageal myotomy is similar to that of myotomy limited to the lower esophageal sphincter with the exception of the need for complete retraction of the lung to allow extension of the myotomy. Proper positioning of the patient is critical in permitting lung retraction. A prone position would be ideal to allow the left lung to fall forward away from the esophagus and facilitate exposure. However,

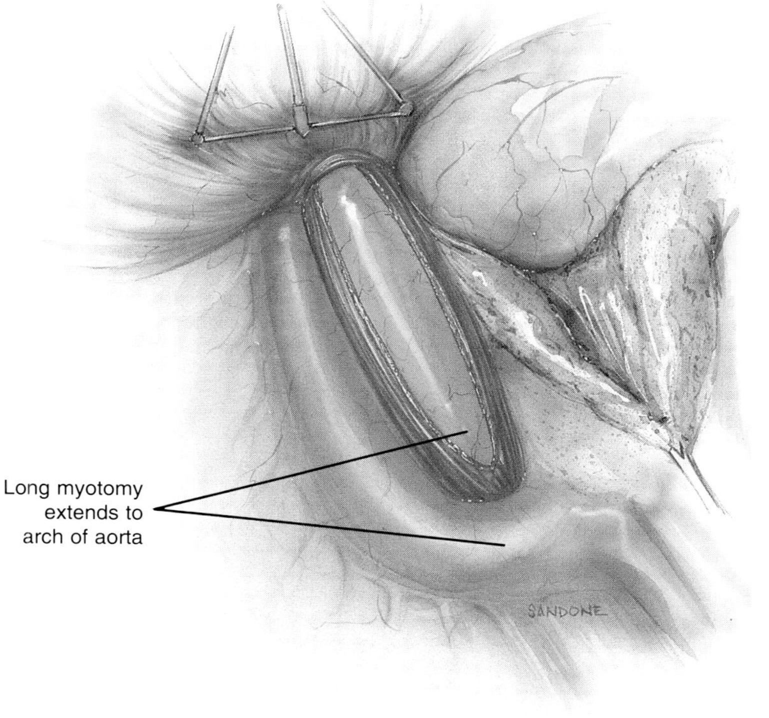

Fig. 6-13. Video thoracoscopic view of long esophageal myotomy at completion of the myotomy.

because of the possible need to convert to open thoracotomy we have been reluctant to place patients in a completely prone position, which would undoubtedly make posterolateral thoracotomy more difficult. For this reason we prefer to place the patient in the right lateral decubitus position and then roll him 45 degrees further toward the prone position. A beanbag and tape are used to secure the patient. The table is rolled the remaining 45 degrees so that the patient ends up nearly prone. Should thoracotomy be necessary, the table can be rolled to the lateral position and thoracotomy performed without difficulty. Prone positioning is the key element, allowing simple retraction of the left lung and thus a long myotomy.

Port placement and the initial dissection are identical to that for myotomy of the lower esophageal sphincter. With suitable lung retraction the myotomy can be performed through all muscle layers, extending distally to the endoscopic gastroesophageal junction and proximal on the esophagus over the distance of the manometric abnormality (Fig. 6-13). The muscle layer is dissected from the mucosa laterally for a distance of 1 cm. Care is taken to divide all minute muscle bands, particularly in the area of the gastroesophageal junction.

The presence of an epiphrenic diverticulum complicates the thoracoscopic procedure. Dissection of the neck of the diverticulum and division via an endoscopic linear stapler may be possible, but it is often difficult to obtain the proper angle of the stapler (see Chapter 8). Once excised, the overlying muscle is closed with interrupted Prolene sutures and the myotomy is then performed on the opposite esophageal wall. At present we do not hesitate to convert to open thoracotomy if any difficulty is encountered in excising the diverticulum. If a midesophageal diverticulum is present, the myotomy is made so that it includes the neck and the diverticulum is inverted and suspended by attaching it to the prevertebral fascia of the thoracic vertebrae.

Results

Open Surgery. Improvements in the results of open myotomy for motor disorders of the esophageal body have paralleled improvements in preoperative diagnosis afforded by manometry.[33] Previous published series report between 40% and 92% symptomatic improvement (Table 6-3), but interpretation is difficult because of the small number of patients involved and the varying criteria for diagnosis of the primary motor abnormality. When this is accurately done, 93% of the patients had effective palliation of dysphagia after a mean follow-up of 5 years and 89% would have the procedure again if it was necessary. Most patients gain or maintain their weight after the operation. Postoperative motility studies show that myotomy reduces the amplitude of esophageal contractions to near zero, eliminating both simultaneous and peristaltic waves. Therefore dysphagia is likely to be ameliorated by the procedure only if the prevalence of simultaneous waves is reduced and, as a consequence, the adverse effect on bolus propulsion exceeds the adverse effect on bolus propulsion caused by the loss of peristaltic wave amplitude. If not, the patient is likely to continue to complain of dysphagia. Thus a delicate balance exists between success and failure of a long esophageal myotomy, emphasizing the importance of preoperative motility studies.

Table 6-3. Summary of results of surgical myotomy for diffuse esophageal spasm

Reference	No. of Patients	Procedure	Symptomatic Results: Good (No.)	Symptomatic Results: Poor (No.)	Follow-Up Period
Ellis et al. (1964)[34]	40	Myotomy	31 (77%)	9 (23%)	1-6.5 yr
Ferguson et al. (1969)[35]	13	Myotomy	12 (92%)	1 (8%)	6 mo–12 yr
Henderson et al. (1974)[36]	17	Myotomy, Belsey	12 (71%)	5 (29%) (2*)	3-48 mo
	5	Myotomy, gastroplasty, Belsey	5 (100%)	0	
Flye and Sealy (1975)[37]	11	Myotomy	11 (100%)	0	Not noted
Leonardi et al. (1977)[38]	11	Myotomy*	10 (91%)	1 (9%)	1-6 yr
Henderson et al. (1987)[39]	20	Myotomy, Belsey	8 (40%)	12 (60%)	8-11 yr
	9	Myotomy, gastroplasty, Belsey	6 (67%)	3 (33%)	7-10 yr
	19	Myotomy, gastroplasty, Nissen	12 (63%)	7 (37%)	2-7 yr
	15	Myotomy, short Nissen	13 (87%)	2 (13%)	1-3 yr
	160		120 (75%)	40 (25%)	

*Myotomy sparing lower esophageal sphincter.

Thoracoscopic Surgery. Reports of thoracoscopic long myotomy for motor disorders of the esophageal body are limited. Shimi et al.[41] have reported their preliminary experience with an extended thoracoscopic distal esophageal myotomy for the treatment of nutcracker esophagus in three patients with symptomatic high-amplitude esophageal peristalsis and chest pain. In this setting the myotomy was extended to the level of the aortic arch. No major morbidity was encountered. Nasogastric tubes were removed the first postoperative day and oral feeding was started on the second postoperative day. Two patients were discharged on postoperative day 4 and one patient on the fifth day. Our experience includes three patients with diffuse esophageal spasm. All showed marked improvement after surgery.

CONCLUSION

Although it is clear that the thoracoscopic treatment of esophageal motor disorders is safe and effective, many questions remain unanswered. Most important, it is not yet clear that the results of endosurgical myotomy will be comparable to open surgery. Excellent long-term results have been demonstrated with open thoracotomy, myotomy, and partial fundoplication, which should serve as the gold standard for comparison of endosurgical techniques. The relative advantages, disadvantages, and benefits of laparoscopic vs. the thoracoscopic approach as well as the addition of an antireflux procedure will require further study.

REFERENCES

1. Waters PF, DeMeester TR. Foregut motor disorders and their surgical management. Med Clin North Am 65:1235, 1981.
2. DeMeester TR, Stein HJ. Surgery for esophageal motor disorders. In Castell DO, ed. The Esophagus. Boston: Little, Brown, 1992, pp 401-439.
3. Eypasch EP, Stein HJ, DeMeester TR, et al. A new technique to define and clarify esophageal motor disorders. Am J Surg 159:144, 1990.
4. Stein HJ, DeMeester TR, Eypasch EP. Ambulatory 24-hour esophageal manometry in the evaluation of esophageal motor disorders and noncardiac chest pain. Surgery 110:75, 1991.
5. Mayberry JF, Atkinson M. Studies on the incidence and prevalence of achalasia in the Nottingham area. Q J Med 56:451, 1985.
6. Mellow MH. Return of esophageal peristalsis in idiopathic achalasia. Gastroenterology 70:1148, 1976.
7. Bianco A, Cagossi M, Scrimieri D, et al. Appearance of esophageal peristalsis in treated idiopathic achalasia. Dig Dis Sci 90:978, 1986.
8. Stein HJ, Feussner H, Eypasch EP, et al. Ambulatory 24-hour manometry in achalasia. Gastroenterology 104:A199, 1993.
9. Little AG, Correnti FS, Calleja JJ, et al. Effect of incomplete obstruction on feline esophageal function with a clinical correlation. Surgery 100:430, 1986.
10. Bonavina L, Nosadinia A, Bardini R, et al. Primary treatment of esophageal achalasia: Long-term results of myotomy and Dor fundoplication. Arch Surg 127:222, 1992.
11. Csendes A, Braghetto I, Mascaro J, et al. Late subjective and objective evaluation of the results of esophagomyotomy in 100 patients with achalasia of the esophagus. Surgery 104:469, 1988.
12. Cassella RR, Brown AL Jr, Sayre GP, et al. Achalasia of the esophagus: Pathologic and etiologic considerations. Ann Surg 160:474, 1964.
13. Bondi JL, Godwin DH, Garnett JM. Vigorous achalasia: Its clinical interpretation and significance. Am J Gastroenterol 58:145, 1972.
14. Richter JE. Surgery or pneumatic dilation for achalasia: A head to head comparison. Gastroenterology 97:1340, 1989.
15. Vantrappen G, Janssens J. To dilate or to operate? That is the question. Gut 24:1013, 1983.

16. Black J, Varbach AM, Collis JL. Results of Heller's operation for achalasia of the esophagus: The importance of hiatal repair. Br J Surg 63:649, 1976.
17. Menzies Gow N, Gummer JW, et al. Results of Heller's operation for achalasia of the cardia. Br J Surg 65:483, 1978.
18. Okike N, Payne WS. Esophagomyotomy versus forceful dilation for achalasia of the esophagus: Results in 899 patients. Ann Thorac Surg 23:119, 1979.
19. Ellis FH Jr, Crozier RE, Watkins E. The operation for esophageal achalasia: Results of esophagomyotomy without an antireflux operation. J Thorac Cardiovasc Surg 88:344, 1984.
20. Sanderson DR, Ellis FH Jr, Olsen AM. Achalasia of the esophagus: Results of therapy by dilation. Chest 58:116, 1970.
21. Ferguson TB, Burford TH. An evaluation of the modified Heller operation in the treatment of achalasia of the esophagus. Ann Surg 152:1, 1960.
22. Belsey R. Functional disease of the esophagus. J Thorac Cardiovasc Surg 52:164, 1966.
23. Jara FM, Toledo Ereya LH, Lewis JH, et al. Long-term results of esophagomyotomy for achalasia of the esophagus. Arch Surg 114:935, 1979.
24. Bjorck S, Dernevik L, Gatzinsky P, et al. Oesophagocardiomyotomy and antireflux procedures. Acta Chir Scand 148:525, 1982.
25. Pai GP, Ellison RG, Rubin JW, et al. Two decades of experience with modified Heller's myotomy for achalasia. Ann Thorac Surg 38:201, 1984.
26. Peyton MD, Greenfield LD, Elkins RC. Combined myotomy and hiatal herniorrhaphy: A new approach to achalasia. Am J Surg 128:786, 1974.
27. Eckardt VF, Aignherr C, Bernhard G. Predictors of outcome in patients with achalasia treated by pneumatic dilation. Gastroenterology 103:1732, 1992.
28. Stipa S, Fegiz G, Iascone C, et al. Heller-Belsey and Heller-Nissen operations for achalasia of the esophagus. Surg Gynecol Obstet 170:212, 1992.
29. Pellegrini C, Wetter LA, Patti M, et al. Thoracoscopic esophagomyotomy. Ann Surg 216:291, 1992.
30. Ferguson TB, Woodbury JD, Roper CL. Giant muscular hypertrophy of the esophagus. Ann Thorac Surg 8:209, 1969.
31. Gillies M, Nicks R, Skyring A. Clinical, manometric, and pathological studies in diffuse oesophageal spasm. Br Med J 2:527, 1967.
32. Castell DO, Richter JE, Dalton CB, eds. Esophageal Motility Testing. New York: Elsevier, 1987.
33. DeMeester TR. Surgery for esophageal motor disorders. Ann Thorac Surg 34:225, 1982.
34. Ellis FH Jr, Olsen AM, Schlegel AF, et al. Surgical treatment of esophageal hypermobility disturbances. JAMA 188:862, 1964.
35. Ferguson TB, Woodbury JD, Roper CL. Giant muscular hypertrophy of the esophagus. Ann Thorac Surg 8:209, 1969.
36. Henderson RD, Ho CS, Davidson JW. Primary motor disorder of the esophagus (diffuse spasm): Diagnosis and treatment. Ann Thorac Surg 18:327, 1974.
37. Flye MW, Sealy WC. Diffuse spasm of the esophagus. Ann Thorac Surg 19:677, 1975.
38. Leonardi HK, Shea JA, Crozier RE, et al. Diffuse spasm of the esophagus: Clinical, manometric, and surgical considerations. J Thorac Cardiovasc Surg 74:736, 1977.
39. Henderson RD, Ryder D, Marryatt G. Extended esophageal myotomy and short total fundoplication repair in diffuse esophageal spasm: Five-year review in 34 patients. Ann Thorac Surg 43:25, 1987.
40. Shimi SM, Nathonson LK, Cuschieri A. Thoracoscopic long oesephageal myotomy for nutcracker oesophagus: Initial experience with a new surgical approach. Br J Surg 79:533, 1992.

Chapter

7

Video-Assisted Laparoscopy for the Treatment of Achalasia

Henrique Walter Pinotti, M.D. • Carlos Eduardo Domene, M.D.
Ary Nasi, M.D. • Marco Aurelio Santo, M.D. • Hilton Telles Libanori, M.D.

STAGING AND MANAGEMENT GUIDELINES

The management of achalasia should be individualized according to the degree of esophageal involvement in each patient. Staging is based on morphologic and functional variables and can be used to assess the degree of esophageal involvement more accurately. Radiologic and manometric studies are used for assessment and patients are classified as follows:

incipient achalasia No esophageal dilatation. Minimal stasis of contrast material and/or radiologic evidence suggestive of motor changes and manometric confirmation of motility abnormalities consistent with achalasia.
intermediate achalasia Esophageal dilatation of 7 cm or less. Barium roentgenographs show the esophagus in its normal position. Manometric studies demonstrate esophageal aperistalsis with amplitudes of contraction >10 cm H_2O.
advanced achalasia Esophageal dilatation of >7 cm and/or a "sigmoid" appearance of the esophagus on x-ray films. Manometric studies reveal esophageal aperistalsis with contraction amplitudes of <10 cm H_2O.

For patients with incipient and intermediate achalasia we recommend a 9 cm cardiomyotomy extending 6 cm into the distal esophagus and 3 cm into the stomach. An antireflux valvuloplasty is also performed, which has been described by Pinotti et al.[1]

Although satisfactory results have been documented in more than 1000 patients with achalasia in whom the open procedure was performed during the past 15 years,[2] video-assisted laparoscopic surgery has opened new vistas. Our technical training and past experience with laparoscopic cholecystectomy since late 1990 have prompted us to pursue laparoscopic cardiomyotomy for the management of megaesophagus.

CLINICAL EXPERIENCE

From April 1991 to February 1993, 25 patients with nonadvanced achalasia underwent laparoscopic cardiomyotomy. There were 17 males and eight females whose ages ranged from 29 to 67 years. The preoperative evaluation included a clinical interview; barium roentgenographs of the esophagus, stomach, and duodenum; manometric studies of the esophagus; esophagogastroduodenoscopy; and abdominal ultrasonography. One patient also had gallstones.

Technique

The procedure is performed under general anesthesia. The surgeon stands between the patient's legs. The assistant on the left controls the video camera. The first assistant and scrub nurse stand on the patient's right side.

Five trocars provide access to the peritoneal cavity (Fig. 7-1). An automatic device is used to insufflate the necessary volume of CO_2 to maintain the intra-abdominal pressure at 14 mm Hg.

The first 10 or 11 mm trocar is used to introduce the laparoscope. The peritoneal cavity is explored and the other trocars are placed under direct vision. A second 10 or 11 mm trocar is introduced for insertion of a liver retractor. This retractor, designed by our service, consists of a hinged metal shaft covered by a soft rubber protector to avoid hepatic injury.

The liver is retracted anteriorly by the first assistant to expose the region of the esophagogastric junction (Fig. 7-2). At this point the third and fourth trocars, 10 or 11 and 5 mm, respectively, are placed for the dissecting forceps. The surgeon holds one of these forceps in each hand. After the esophagogastric junction is dissected and the distal esophagus isolated, a supraumbilical incision is made to introduce and position an esophageal retractor designed by our service. This retractor, also designed by our service, is useful for pulling the esophagus caudally, allowing exposure of the distal esophagus. It also permits slight rotation of the esophagus to simplify execution of the valvuloplasty (Fig. 7-3).

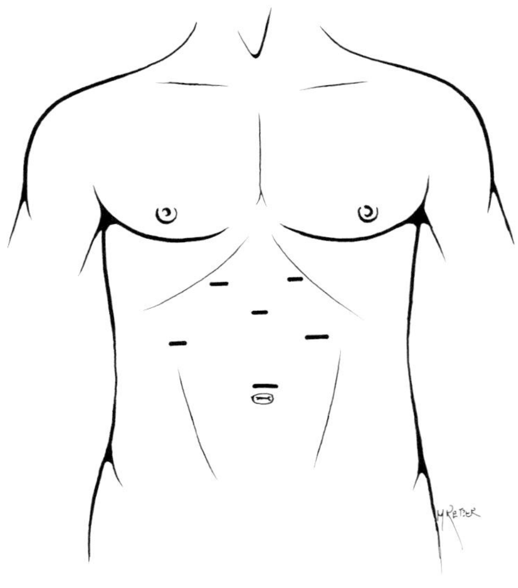

Fig. 7-1. Location of ports for the abdominal approach.

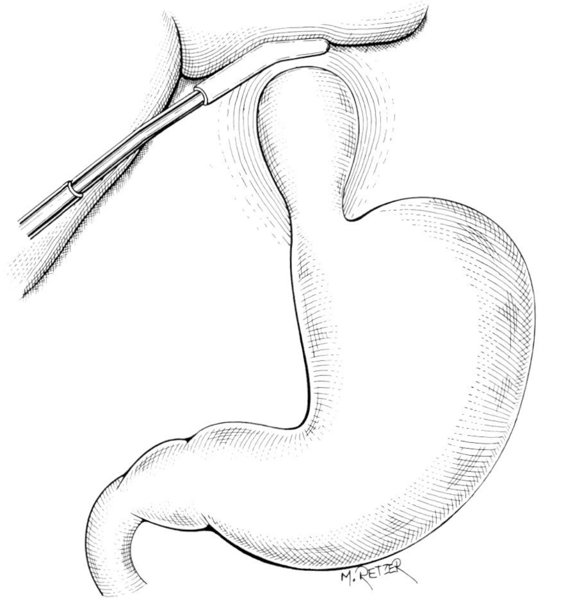

Fig. 7-2. Retraction of the liver.

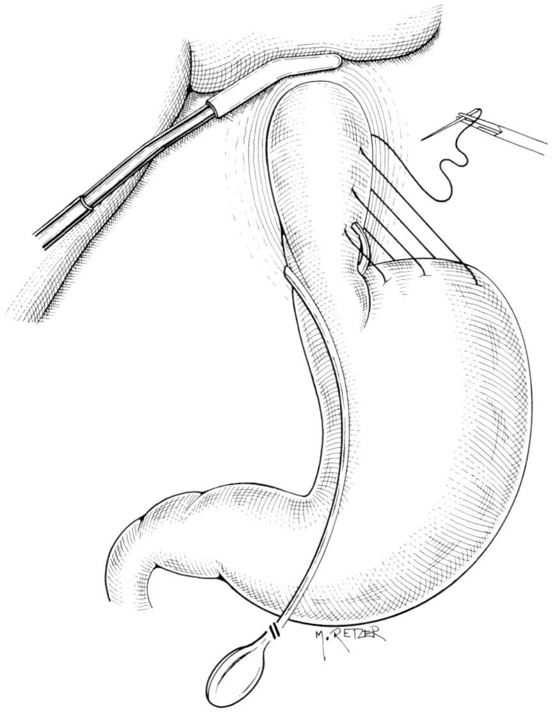

Fig. 7-3. The first suture line fixes the gastric fundus to the posterior region of the esophagus.

The esophageal retractor is positioned and traction is applied toward the patient's feet in a caudal direction with counterclockwise rotation, allowing construction of the valvuloplasty. The gastric fundus is sutured with a continuous suture to the posterior region of the distal esophagus for about 6 cm (Fig. 7-3). The esophageal retractor can then be released slightly to facilitate the next suture line (Fig. 7-4).

After the two suture lines of the valvuloplasty (one in the posterior and the other in the left lateral region of the esophagus) are completed, the cardiomyotomy is begun. The adventitia and muscle layers of the distal 6 cm of the esophagus and the serosa and muscle layers of a 3 cm length of the proximal stomach are cut, resulting in a 9 cm myotomy. Fragments of the cut layers are resected so that a cardiomyotomy as well as a cardiomyectomy is performed (Figs. 7-5 and 7-6).

The resected strip is sent for histopathologic study. After the integrity of the exposed mucosa is checked, the counterclockwise traction on the esophageal retractor is released and the third and last suture is placed on the gastric fundus, now on the right margin of the cardiomyectomy (Figs. 7-7 and 7-8). Cardiomyectomy without a valvuloplasty was performed in the first three patients in our series.

Results

The procedure was successfully completed in all patients without the need to convert to the open technique. Intraoperative complications included two cases of perforation of the esophageal mucosa and two cases of subcutaneous cervical emphysema. It should be mentioned that these problems occurred in the first four patients in this

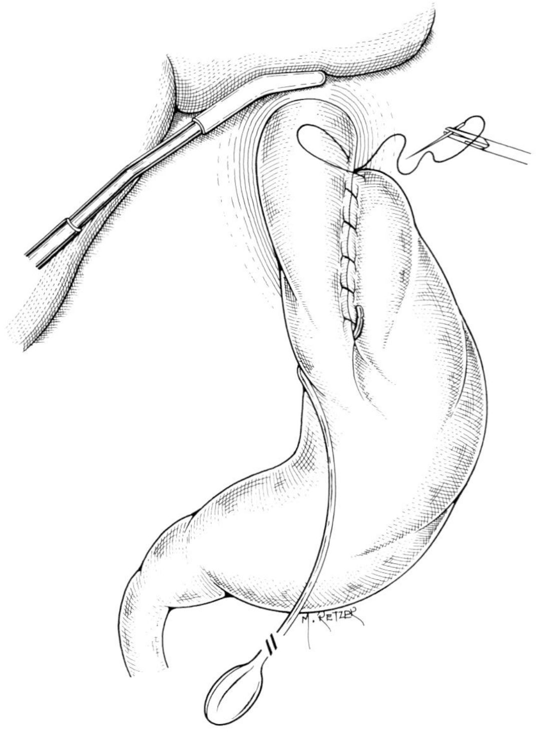

Fig. 7-4. The second suture line secures the gastric fundus to the esophagus.

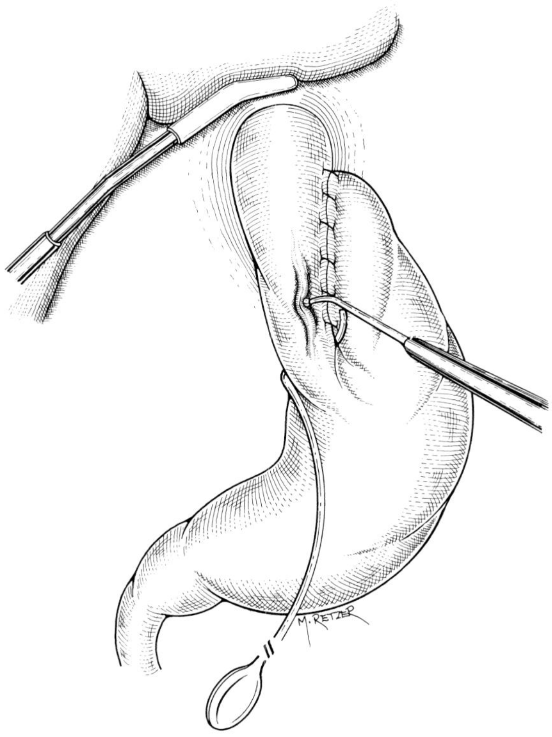

Fig. 7-5. The cardiomyectomy is begun at the gastroesophageal junction.

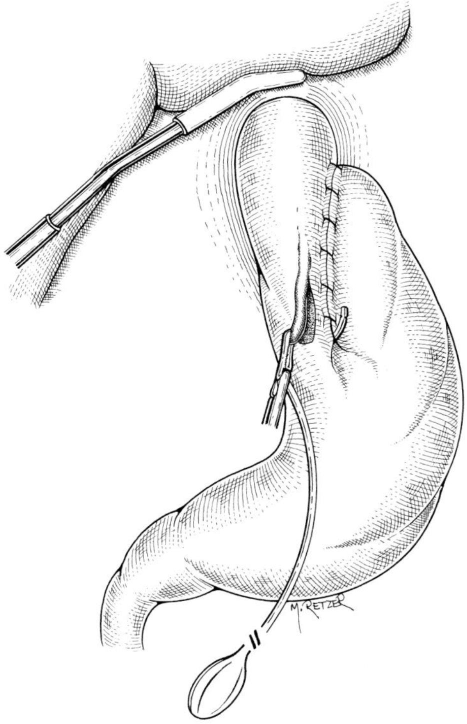

Fig. 7-6. A small strip of esophageal muscle is removed, creating a cardiomyectomy not simply a cardiomyotomy.

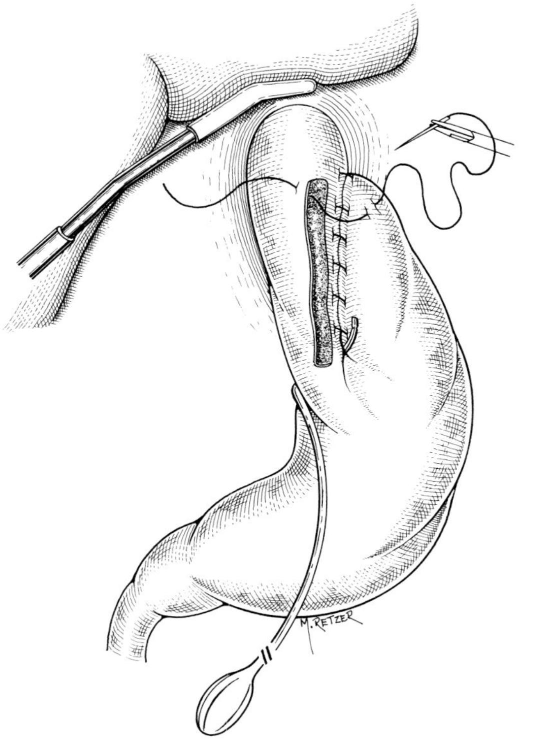

Fig. 7-7. The third suture line connects the gastric fundus to the right margin of the myectomy, covering it completely.

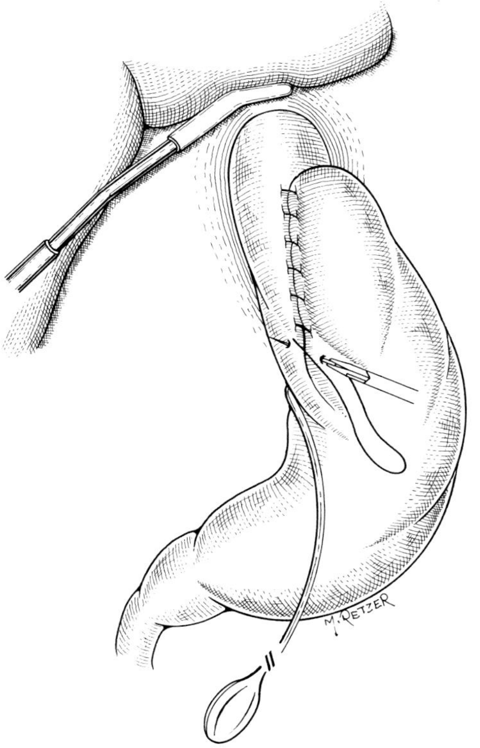

Fig. 7-8. The third suture line lateral to the right edge of the cardiomyectomy completes the procedure.

series. After the technique was refined, the esophageal and liver retractors were modified, and the first two suture lines for the valvuloplasty were placed prior to the cardiomyectomy, we no longer encountered these problems.

The mucosal perforations were closed with a continuous mucomucosal suture and protected by wrapping the suture line with the gastric fundus during the valvuloplasty and placement of a Penrose drain. Subcutaneous emphysema was treated by reducing the intraperitoneal pressure. The region of the emphysema was carefully observed by the anesthetist; it eventually stabilized during the operation and regressed completely postoperatively.

A small esophageal fistula developed in one of the patients with an esophageal perforation. It was suspected because of the characteristic drainage and confirmed by barium swallow. The fistula closed spontaneously after 7 days of fasting and parenteral feeding, and the patient's recovery was satisfactory. This was the only postoperative complication observed.

Although 21 of the 25 patients could have been discharged 48 hours postoperatively, they were not released so that we could perform further clinical evaluation and carry out initial functional assessment.

Immediate functional results were assessed by clinical interviews, barium x-ray studies, and manometric studies. The initial interview and x-ray studies took place after oral feeding was first resumed and the manometric studies 7 to 10 days postoperatively.

Alleviation of dysphagia and patient satisfaction with the results were noted in all cases at the first clinical interview. The contrast material for the x-ray evaluation passed more easily to the stomach in all patients.

Esophageal manometry was performed in 23 patients preoperatively and 24 postoperatively. The mean lower esophageal sphincter pressure was reduced from 50 cm H_2O preoperatively to 23 cm H_2O postoperatively.

The patients are still being followed clinically to assess the results over the long term. At follow-up ranging from 6 to 28 months more than 90% of patients have less difficulty in swallowing.

Five patients still have some degree of residual dysphagia with solid foods despite improvement. Nineteen subjects no longer complain of dysphagia, and dysphagia improved temporarily in one patient but returned 10 months later with the same intensity as before the operation.

One patient who underwent cardiomyectomy only has symptoms suggestive of gastroesophageal reflux. His symptoms are presently controlled by sleeping with the head elevated, dietary restrictions, and periodic use of H_2-blocking agents.

CONCLUSION

The growing experience with video-assisted laparoscopy and the rapid design and development of instrumentation have extended the applications. Complex procedures requiring extensive dissection and resection are now being performed.

Because of these advances and accumulated experience, we elected to use a laparoscopic approach for the treatment of nonadvanced achalasia. The operation is much the same as the open procedure but without the inherent morbidity associated with the classic technique.

Our limited experience to date is encouraging. The low rate of interoperative and postoperative complications demonstrates the safety of the procedure. This factor added to the satisfactory results achieved over the short and medium term attest to the value of this modality. A longer period of clinical observation is required before the results of the operation can be fully assessed.

The growing experience of the team and the development of techniques and equipment for suturing and proper retraction of the liver and esophagogastric junction have decreased the operative time considerably and it is gradually approaching that required for conventional surgery.

Functional results are comparable to those achieved with the open procedure. Laparoscopic cardiomyotomy represents a valuable management alternative that is safe and effective and is associated with a shorter recovery period, better cosmetic results, a more rapid return to normal activities, reduced postoperative pain, and fewer complications.

REFERENCES

1. Pinotti HW, Gama-Rodrigues JJ, Ellenbogen G, Raia A. Nova técnica no tratamento cirúrgico do megaesôfago. Esofagocardiomiomia associada a esofagofundogastropexia. Rev Goiania Med 20:1, 1974.
2. Ellenbogen G. Megaesôfago não avancado. Tratamento pela cardiomiectomia associada a esofagofundogastropexia. Avaliacão clínica, morfológica e funcional dos seus resultados. Thesis. Faculdade de Medicina da Universidade de São Paulo, 1979.

Chapter

8

Thoracoscopic Resection of Epiphrenic Esophageal Diverticula

Alberto Peracchia, M.D. • Luigi Bonavina, M.D.
Riccardo Rosati, M.D. • Stefano Bona, M.D.

Acquired diverticula occurring in the lower 10 cm of the esophagus are relatively uncommon, representing about 20% of most large published series of esophageal diverticula.[1] These "pulsion" diverticula usually develop from the right side of the esophagus and are thought to be associated with or even caused by an underlying esophageal motor disorder. This has led to the belief that an esophagomyotomy is necessary for relieving all potential esophageal obstructions and for preventing early and late complications of diverticulectomy such as esophageal leak and recurrent pouch formation.[2] According to some authors, the myotomy should encompass the gastric cardia to ensure that functional obstruction is eliminated and should be combined with a Belsey antireflux repair.[3]

Controversy persists as to whether all patients with an epiphrenic diverticulum should be offered surgery since symptoms can be minimal regardless of the size of the pouch and an esophageal motility disorder is not always documented. On the other hand, a formal thoracotomy is a major surgical procedure associated with significant postoperative pain and often a prolonged hospital stay and recovery period.

Recent advances in minimally invasive surgery have renewed interest in the surgical treatment of benign esophageal disorders. Minimally invasive procedures markedly shorten the hospital stay and recovery period largely by reducing the severity of incisional pain. Lower health care costs and a more satisfactory cosmetic result are added dividends.

INDICATIONS AND ADVANTAGES

Surgical treatment of pulsion diverticula of the thoracic esophagus is usually indicated since the pouch tends to increase in size over time and interferes with esophageal emptying. Even in patients who are asymptomatic an epiphrenic diverticulum may cause pulmonary fibrosis secondary to aspiration.[4] Achalasia is rarely associated with an epiphrenic diverticulum in our experience. If present, treatment of the underlying disorder is required for palliation of dysphagia.

Although surgical treatment of epiphrenic diverticula remains controversial, most esophageal surgeons agree that the ideal operation includes diverticulectomy, myotomy, and antireflux repair via a thoracic approach. The right thoracic approach is preferred for distal diverticula, regardless of their orientation. The esophagus is mobilized so that it can be rotated to visualize a left-sided diverticulum. Once the neck of the diverticulum is isolated and stapled, a myotomy is performed on the opposite side of the esophagus.

Recent studies have challenged this thinking. Some authors believe myotomy should be performed only in selected patients based on the results of esophageal manometry.[5] Moreover, extending the myotomy to the cardia in patients with a normal sphincter can potentially cause gastroesophageal reflux.[6]

We have applied these generally accepted management criteria to the minimally invasive surgical approach. In patients with documented sphincter abnormalities we have performed pneumatic dilation of the cardia preoperatively in an effort to reduce the outflow resistance to esophageal transit. Our preliminary experience shows this approach has been satisfactory with the exception of one patient in whom reflux symptoms developed.

The advantage of the thoracoscopic approach is that the right-sided diverticulum can be dissected and resected quite easily through the right side of the chest with minimal operative trauma. In the rare patient with a left-sided diverticulum a myotomy and fundoplication should be performed using a left thoracoscopic approach. Avoiding the trauma of thoracotomy is a substantial benefit to the patient with benign esophageal disease. Although thoracoscopic resection of epiphrenic diverticula is feasible, we recommend careful patient selection based on preoperative esophageal function studies. If necessary, pneumatic dilation of the cardia should be performed. A longer follow-up is needed to evaluate the long-term results of this innovative approach.

TECHNIQUE

The technique of thoracoscopic diverticulectomy has been developed based on the pathophysiology of the disease. To overcome the intrinsic limitations of the thoracoscopic approach, that is, the difficulty in performing a myotomy and a Belsey fundoplication through a right thoracoscopy or in approaching the pouch from the left side, we used pneumatic dilation of the cardia preoperatively in patients with manometric abnormalities of the lower esophageal sphincter.

A general anesthetic is administered via double-lumen endotracheal intubation. The patient is placed in the left recumbent position as for a right posterolateral thoracotomy. Four trocars are placed in the intercostal spaces to allow dissection and subsequent resection of the diverticulum (Fig. 8-1, *A*) The first 10 mm trocar is introduced in the fifth intercostal space at the midaxillary line; two other 5 mm trocars are inserted in the fifth or sixth interspaces, one on the anterior and one on the posterior axillary line. A fourth 10 mm port is placed in the sixth or seventh intercostal space and is used initially for a lung retractor.

For diverticula located in the very distal thoracic esophagus, the dissection should proceed from above to below; for more proximal diverticula, the position of the instruments is altered slightly to permit dissection from a more favorable angle (Fig. 8-1, *B*).

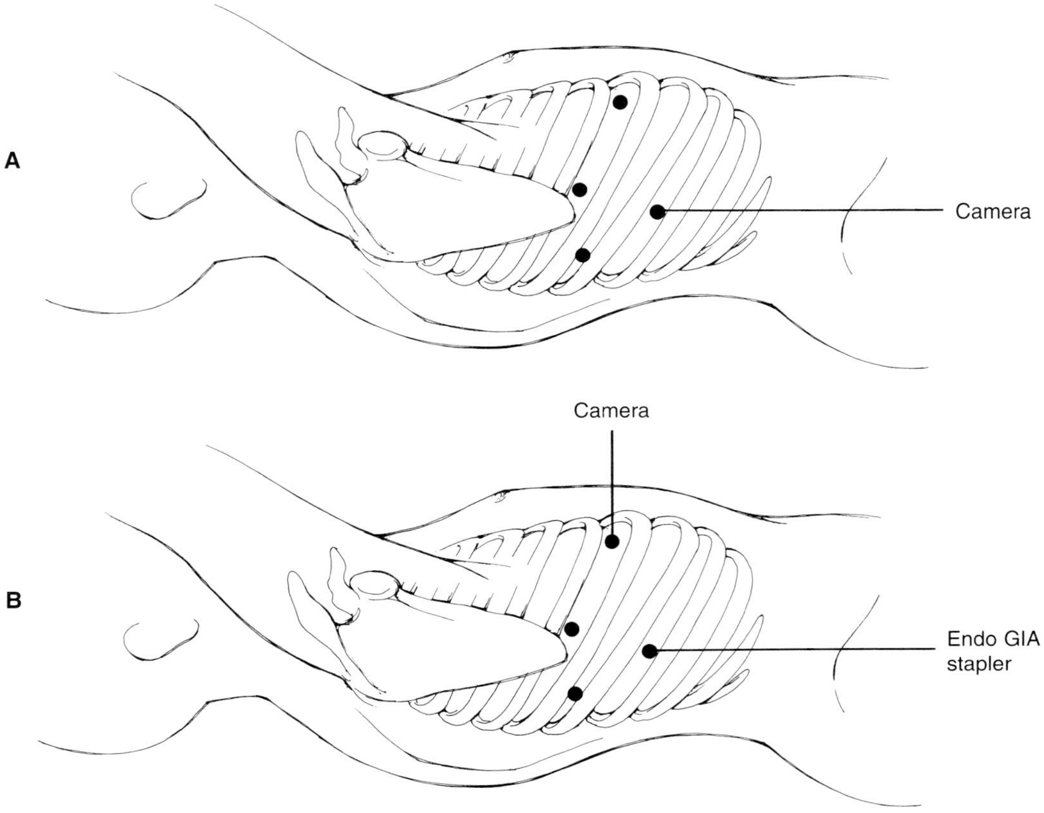

Fig. 8-1. A, Port positioning for dissection of more proximal diverticulum. **B,** Camera repositioned for resection of diverticulum with an Endo GIA stapler.

Moderate insufflation and transillumination through an endoluminal esophagoscope often facilitates both dissection and resection of the diverticulum. The inferior pulmonary ligament is divided using a coagulating hook and/or scissors. The mediastinal pleura overlying the diverticulum should be incised gently; care must be taken not to damage the mucosa, which is very thin at this level (Fig. 8-2).

A Babcock clamp is placed on the pouch and mild traction is used to facilitate sharp dissection of the neck. Gentle dissection of the neck is essential to preserve the integrity of the muscular fibers for reapproximation at the end of the procedure (Fig. 8-3).

The limits of the diverticular neck can be checked from the endoluminal site with the esophagoscope. At this point an endoscopic stapler can be introduced from above or below, depending on the location of the pouch, and the base of the diverticulum divided and closed keeping the angle with the esophagus as small as possible (Fig. 8-4). This is a crucial step in preventing the formation of a pseudodiverticular blind pouch. One or more firings of the stapler may be necessary. Gentle upward traction on the residual pouch during the application of the first row of staples can make the application of the second row easier. The esophagoscope is used to check the placement of the stapler after closure of the jaws as well as to check the integrity of the suture line after the diverticulum is resected and removed.

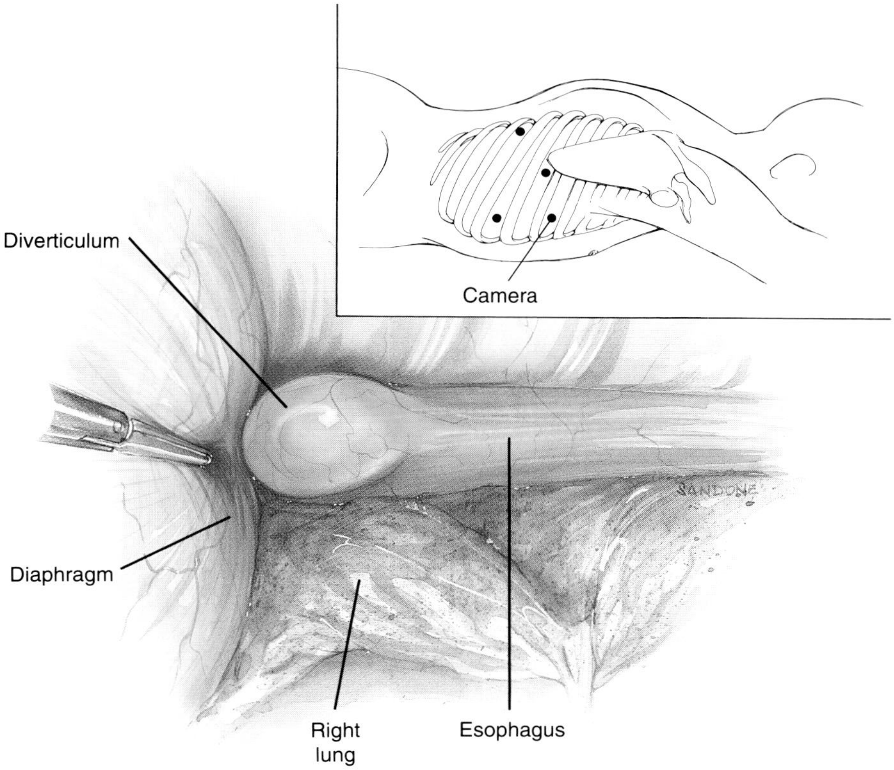

Fig. 8-2. Thoracoscopic view of an epiphrenic diverticulum. Inset: Camera positioned in lower trocar.

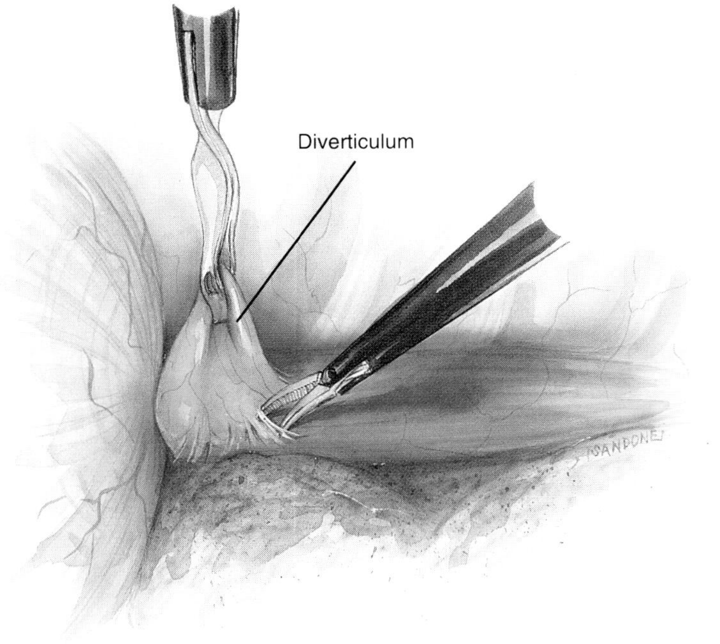

Fig. 8-3. Dissection of epiphrenic diverticulum through a right thoracoscopic approach. (The camera is between the two operating instruments.)

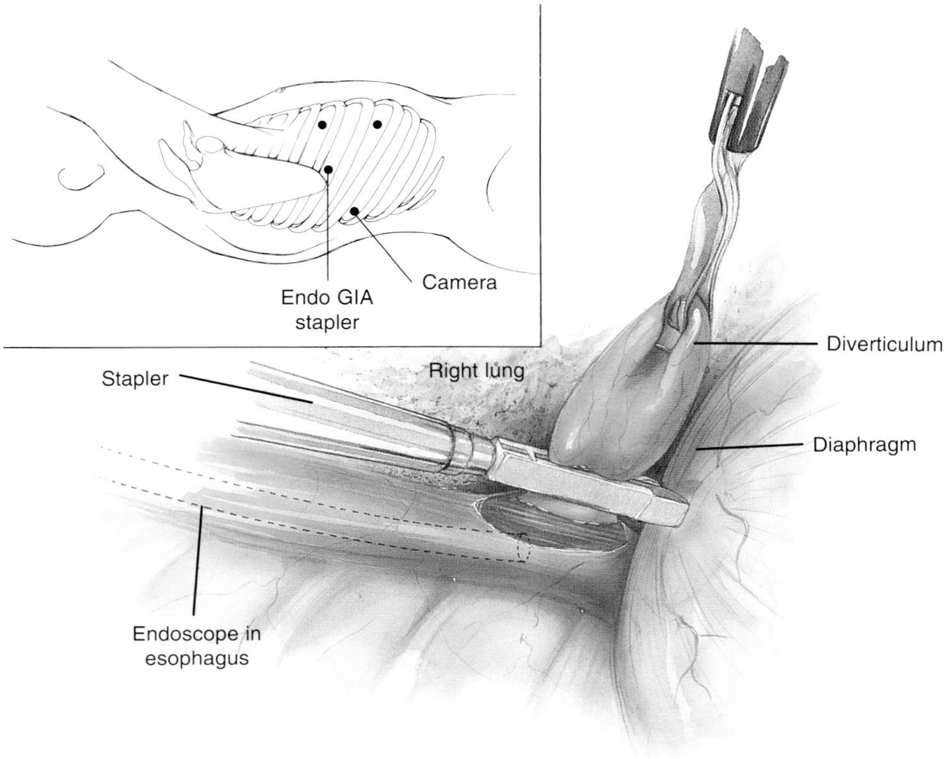

Fig. 8-4. The camera is moved to allow the endoscopic linear stapler to be properly applied to the neck of the diverticulum.

The muscular edges of the esophageal wall are approximated with either interrupted or running sutures to protect the staple line (Fig. 8-5). A nasogastric tube is placed and the pleural cavity irrigated with warm saline solution. A chest tube is placed through the lowest trocar site at the end of the operation.

We perform a Gastrografin swallow on the fourth postoperative day after the nasogastric tube has been removed. The patient is placed on a liquid diet and discharged on the sixth postoperative day.

CLINICAL EXPERIENCE

Thirty-seven patients have undergone surgical treatment for pulsion diverticula of the thoracic esophagus at our institution since 1976. From November 1991 through June 1993, thoracoscopic resection of esophageal diverticula was attempted in eight symptomatic patients, seven men and one woman whose mean age was 54 years (range 42 to 77 years). Six patients complained of intermittent dysphagia, four of regurgitation of food, and one of nocturnal cough. The diverticula were located along the right lateral wall of the esophagus in all but one patient and ranged in size from 4 to 10 cm. None of the patients showed signs of endoscopic esophagitis or abnormal gastroesophageal reflux on 24-hour pH monitoring. Esophageal manometry showed a hypertensive (basal pressure >30 mm Hg) and/or an incompletely relaxed

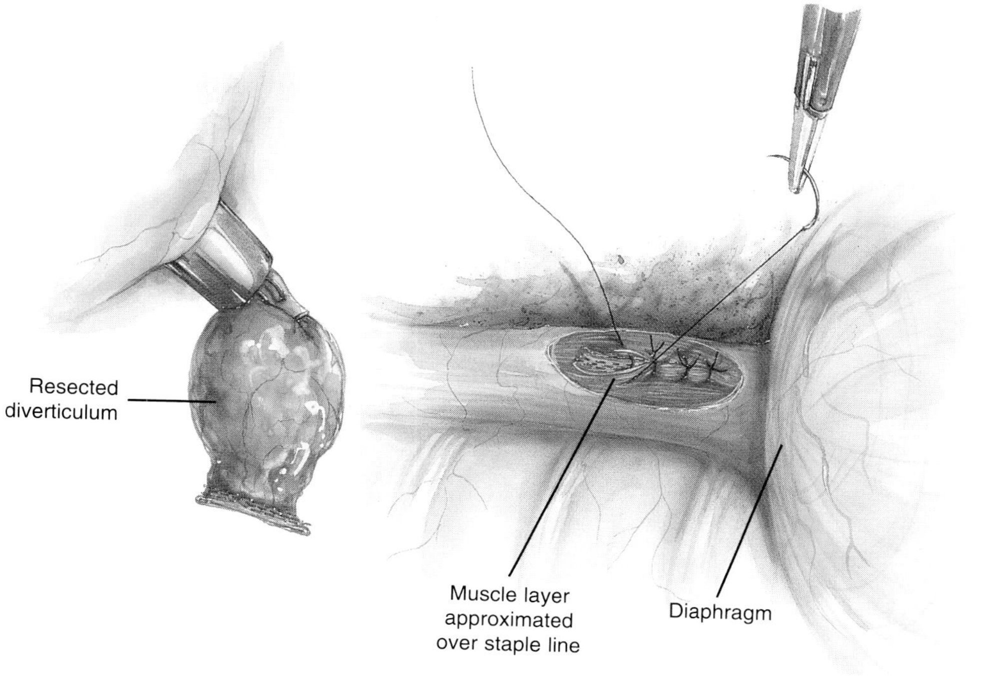

Fig. 8-5. After diverticulectomy, the muscle layer edges are approximated with interrupted sutures.

(residual pressure >20 mm Hg) lower esophageal sphincter in five of the eight patients. In these patients, preoperative pneumatic dilation of the cardia was performed using a 30 mm Rigiflex balloon inflated up to 10 psi for 1 minute. A marked reduction of lower esophageal sphincter pressure (to <20 mm Hg) was manometrically recorded 1 week later in these patients.

In two patients, one of whom had a left-sided diverticulum, the thoracoscopic procedure was converted to a thoracotomy because of failure to collapse the lung.

The operative time for thoracoscopic resection averaged 3.5 hours. Minor bleeding from a trocar site was noted in one patient and resolved with conservative treatment. In another patient a leak from the staple line occurred despite preoperative pneumatic dilation of the cardia. Conservative treatment consisting of repeat pneumatic dilation, nasogastric aspiration, and antibiotics failed and surgical revision was required.

Clinical results are satisfactory in five of the six patients at follow-up of 8 to 22 months. One patient complains of heartburn (responsive to treatment with H_2 blockers) and shows abnormal esophageal acid exposure on 24-hour pH monitoring.

REFERENCES

1. Postlethwait R. Surgery of the Esophagus. New York: Appleton-Century-Crofts, 1979.
2. Debas H, Payne W, Cameron A, Carlson H. Physiopathology of lower esophageal diverticulum and its implication for treatment. Surg Gynecol Obstet 151:593-600, 1980.
3. Evander A, Little A, Ferguson M, Skinner D. Diverticula of the mid and lower esophagus: Pathogenesis and surgical management. World J Surg 10:820-828, 1986.

4. Altorki N, Sunagawa M, Skinner D. Thoracic esophageal diverticula: Why is operation necessary? J Thorac Cardiovasc Surg 105:260-264, 1993.
5. Streitz J, Glick M, Ellis F. Selective use of myotomy for treatment of epiphrenic diverticula. Arch Surg 127:585-588, 1992.
6. Favre J, Baulieux J, Ducerf C, Rat P, Haas O, Sala J. Traitement chirurgical des diverticules de l'oesophage thoracique. Chirurgie 116:786-790, 1990.

Part

III

Gastroesophageal Reflux

Chapter

9

Fundamentals of Antireflux Surgery

Ross M. Bremner, B.Sc., M.B., B.Ch.
Cedric G. Bremner, M.B., B.Ch., Ch.M., F.R.C.S.(Eng), F.R.C.S.(Ed)
Jeffrey H. Peters, M.D. • Tom R. DeMeester, M.D.

HISTORICAL PERSPECTIVE

Gastroesophageal reflux disease was not recognized as a significant clinical problem until the mid-1930s and was not identified as a precipitating cause of esophagitis until after World War II.[1] Initially the symptoms of gastroesophageal reflux were associated with hiatal hernia, leading to the conclusion that the hernia itself caused the symptoms. It thus seemed reasonable that this condition could be cured by surgical reduction of the hernia with simple closure of the crura. Consequently, hiatal hernia became an indication for surgery that often yielded poor results. Since esophageal function studies were unavailable and rigid endoscopy was performed with difficulty, the reasons for failure were not understood. It was not until much later that the relationship between hiatal hernia and reflux was identified.

Allison[2] was the first to accurately describe the connection between symptoms of hiatal hernia and gastroesophageal reflux, clearly demonstrating that the function of the cardia must be improved rather than simply reducing the hernia. The Allison repair introduced in 1951 represented the first effort in this direction. He emphasized that the gastroesophageal junction must be placed in its normal intra-abdominal position to improve its function. Although repair was associated with a high incidence of recurrence, Allison[3] was justly credited with initiating the modern era of antireflux surgery.

Experience with the Allison repair demonstrated that symptoms of reflux were relieved when the gastroesophageal junction remained in the intra-abdominal position. Consequently, procedures were designed to place and anchor the lower esophagus more effectively in the abdomen. Initially these operations were basically various forms of gastropexy in which the stomach was pulled down in the abdomen whether the esophagus was herniated or not. The stomach was then attached to the anterior abdominal wall or to any posterior peritoneal structure that seemed strong enough to maintain it in an intra-abdominal position. Consequently, the gastropexies became dislodged and reflux symptoms returned.[4,5] The most popular of these operations was the Hill procedure, which anchored the gastroesophageal junction posteriorly to the median arcuate ligament.[6]

With the exception of the Hill procedure, these operations did not withstand the test of time and were gradually abandoned. The Belsey Mark IV repair[7] and Nissen fundoplication[8,9] incorporated a portion of the distal esophagus into the stomach so that it was subject to the intra-abdominal pressure transmitted by the gastric conduit. In essence, the Belsey Mark IV procedure is a partial fundoplication that places a 280-degree envelope of gastric fundus over the distal esophagus. The Nissen procedure is a complete fundoplication that places a 360-degree envelope of gastric fundus over the distal esophagus.

It soon became apparent that simply wrapping the stomach around the lower esophagus and sewing it in place would not result in a successful Nissen fundoplication. Determining how tight and how long to make the fundoplication, what portion of the stomach to use, and what conditions contraindicate the operation requires judgment and experience. Poor surgical technique and improper patient selection have resulted in a number of postoperative symptoms.[10] If the fundoplication is too long or the esophagus is wrapped rather than enveloped by the fundus, permanent dysphagia or odynophagia may result. Such a fundoplication precludes physiologic belching and vomiting. Instead of surgeons focusing on improving their technique, a variety of partial fundoplications have been introduced to avoid these problems, usually by covering either the anterior or posterior wall of the distal esophagus with the stomach. These necessitate suturing the fundus of the stomach to the esophagus. This suture line is subject to high stress levels and as a consequence has limited durability. Although partial fundoplication procedures are successful in preventing reflux and permitting physiologic belching, they disrupt with distressing frequency.

The most durable of the partial fundoplications is the Belsey Mark IV operation. In this procedure the attachment of the esophagus to the stomach is more extensive than that advocated for other partial fundoplications, and the procedure is performed transthoracically so that the esophagus can be adequately mobilized to construct the repair without undue tension. The primary drawback of the Belsey Mark IV procedure is that the antireflux protection is not as predictable as with a complete Nissen fundoplication. This is in large part a reflection of the skill of the surgeon since the nuances of the Belsey procedure are difficult to teach and there is less margin for error. In experienced hands the success rate with the Belsey operation appears similar to that with the Nissen procedure.

The lessons learned from the past have paved the way for improvements in antireflux surgery. Now excellent results can be achieved in the majority of patients given proper patient selection and meticulous attention to technique. It is hoped that those performing minimally invasive surgery who are not familiar with the history of antireflux surgery will not repeat the mistakes of the past.

MEDICAL THERAPY

Gastroesophageal reflux disease is such a common condition that most patients with mild symptoms manage well with self-medication. If symptoms of heartburn are present in the absence of obvious complications, patients can reasonably be placed on 8 to 12 weeks of simple antacid therapy before undergoing extensive investigations. In many situations this successfully relieves the symptoms. Patients should be advised to elevate the head of their bed; avoid tight clothing; eat small, frequent meals; avoid eating their nighttime meal shortly before retiring; lose weight; and avoid alcohol, cigarettes, coffee, and peppermints, which may aggravate the symptoms. Alginic acid used in combination with simple antacids may augment symptomatic relief by creating a physical barrier to reflux as well as reducing acid. Alginic acid reacts with sodium bicarbonate in the presence of saliva to form a highly viscous solution that floats like a raft on the surface of the gastric contents. When reflux occurs, this protective layer is refluxed into the esophagus and acts as a protective barrier against the noxious gastric contents. Medications to promote gastric emptying such as metoclopramide, domperidone, or cisapride have been of little value.

The second phase of medical therapy in patients with persistent symptoms is acid suppression by the use of H_2 blockers. In high doses they reduce gastric acidity by 70% to 80%. This treatment, however, cures esophagitis in only about 50% of patients after an 8-week course of therapy. The new hydrogen potassium proton pump inhibitor omeprazole, which can totally prevent gastric acid secretion, causes an almost complete disappearance of symptoms and results in a greater than 75% healing rate in patients with mild esophagitis and a 50% healing rate in patients with severe esophagitis after a 12-week course of therapy. These medications, however, should not be continued over the long term because of the cost and the potential for complications secondary to the alkaline component of the reflux gastric juice while symptoms are being masked by therapy. Unfortunately, within 6 months of discontinuing any form of medical therapy for gastroesophageal reflux disease, 80% of patients have a recurrence of symptoms since acid suppression therapy does not correct the underlying defect, that is, the mechanically defective sphincter.

All patients whose symptoms persist despite simple antacid therapy should undergo endoscopy to determine if esophagitis, stricture, or Barrett's esophagus is present. They are then placed on H_2 or omeprazole therapy. If their symptoms disappear completely after 12 weeks of therapy, the medication should be discontinued and the patient observed. If their symptoms recur within 4 weeks, they should undergo manometric studies and 24-hour foregut pH monitoring. If repeat endoscopic studies indicate persisting complications, these patients should also undergo further study. Depending on the results of the tests, further intensive medical therapy may be instituted or patients may be considered for surgical therapy. Patients whose symptoms do not recur within 4 weeks and who are free of complications of the disease should be monitored and treated intermittently as needed.

SURGICAL CONSIDERATIONS

Antireflux surgery is one of the most commonly performed foregut procedures, reflecting the prevalence of gastroesophageal reflux disease in Western society.[11] Gastroesophageal reflux disease is a symptomatic foregut abnormality caused by increased esophageal exposure to gastric juice. Before the decision is made to treat the disease surgically, increased exposure of the esophagus to acid must be documented to be the underlying cause of the patient's symptoms, the physiologic basis for the acid exposure determined, and the patient screened to see if he would benefit from a surgical antireflux procedure.

Documentation of Increased Esophageal Acid Exposure

Symptoms are an unreliable guide to the patient's underlying problem. The symptoms of diseases of different foregut organs overlap, and patients with reflux disease may present with atypical symptoms such as asthma or chronic cough.[12] Endoscopic evidence of mucosal injury such as esophagitis, stricture, or Barrett's esophagus will confirm reflux disease only in those patients with complications, which constitutes only about 60% of all patients with gastroesophageal reflux disease.[13] Also, in approximately 10% of patients with esophagitis, esophageal acid exposure is not abnormal; mucosal injury has originated from another source such as pill damage or infection.[11] Radiologic studies and the standard acid reflux test are also noted for their poor diagnostic sensitivity and specificity. The only reliable method of detecting abnormal exposure of the esophagus to gastric juice is 24-hour pH monitoring.[14] Furthermore, it serves as a "physiologic Bernstein test" by correlating pH events and patient symptoms in the physiologic environment of outpatient monitoring. A "symptom index" that uses this correlation to specifically link the patient's symptoms to changes in intraesophageal pH has been reported.[15,16]

Identifying the Cause of Increased Esophageal Acid Exposure

Although useful for measuring the esophageal exposure to gastric juice and diagnosing the presence of gastroesophageal reflux disease, 24-hour pH monitoring does not identify the underlying cause of increased exposure, which needs to be determined before a therapeutic approach is selected. The antireflux mechanism in humans consists of three components: the lower esophageal sphincter, which acts as a valve between the esophagus and the stomach; the worm-drive pump of the esophageal body, which together with the neutralizing activity of swallowed saliva acts to clear reflux from the esophageal lumen[17]; and the gastric reservoir.

Who Should Undergo Esophageal Function Studies?

Although most patients with gastroesophageal reflux disease have a mechanically defective sphincter (defined as a sphincter with a manometric resting pressure of <6 mm Hg, a total length of <2 cm, or an intra-abdominal length of <1 cm), this is not always the case.[18] A mechanically defective sphincter must be documented since antireflux surgery is designed to correct this problem. However, up to 35% of patients with increased esophageal acid exposure do not have an incompetent valve. This group of patients may have a defective esophageal pump that results in poor clearance of physiologic reflux or a gastric abnormality such as gastric dilatation, delayed gastric emptying, or gastric hypersecretion that may result in increased quantities or an increased concentration of refluxed acid. In these patients an antireflux procedure in the face of a normal valve is misguided since improving sphincter function when the underlying problem is an abnormality of the esophageal body or gastric reservoir will only exacerbate problems. This emphasizes the importance of preoperative manometry in assessing esophageal body function. Manometry measures lower esophageal sphincter characteristics and assesses esophageal body motility. This test is essential before performing surgery to ascertain that the sphincter is deficient and to ensure that the esophageal pump mechanism is adequate and has not been destroyed by long-term gastroesophageal reflux.

Careful selection of patients for antireflux surgery is key to a successful outcome and the patient's well-being. Since it is not practical to perform manometry

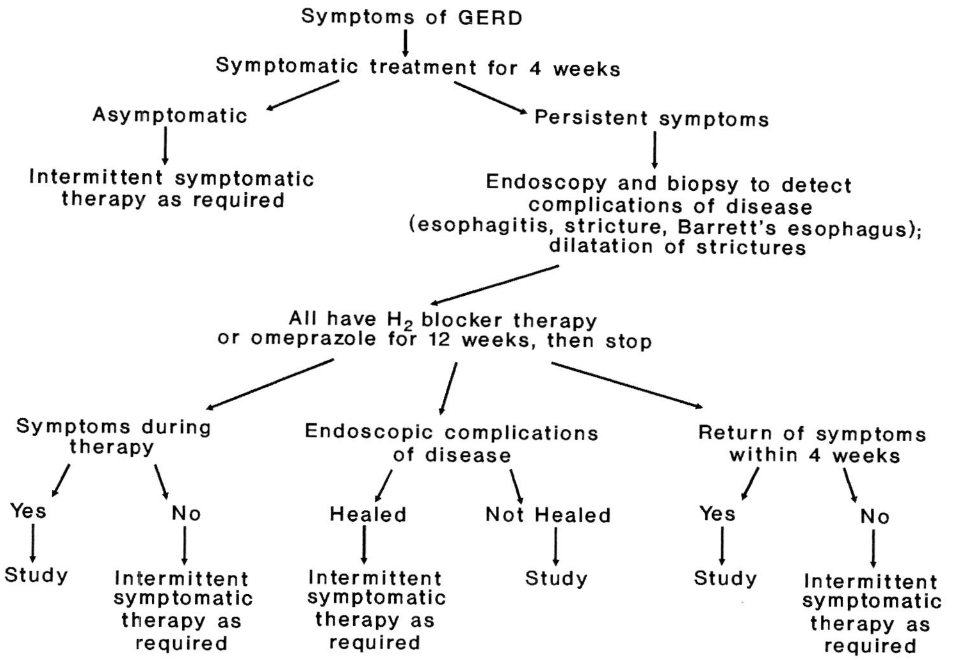

Fig. 9-1. Algorithm for selecting patients with gastroesophageal reflux disease for further study.

and 24-hour pH monitoring on all patients who complain of symptoms suggestive of reflux disease, a selective approach to esophageal function studies is outlined in Fig. 9-1.

Indications for Surgery

Many patients with gastroesophageal reflux disease will respond to simple changes in lifestyle and intermittent antacid therapy. Surgery is reserved for those patients who do not respond to medical therapy (i.e., remain symptomatic, fail to heal, or develop complications while taking medications) and for those patients who become medication dependent. Unfortunately, the results of inappropriate and poorly executed antireflux surgery have made many physicians wary of recommending major surgery for a benign disease. We emphasize that surgery should be performed only in properly selected patients. The criteria for selection are:

1. Persistent or recurrent symptoms and/or complications after 8 to 12 weeks of intensive acid suppression therapy
2. Increased esophageal exposure to gastric juice documented by 24-hour esophageal pH monitoring
3. Presence of a mechanically defective lower esophageal sphincter on manometric studies
4. Adequate esophageal body motor function[19]

Patients who present with complications of reflux disease (esophagitis, stricture, or Barrett's esophagus) are less likely to respond to medical therapy. Although some

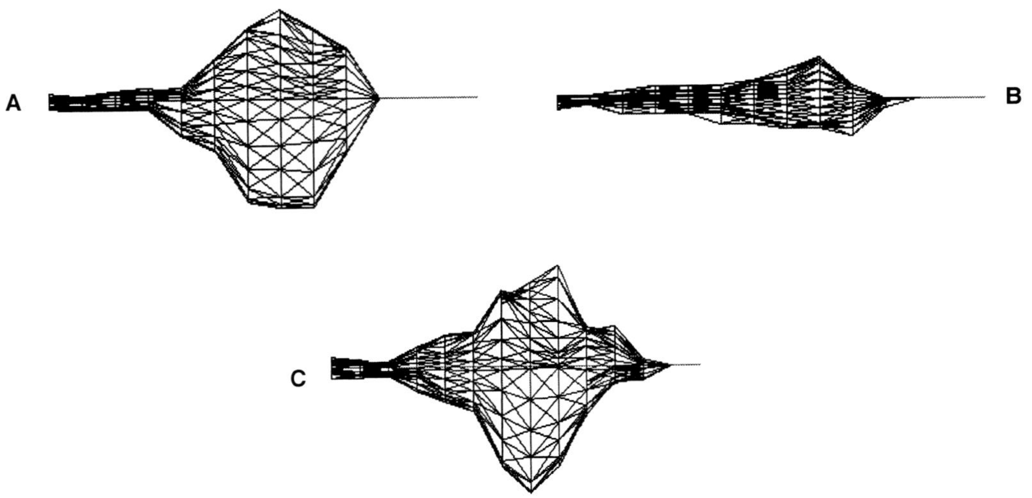

Fig. 9-2. Three-dimensional lower esophageal sphincter pressure profile in a normal volunteer **(A)** and a patient with a mechanically defective sphincter before **(B)** and 1 year after **(C)** Nissen fundoplication. (From DeMeester TR, Stein HJ. Surgical treatment of gastroesophageal reflux disease. In Castell DO, ed. The Esophagus. Boston: Little, Brown, 1992, p 619.)

patients with esophagitis respond well to a short course of medical therapy, it is estimated that at least 45% will relapse after treatment is discontinued.[20] At least 20% of patients with esophagitis will develop a more serious complication such as stricture or Barrett's esophagus after 6 years or more of follow-up.[21] Similar findings were observed in a large multicenter prospective study in which 8% of patients with gastroesophageal reflux disease developed a stricture within a year despite control of symptoms with intermittent or intensive medical therapy.[22] Patients with complicated reflux disease were shown by this large study to be more adequately treated by surgical than medical therapy.[23] The case for surgical intervention in the group of patients who present with complications is well made. On the other hand, a significant subgroup of patients without mucosal complications will benefit from surgical intervention. Chronic medication or severe lifestyle and dietary restrictions that are sometimes required to control symptoms of reflux cannot be considered ideal management. In this situation surgical therapy has been shown to be preferable with regard to long-term patient convenience and cost effectiveness.[24] Yet another group of patients in whom surgery is indicated are those presenting with predominantly respiratory symptoms that are most often caused by chronic aspiration of refluxed gastric contents. Antisecretory therapy in these patients will result in continued pulmonary damage from uncontrolled gastroesophageal reflux.[25]

Antireflux surgery is the only treatment that will correct the underlying defect—the mechanically defective lower esophageal sphincter (Fig. 9-2). There is increasing concern that medical therapy directed at reduction of gastric acid secretion may not prevent ongoing esophageal mucosal damage since reflux of gastric contents continues unabated even though the acid content is reduced. Although the acid may be the primary cause of heartburn, there is growing evidence that gastroesophageal reflux

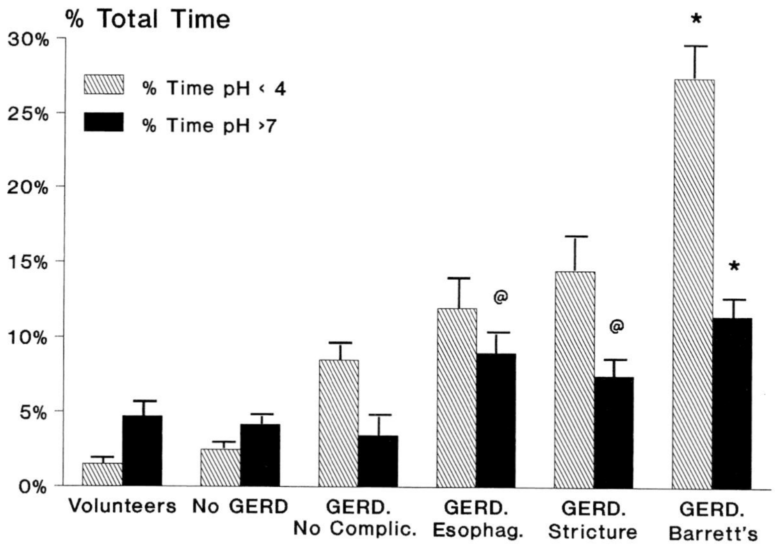

Fig. 9-3. Esophageal acid and alkaline exposure expressed as percent total time pH <4 and pH >7. * = $p < 0.01$ vs. patients with no complication; @ $p < 0.05$ vs. patients with no complications. (From Stein HJ, Barlow AP, DeMeester TR, et al. Complications of gastroesophageal reflux disease: Role of the lower esophageal sphincter, esophageal acid and acid/alkaline exposure, and duodenogastric reflux. Ann Surg 216:35, 1992.)

containing duodenal juice may cause serious esophageal mucosal damage. Bile has been noted to be present in the stomachs of patients with complicated Barrett's esophagus, and others have shown that bile, indeed, refluxes into the esophagus in this group of patients.[26-28] We have also shown that there is greater esophageal alkaline exposure in patients with complicated Barrett's esophagus (stricture, ulceration, or dysplasia) vs. noncomplicated Barrett's esophagus.[29] Our more recent work has also shown a linear correlation between the incidence of complications of gastroesophageal reflux and the degree of alkaline reflux (Fig. 9-3).[30]

A further concern is that the esophageal body function deteriorates with increasing severity of mucosal damage if reflux is not corrected (Fig. 9-4). Although peristalsis is somewhat improved by fundoplication, this is not the case if esophageal motor function has been significantly compromised (Fig. 9-5).[31] Since many patients with gastroesophageal reflux are not referred for surgery until late in the course of the disease, changes in esophageal body function further challenge a satisfactory surgical result. Early surgical intervention when properly indicated offers excellent symptomatic results, protects against the mucosal complications of reflux disease, and preserves normal body function.

To evaluate the success of antireflux surgery the results of 100 consecutive primary Nissen fundoplications performed for uncomplicated reflux disease over a 13-year period were assessed.[32] The actuarial success rate in controlling reflux symptoms was 91% at 10 years. From the patient's perspective, 90% were satisfied with the operation and 92% would undergo the operation again if the decision were to be made over.

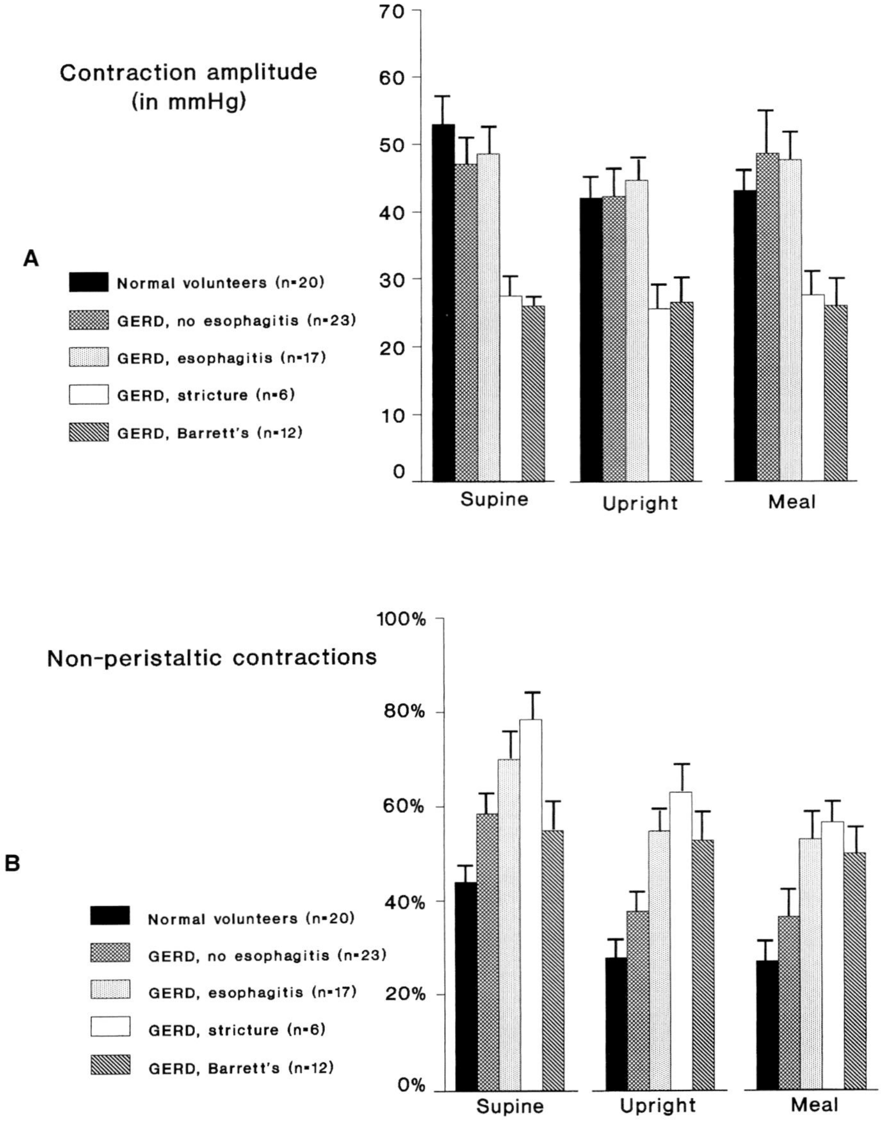

Fig. 9-4. Median contraction amplitude **(A)** and frequency of nonperistaltic contractions **(B)** on 24-hour ambulatory esophageal motility monitoring in patients with gastroesophageal reflux disease and various degrees of mucosal injury. (From Stein HJ, Eypasch EP, DeMeester TR, et al. Circadian esophageal motor function in patients with gastroesophageal reflux disease. Surgery 108:773, 1990.)

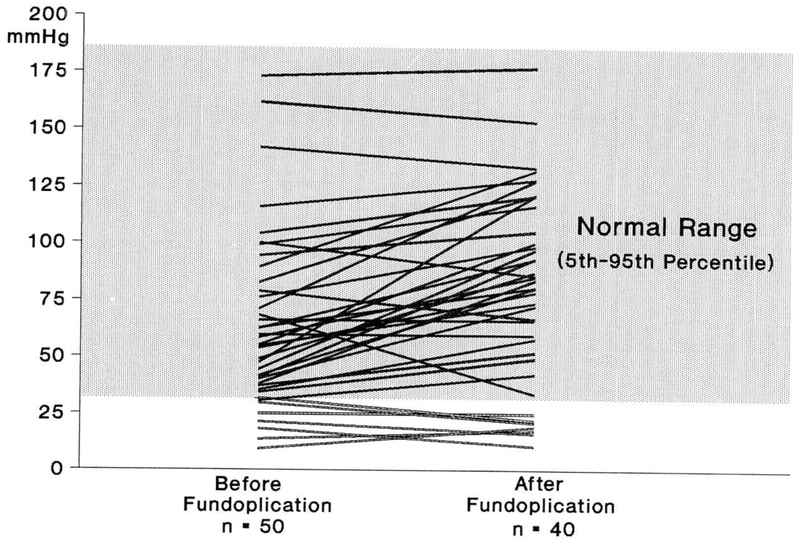

Fig. 9-5. Mean amplitude of contractions of the lower esophagus in patients before and after Nissen fundoplication. No improvement was noted in patients who had a preoperative mean contraction amplitude in the distal esophagus <35 mm Hg. (From Stein HJ, Bremner RM, Jamieson J, et al. Effect of Nissen fundoplication on esophageal motor function. Arch Surg 127:788, 1992. Copyright 1992, American Medical Association.)

PATIENT SELECTION FOR LAPAROSCOPIC NISSEN FUNDOPLICATION

The short-term success of laparoscopic Nissen fundoplication has been well documented.[33] Since the laparoscopic procedure is basically the same as the open procedure, the long-term results are expected to be comparable.

A laparoscopic approach can be used in most patients who are candidates for an antireflux procedure. As with laparoscopic cholecystectomy, many of the contraindications that were previously thought to be absolute are now seen by many to be relative. Contraindications to the laparoscopic antireflux procedure include those common to all laparoscopic procedures, such as previous upper abdominal surgery, severe obstructive pulmonary disease, a major bleeding disorder, and possibly pregnancy. Patients with severe coagulopathies or with portal hypertension may pose problems, and should surgery be indicated in these patients, it is probably a wiser course to use the open technique rather than have to convert the procedure later. Bleeding as a consequence of elevating and retracting the liver from the hiatus using the currently available liver fans or retractors can be problematic even in the absence of a bleeding diathesis.

Relatively little data are available on the long-term effects of laparoscopy on the fetus, although it appears that cholecystectomy can be safely performed up to the end of the second trimester. It would remain prudent, however, to delay a laparoscopic antireflux procedure until after childbirth, especially since the severity of reflux may lessen in the postpartum period.

Obesity was previously considered a relative contraindication to laparoscopy, but it has since been shown that laparoscopic cholecystectomy can be performed safely in all but extremely obese patients in whom the instruments may not be long enough to reach the area of dissection.[34] However, obesity may prove to be a relative indication for the laparoscopic approach since better exposure and visualization of the hiatal area can be achieved.

Some factors may be even more important when considering a laparoscopic antireflux repair. These include esophageal body motility, esophageal length, and a previous antireflux procedure.

Esophageal Body Motility

We have found that a global loss of motility of the esophageal body, that is, contraction amplitudes less than the 5th percentile of normal in the lower three fifths of the esophagus, precludes the performance of a full 360-degree fundoplication such as the Nissen procedure. In this situation complete fundoplication provides a relative outflow obstruction in the face of poor contractions and dysphagia is likely to result. For these patients we have suggested a partial fundoplication such as a Belsey Mark IV repair, which causes less of an obstruction but carries a slightly greater risk of postoperative reflux. Since the Belsey procedure is performed through the chest, the minimally invasive approach is more complex. Some centers are performing modified partial fundoplications or cardiopexies laparoscopically, but it remains to be seen whether these procedures can produce a good outcome in patients with poor motility.[35] Until further data are available, we believe the laparoscopic approach should be avoided if esophageal body motility is significantly compromised. This group of patients includes those with strictures since they usually have severely altered motility often associated with marked esophageal shortening and large hiatal hernias.[36]

The effects of a nonspecific motility disorder on the outcome of Nissen fundoplication have only recently been investigated. Evaluation of the results in an additional series of 100 patients who had a primary Nissen fundoplication for gastroesophageal reflux disease showed that good results are independent of the presence of a nonspecific motor abnormality, providing that patients with a motor disorder such as achalasia or diffuse esophageal spasm or a global loss of motor function are excluded[37] (Fig. 9-6). These results probably relate to the short, loose fundoplication that we perform. Since exactly the same repair can be achieved laparoscopically, we believe the same results can be expected with the laparoscopic approach.

Esophageal Length

It is well known that a short esophagus is often associated with gastroesophageal reflux disease, as in patients with stricture formation, a large hiatal hernia, or Barrett's esophagus, but it is also found in those with lesser degrees of disease. We recently compared esophageal length in patients with reflux disease of different severities with that in normal subjects using a nomogram that correlates patient height with esophageal length (Fig. 9-7). We found that the esophagus shortens in reflux disease even in the absence of mucosal damage, but the shortening is

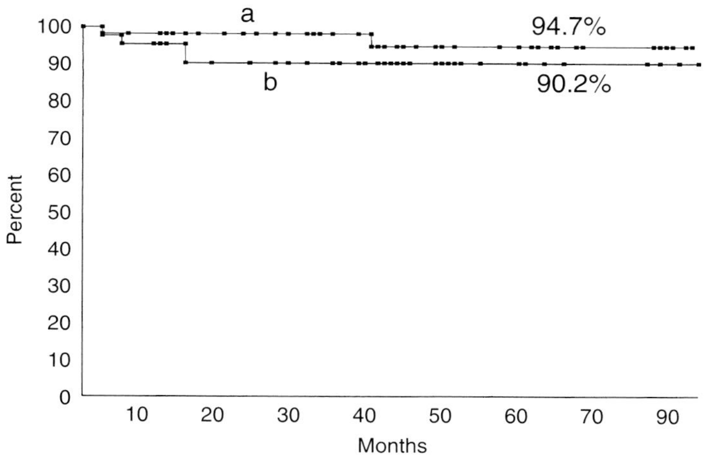

Fig. 9-6. Recurrence of heartburn or regurgitation over an 8-year period in 100 patients. There is no significant difference in outcome for patients with *(a)* and without *(b)* a nonspecific motor disorder of the esophageal body. (From Bremner RM, DeMeester TR, Crookes PF, et al. The effect of symptoms and nonspecific motility abnormalities on surgical therapy for gastroesophageal reflux disease. J Thorac Cardiovasc Surg [in press].)

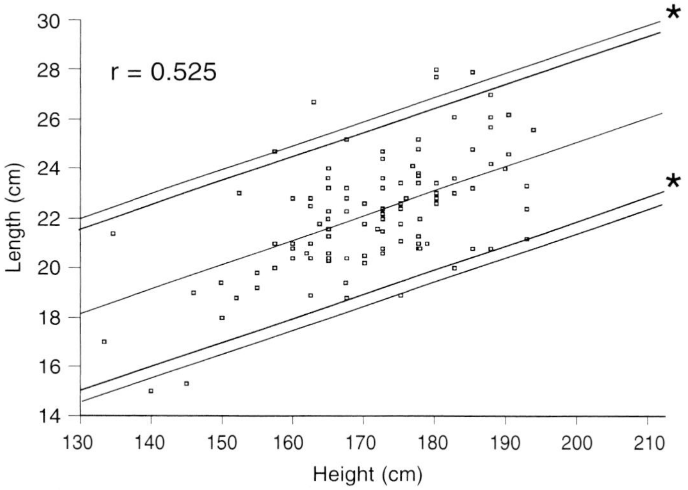

Fig. 9-7. Nomogram relating subject height to esophageal length based on manometric measurements in 111 normal volunteers. This nomogram enables more accurate detection of esophageal shortening in patients with gastroesophageal reflux disease prior to surgical therapy. Asterisks represent 90th and 95th percentile confidence intervals.

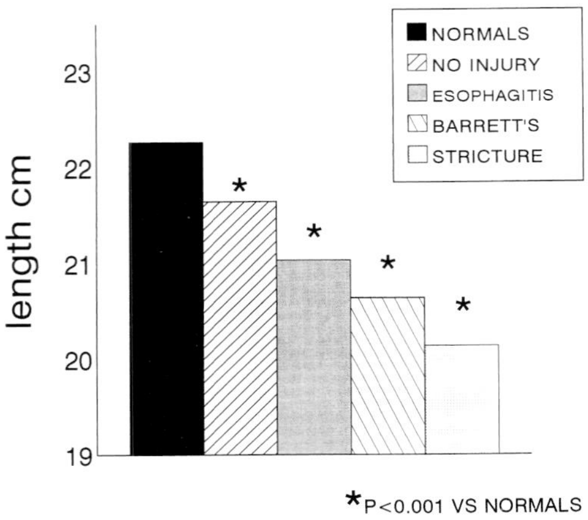

Fig. 9-8. Length of esophagus in patients with gastroesophageal reflux disease compared to normal subjects. Esophageal length progressively shortens as complications of the disease become more severe. Data from 24-hour pH monitoring and endoscopy in 172 patients, 74 with no mucosal injury, 42 with esophagitis, 25 with Barrett's esophagus, and 31 with stricture.

greater with increasing degrees of mucosal damage[38] (Fig. 9-8). In antireflux surgery a short esophagus makes it impossible to reduce the lower esophagus into the abdomen, an essential part of the operation. If the fundoplication is performed around the upper stomach, a so-called slipped Nissen fundoplication will result. Consequently, the success of the Nissen procedure depends on the ability to reduce the lower esophagus into the abdomen; this becomes more difficult when performed laparoscopically without the aid of the surgeon's fingers. Complete esophageal mobilization by the thoracic approach and an esophageal lengthening procedure such as the Collis gastroplasty for severe esophageal shortening are procedures that cannot yet be performed laparoscopically. How can we predict which patients will have an esophagus that is too short to be easily reduced laparoscopically? Usually a large hernia seen on a barium esophagogram that does not reduce spontaneously with the patient in the upright position predicts a difficult reduction of the hernia laparoscopically and a probable short esophagus. We also suggest that if the esophageal length, as measured manometrically, is below the 5th percentile of normal the laparoscopic approach be avoided. Furthermore, we encourage surgeons who are having difficulty reducing a hernia and the lower esophagus laparoscopically to convert to an open procedure.

Previous Surgery

Redo antireflux surgery generally yields poorer results than primary surgery.[39] This, as well as the scarring and adhesions that occur with esophageal and gastric surgery, precludes the laparoscopic approach to antireflux surgery. Although there is no evidence to support this as yet, it is generally agreed that redo surgery should be performed using the open approach. Whether laparoscopic redo surgery is prudent in patients who have had a primary open repair is as yet unknown, although it is obvious that this would be a far greater technical undertaking than operating on a virgin gastroesophageal junction. Nonetheless, as surgeons become more adept at laparoscopic techniques and as the instrumentation continues to improve, this too may become a possibility in the future.

PRINCIPLES OF SURGICAL THERAPY

The primary goal of antireflux surgery is to reestablish the competency of the cardia by mechanically improving its function while preserving the patient's ability to swallow normally, to relieve gaseous distention through belching, and to vomit when necessary. Regardless of the choice of procedure, this goal can be achieved if five principles in reconstructing the cardia are observed.

1. The operation should restore the pressure of the distal esophageal sphincter to a level twice the resting gastric pressure (i.e., 12 mm Hg for a gastric pressure of 6 mm Hg) and its length to at least 3 cm. This can be achieved by buttressing the distal esophagus with the fundus of the stomach. Preoperative and postoperative esophageal manometric measurements have shown that the resting sphincter pressure and the overall sphincter length can be surgically augmented and that the change in length is a function of the degree of gastric wrap around the esophagus.

2. An adequate length of the distal esophageal sphincter should be placed in the positive pressure environment of the abdomen so that its response to changes in intra-abdominal pressure is ensured. The permanent restoration of 1.5 to 2 cm of abdominal esophagus in a patient whose sphincter pressure has been augmented to twice the resting gastric pressure will maintain the competency of the cardia. All three of the popular antireflux procedures increase the length of the sphincter exposed to abdominal pressure by an average of 1 cm. However, when poorly performed, an operation may result in a reduction of length of the abdominal sphincter. Increasing the length of the sphincter will improve competency only if it can respond to the challenges of the intra-abdominal pressure. Thus creation of a conduit that will ensure the transmission of intra-abdominal pressure changes around the abdominal portion of the sphincter is essential to a successful surgical repair. The Nissen and Belsey fundoplications fulfill this goal.

3. The operation should allow the reconstructed cardia to relax on deglutition. In normal swallowing a vagally mediated relaxation of the distal esophageal sphincter and the gastric fundus occurs. The relaxation lasts for approximately 10 seconds and is followed by a rapid recovery to its former tonicity. To ensure relaxation of the sphincter only the fundus of the stomach should be used to buttress the sphincter since it is known to relax in concert with the sphincter[40]; the gastric wrap should be properly placed around the sphincter without incorporating a portion of the stomach or be placed around the stomach itself since the body of the stomach does not relax on swallowing; and the vagal nerves should be preserved intact during dissection of the thoracic esophagus.

4. The fundoplication should not increase the resistance of the relaxed sphincter to a level that exceeds the peristaltic power of the body of the esophagus. The resistance of the relaxed sphincter depends on the degree, length, and diameter of the gastric fundic wrap and on the variations in intra-abdominal pressure (Fig. 9-9). A 360-degree gastric wrap should be no longer than 2 cm and constructed over a 60 F bougie. This will ensure that the relaxed sphincter will have an adequate diameter with minimal resistance. This is not necessary when constructing a partial wrap.

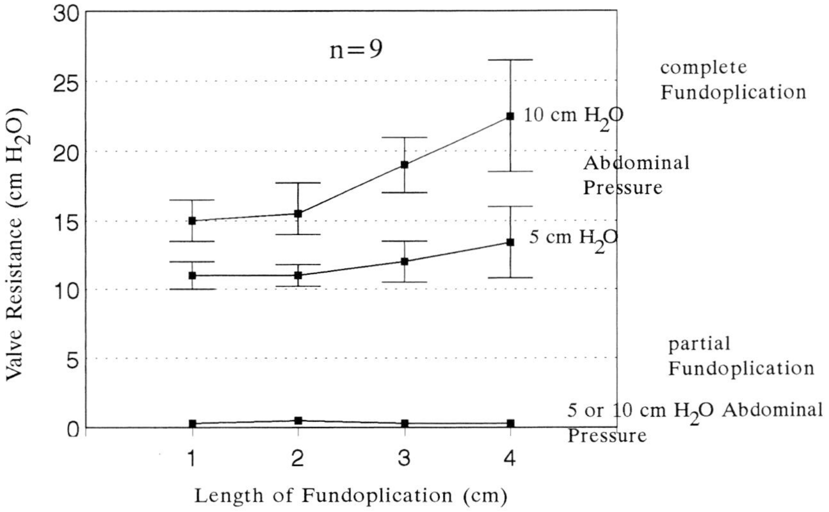

Fig. 9-9. Comparison of outflow resistance for various lengths of complete and partial fundoplications. Experiments were performed in vitro with fresh human esophagogastric specimens and controlled for either 5 or 10 cm of abdominal pressure. Values are expressed as mean ± SEM.

5. The operation should ensure that the fundoplication can be placed in the abdomen without undue tension and maintained there by approximating the crura of the diaphragm above the repair. Leaving the fundoplication in the thorax converts a sliding hernia into a paraesophageal hernia with all the complications associated with that condition.[41] Maintaining the repair in the abdomen under tension predisposes to an increased incidence of recurrence. This is observed in patients with stricture or Barrett's esophagus and is probably caused by an inflammatory process that shortens the esophagus. Lengthening the esophagus by gastroplasty and constructing a partial fundoplication will resolve this problem.

Complications of Increased Esophageal Exposure to Gastric Juice

Complications of gastroesophageal reflux result from the damage inflicted by gastric juice on the esophageal mucosa or respiratory epithelium and changes caused by their subsequent repair and fibrosis. Complications due to repetitive reflux include esophagitis, stricture, and Barrett's esophagus; repetitive aspiration results in progressive pulmonary fibrosis. The severity of complications is directly related to the prevalence of a mechanically defective sphincter. The occurrence of a mechanically defective sphincter in 42% of patients without complications suggests that this is a primary cause and not secondary to inflammation or tissue damage. A mechanically defective sphincter allows unrestricted reflux of gastric juice into the esophagus and overwhelms its normal clearance mechanisms. This leads to mucosal injury and progressive deterioration of esophageal contractility, particularly in patients with stricture and Barrett's esophagus, and regurgitation into the pharynx with aspiration.

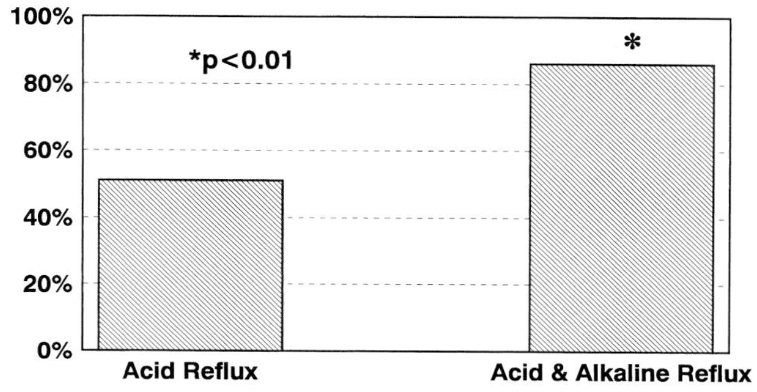

Fig. 9-10. Prevalence of complications in patients with gastroesophageal reflux disease who have only an acid or combined acid/alkaline component. (From Stein HJ, Barlow AP, DeMeester TR, et al. Complications of gastroesophageal reflux disease: Role of the lower esophageal sphincter, esophageal acid and acid/alkaline exposure, and duodenogastric reflux. Ann Surg 216:40, 1992.)

Composition of the Refluxate

The observation that complications of gastroesophageal reflux can occur in patients with a mechanically normal sphincter and that some patients with a mechanically defective sphincter are free of complications indicates that factors other than a mechanical defect such as the composition of the refluxed gastric juice are implicated in the development of complications. Refluxed acid gastric juice has generally been regarded as the primary damaging agent in gastroesophageal disease. Recent studies have shown that the presence and severity of reflux complications (i.e., stricture and Barrett's esophagus) are related to a mechanically defective sphincter and increased esophageal exposure to both acid and alkali.[42] Combined esophageal and gastric pH monitoring shows that the alkaline component results from excessive reflux of duodenal contents through the stomach and into the distal esophagus. The prevalence of complications of gastroesophageal reflux disease in patients with acid/alkaline reflux as compared with those with acid reflux only supports this observation (Fig. 9-10). In those with acid reflux only, complications are unusual if these patients have a mechanically normal sphincter and are somewhat more frequent if they have a mechanically defective sphincter. In contrast, complications are almost always present in patients who have a mechanically defective sphincter and an acid reflux with an alkaline component (Fig. 9-11). In addition to the prevalence of complications, the severity of the complications progressively increases in patients with a defective sphincter and acid/alkaline reflux. Patients with a normal lower esophageal sphincter and acid reflux were more likely to have esophagitis or no complications, whereas those with a mechanically defective sphincter and acid/alkaline reflux were more likely to have a stricture or Barrett's esophagus.

Our current understanding of the role that various ingredients in gastric juice play in the development of reflux complications is based on the elegant studies of Johnson and Harmon.[43] Hydrogen ion injury of the esophageal squamous mucosa occurs only at a pH of 2. In acid refluxate the enzyme pepsin appears to be the major injurious agent. Reflux of bile and pancreatic enzymes into the stomach can either protect or augment esophageal mucosal injury. For instance, the reflux of duodenal contents into the stomach may prevent the development of peptic esophagitis in a

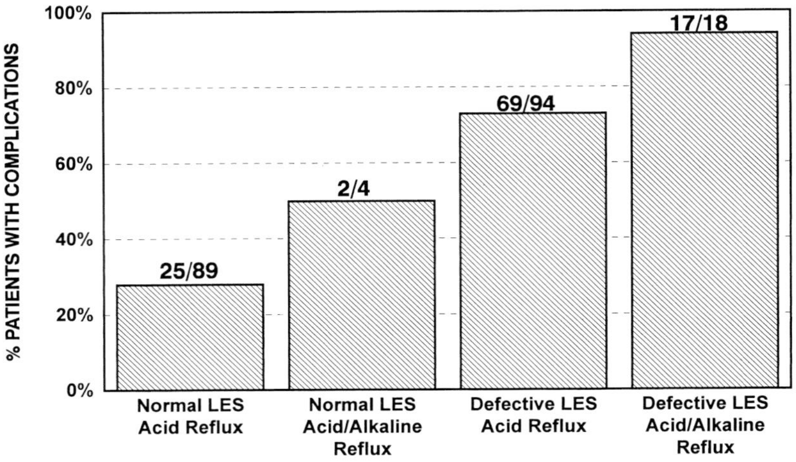

Fig. 9-11. Prevalence of complications in patients with gastroesophageal reflux disease who have acid or acid/alkaline reflux with or without a mechanically defective lower esophageal sphincter. * = $p < 0.01$ vs. patients with a lower esophageal sphincter; @ = $p < 0.05$ vs. patients with acid reflux and a defective lower esophageal sphincter.

patient whose gastric acid secretion content is predominantly acid because the bile salts attenuate the injurious effect of pepsin and the acid inactivates the trypsin. Such a patient would have bile-containing acid gastric juice that would irritate the esophageal mucosa when refluxed but would cause less esophagitis than if the acid gastric juice contained pepsin. In contrast, the reflux of duodenal contents into the stomach of a patient with limited gastric acid secretion can result in esophagitis since the intragastric alkaline environment would support optimal trypsin activity, and the soluble bile salts with a high pk_a would potentiate the enzyme effect. Hence duodenal/gastric reflux and the acid secretory capacity of the stomach interrelate by altering the pH and the enzymatic activity of the refluxed gastric juice to modulate the injurious effects of enzymes on the esophageal mucosa.[44]

Similarly, the disparity in injury, that is, mucosal barrier abnormalities caused by acid and bile alone as opposed to gross esophagitis caused by pepsin and trysin, explains the poor correlation between the symptom of heartburn and endoscopic esophagitis. The reflux of acid gastric juice contaminated with duodenal contents could break the esophageal mucosal barrier, irritate nerve endings in the papillae close to the luminal surface, and cause severe heartburn. Despite the presence of intense heartburn, the bile salts present can inhibit pepsin, the acid pH will inactivate trypsin, and the patient will have little or no gross evidence of esophagitis. In contrast, the patient who refluxes alkaline gastric juice may have minimal heartburn because of the absence of hydrogen ions in the refluxate but may show evidence of esophagitis on endoscopic examination because of the bile salt potentiation of trypsin activity on the esophageal mucosa. Gotley et al.[45] have performed aspiration studies that confirm the presence of conjugated bile acids in gastric aspirates after gastrectomy in patients with refractory reflux esophagitis. It is important to note that analysis also demonstrated the presence of trypsin in association with bile acids; the trypsin concentrations followed time patterns similar to those observed for bile acids. Consequently, changing the pH of refluxed duodenogastric juice from acid to

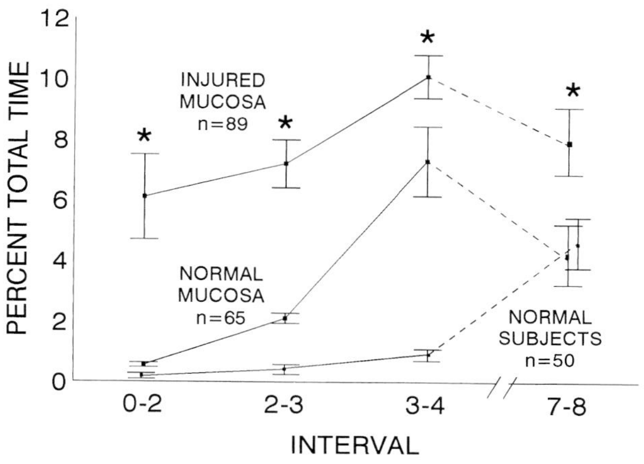

Fig. 9-12. Mean percent time of esophageal exposure to different pH intervals for normal subjects and patients with normal or injured mucosa. Normal values are included for reference. * = $p < 0.01$ vs. no injury. Data are expressed as mean ± SEM. (From Bremner RM, Crookes PF, DeMeester TR, et al. Concentration of refluxed acid and esophageal mucosal injury. Am J Surg 164:522, 1992.)

alkaline by the administration of H_2 blockers or proton pump inhibitors may intensify the mucosal injury while alleviating the symptom of heartburn. This is supported by recent clinical studies that indicate alkaline reflux is associated with the development of mucosal injury (Fig. 9-12).[30] This suggests that the combination of duodenogastric reflux and gastroesophageal relux may be more detrimental than gastroesophageal reflux alone.

Sequelae of Mucosal Injury

When the composition of the refluxed gastric juice is such that sustained or repetitive esophageal injury occurs, two sequelae can result. First, a luminal stricture can develop from submucosal and eventually intramural fibrosis. Second, Barrett's esophagus can develop by replacement of destroyed squamous mucosa with columnar epithelium.[46] The columnar epithelium is resistant to acid and is associated with the alleviation of heartburn. Endoscopy shows that changes attributable to Barrett's esophagus can be quiescent or associated with complications of esophagitis, stricture, Barrett's ulceration, and dysplasia. Clinical evidence suggests that the complications associated with Barrett's esophagus may be due to the continuous irritation caused by refluxed alkalinized duodenogastric juice.[29] Most important, metaplastic Barrett's epithelium may become dysplastic and progress to adenocarcinoma with an incidence predicted to be between 0.5% and 10% but is as yet unconfirmed.[47]

An esophageal stricture can be associated with severe esophagitis or Barrett's esophagus.[48] In the latter case it occurs at the site of maximal inflammatory injury (i.e., the columnar-squamous epithelial interface). As the columnar epithelium advances into the area of inflammation, the inflammation extends higher into the proximal esophagus and the site of the stricture moves progressively up the esophagus. In patients who have a stricture in the absence of Barrett's esophagus the presence of gastroesophageal reflux should be documented before the stricture is ascribed to reflux esophagitis. In patients with normal acid exposure the stricture may be attributed to drug-induced chemical injury resulting from lodgment of a capsule or tablet in the distal esophagus.[49] In such patients dilation usually corrects the symptom of dysphagia. Heartburn, which may have occurred only because of the chemical injury, need not be treated. Drug-induced injuries may also occur in patients who have underlying esophagitis and a distal esophageal stricture secondary to gastroesophageal reflux. In this situation a long stringlike stricture progressively develops as a result of repetitive caustic injury from capsule or tablet lodgment on top of an initial reflux stricture. These strictures are often resistant to dilation.

When the refluxed gastric juice is of sufficient quantity, it can reach the pharynx and potentially result in pharyngeal tracheal aspiration, causing symptoms of repetitive cough, choking, hoarseness, and recurrent pneumonia.[50] This is an often unrecognized complication of gastroesophageal reflux disease since either pulmonary or gastrointestinal symptoms may be predominant and the physician's attention may focus on one to the exclusion of the other. Clinical studies have identified three significant factors in these patients. First, the loss of respiratory epithelium secondary to the aspiration of gastric contents can take up to 7 days to recover and may give rise to a chronic cough between episodes of aspiration. If the patient is examined at this time, the cough may not be related to a reflux episode. Second, an esophageal motility disorder is observed in 75% of patients with reflux-induced aspiration and is believed to promote the aboral movement of the refluxate toward the pharynx. Finally, in patients with increased esophageal acid exposure the respiratory symptoms have a high probability of being caused by aspiration if the pH is below 4 for 3% of the time in the cervical esophagus.[51]

SURGICAL TREATMENT OF COMPLICATED GASTROESOPHAGEAL REFLUX DISEASE

Barrett's Esophagus

In 1950 Barrett described the condition in which the tubular esophagus is lined with columnar epithelium rather than squamous epithelium. He incorrectly believed it to be congenital in origin. We now know that this acquired abnormality occurs in 7% to 10% of patients with gastroesophageal reflux disease and represents the end stage of the natural history of this disease. It is distinctly different from the congenital condition in which islands of mature gastric columnar epithelium are found in the upper half of the esophagus.

In the spectrum of gastroesophageal reflux disease, Barrett's esophagus is characterized by a profound mechanical deficiency of the lower esophageal sphincter, severe impairment of esophageal body function, and marked esophageal acid exposure. Gastric hypersecretion occurs in 44% of patients.

The typical complications of Barrett's esophagus include ulceration of the columnar-lined segment, stricture formation, and a dysplasia cancer sequence. The ulceration is unlike the erosive ulceration of reflux esophagitis in that it more closely resembles peptic ulceration in the stomach or duodenum and has the same propensity to bleed, penetrate, or perforate. The strictures found in Barrett's esophagus occur at the squamous-columnar junction and are typically higher than peptic strictures in the absence of Barrett's esophagus. The risk of adenocarcinoma developing in Barrett's mucosa is variously estimated at 1 in 50 patient years to 1 in 400 patient

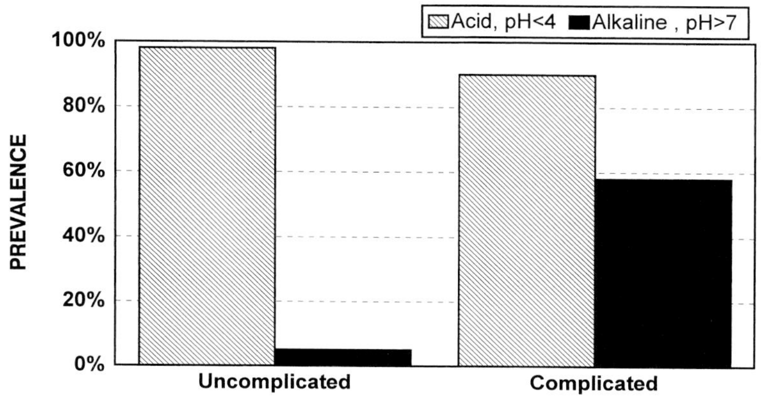

Fig. 9-13. Acid and alkaline exposure in patients with Barrett's esophagus with and without complications. Data are expressed as mean ± SEM. (From Attwood SE, DeMeester TR, Bremner CG, et al. Alkaline gastroesophageal reflux: Implications in the development of complications in Barrett's columnar-lined esophagus. Surgery 106:764, 1989.)

years, but even the most conservative estimates exceed the risk in the general population by 40 times. Most cases of adenocarcinoma of the esophagus occur in Barrett's esophagus. Conversely, approximately one third of the patients with Barrett's esophagus have a malignancy at the time of presentation.

The development of complications is related to the nature of the refluxed gastric juice, particularly when there is an alkaline component, because of excessive duodenogastric reflux (Fig. 9-13). Nearly 60% of patients with complications of Barrett's esophagus have abnormal esophageal alkaline exposure as compared with 6% of patients without complications. The columnar mucosal insensitivity resulting from repetitive injury may be important in progression of severe tissue damage without exacerbating the patient's symptoms.

The approach to the patient with suspected Barrett's esophagus starts with a barium roentgenogram and upper gastrointestinal endoscopy. The esophagram may show a hiatal hernia; if it fails to reduce when the patient is in the upright position, the esophagus may be shortened. A high esophageal stricture or a penetrating ulcer may also be demonstrated. Barrett's esophagus is recognized endoscopically by the appearance of gastric-type mucosa extending 2 cm or more into the tubular esophagus. Smaller segments of Barrett's mucosa have been discovered on biopsy and are prone to the same risks. The columnar mucosa may be in the form of a tongue rather than circumferential. The endoscopic diagnosis must be confirmed histologically. To avoid sampling errors we recommend at least two biopsies for every 1 cm interval along the length of Barrett's segment. The most important features are the presence of intestinalization of the mucosa and high- or low-grade dysplasia.

Patients at low risk for developing complications and those whose symptoms are readily controlled by medication are suitable candidates for medical therapy. H_2 blockers and omeprazole often bring symptomatic improvement, especially if hypersecretion of acid is the cause. Healing of ulcers and stabilization of strictures are not as reliably achieved. The value of prokinetic agents such as bethanechol or cisapride is usually minimal because of the loss of esophageal body function. However, it must be remembered that medical treatment does not correct the underlying defective sphincter and therefore does not reduce the reflux of alkalinized gastric juice or prevent aspiration. Indeed, the symptomatic relief may allow tissue damage to progress unnoticed. For this reason, surgery may be indicated earlier in the course of the disease.

In uncomplicated Barrett's esophagitis, esophageal body function can be diminished but patients are less frequently referred for surgery. Patients with complicated Barrett's esophagus are more often referred for surgery. In these patients esophageal damage dictates a modification of the operative strategy because of the shortened esophageal body, loss of peristaltic propulsive force, stricture formation, and large ulcers. A transthoracic approach is recommended for these patients so that the infra-aortic esophagus can be completely mobilized and a Collis gastroplasty can be performed if shortening of the esophagus persists despite full mobilization. It also enables the surgeon to deal more effectively with mediastinal inflammation secondary to a penetrating ulcer, which poses the risk of creating a full-thickness defect in the esophagus after mobilization. If this occurs, esophageal replacement is usually necessary.

In view of the fact that Barrett's esophagus is a premalignant condition, there is a strong theoretical rationale for reversing the underlying cause by performing antireflux surgery before a malignancy develops. The goal of antireflux surgery is not regression of Barrett's epithelium but rather to prevent progression of the disease. The few reports of regression of Barrett's epithelium after surgery may be an artefact related to surgical relocation of the esophagogastric junction. Despite the lack of regression, a growing body of evidence attests that fundoplication protects against dysplasia and invasive malignancy. Although in some cases cancer has developed after antireflux surgery, the absence of preexistent dysplasia or the efficacy of the particular operative procedure in reducing 24-hour esophageal acid exposure to normal levels has not been documented. Based on a long-term registry of patients with Barrett's epithelium who do not have dysplasia on entry, it was recently reported that dysplasia and cancer developed in 19.7% and 1.3%, respectively, of patients undergoing medical therapy.[52] In those who underwent fundoplication, dysplasia developed in 3.4% and none developed cancer. These data support surgery as a prophylactic measure in patients with a segment of Barrett's mucosa who are free of dysplasia. The effect of antireflux surgery on low-grade dysplasia is unknown. The situation is more clear cut when high-grade dysplasia is discovered on biopsy. If the diagnosis is confirmed by two knowlegeable pathologists, esophagectomy is recommended since 50% of such specimens exhibit evidence of early invasive carcinoma.

Stricture

A patient with a mechanically defective sphincter who develops a stricture while on acid suppression therapy is considered to be a treatment failure and a surgical antireflux procedure is indicated. Before the operation malignancy should be excluded and the stricture progessively dilated using up to a 60 F bougie. Three factors should be considered in the management of these patients: their response to dilation, assessment of the esophageal length by endoscopy or barium swallow, and the adequacy of esophageal contractility on motility studies. If dysphagia is relieved, the amplitude of esophageal contractions is satisfactory, and the length of the esophagus is adequate, a total fundoplication can be performed. In a patient with adequate esophageal length in whom dysphagia persists or esophageal contractility is compromised, a partial fundoplication is indicated. In either of these situations, if the esophagus is shortened by the disease process, gastroplasty and partial fundoplication should be performed. When esophageal acid exposure is normal in a patient with stricture, a drug-induced injury is the likely cause and dilation is often all that is necessary.

Atypical Reflux Symptoms

Chronic respiratory symptoms such as chronic cough, recurrent pneumonia, episodes of nocturnal choking, and waking up with gastric contents in the mouth or on the pillow may also indicate the need for surgical intervention. Chest roentgenograms in patients suffering from repetitive pulmonary aspiration secondary to gastroesophageal reflux often show signs of pleural thickening, bronchiectasis, and chronic interstitial pulmonary fibrosis. If 24-hour pH monitoring confirms the presence of increased esophageal acid exposure and manometry shows a mechanical defect of the lower esophageal sphincter and normal esophageal body motility, an antireflux procedure can be expected to produce good results. Usually, however, these patients have a nonspecific motor abnormality of the esophageal body that tends to propel the refluxed material toward the pharynx. In some patients the motor abnormality will disappear after a surgical antireflux procedure. In others the motor disorder will persist and contribute to postoperative aspiration of swallowed saliva and food. Consequently, the results of an antireflux procedure in patients with a motor disorder of the esophageal body are variable.

Chest pain is an atypical symptom of gastroesophageal reflux and is often confused with coronary artery disease. In 50% of the patients in whom a cardiac etiology has been excluded, increased esophageal acid exposure is the cause of the chest pain. An antireflux procedure will relieve the chest pain more consistently than medical therapy.

Dysphagia, regurgitation, and/or chest pain on eating when endoscopic and esophageal function studies are normal can be an indication for an antireflux procedure. These symptoms are usually related to a large paraesophageal hernia, an intrathoracic position of the stomach, or a small hiatal hernia with a narrow diaphragmatic hiatus. A Schatzki ring may be present in the latter case. All these conditions are easily identified on an upper gastrointestinal roentgenographic barium examination performed by a knowledgeable radiologist. These patients may not experience heartburn since the lower esophageal sphincter is usually normal and reflux of gastric acid into the esophagus does not occur. Surgical repair of the hernia usually includes an antireflux procedure since surgical dissection can destroy the competency of the cardia. If a Schatzki ring is identified in a patient with dysphagia, a hiatal hernia, or a normal size hiatus and normal esophageal acid exposure, dilation with a 60 F bougie is usually effective without the need for surgery.

Scleroderma

Gastroesophageal reflux in association with scleroderma poses special problems because of the complete absence of the lower esophageal sphincter and contractility in the distal esophagus. Intensive medical therapy is called for initially until symptoms of severe esophagitis can no longer be controlled. At that point a Belsey Mark IV partial fundoplication and gastroplasty will reduce esophageal acid exposure but will not return it to normal. Gastroplasty is necessary to correct the shortened esophagus that is a consequence of the disease. Excellent to good results are noted in approximately 50% of patients. If the esophagitis is severe or a previous antireflux procedure has failed, delayed gastric emptying is the probable cause. In these cases gastric resection with a Roux-en-Y esophagojejunostomy and a Hunt-Lawrence pouch is the best option.

Previous Gastric Surgery

A mechanically defective sphincter after vagotomy and gastric resection or pyloroplasty can permit reflux of gastric and pancreaticobiliary secretions into the esophagus, causing symptoms of regurgitation and pulmonary aspiration. Heartburn may also be present. Esophagitis can be seen on endoscopic exploration and is usually mild. Medical therapy designed to control both acid and alkaline reflux usually fails, and a bile-diverting procedure without reconstruction of the cardia is of little benefit in preventing the symptoms of aspiration and may contribute to delayed gastric emptying. If a resection has been performed, a simple antireflux procedure may prove difficult. Usually a gastric resection with a Roux-en-Y esophagojejunostomy and a Hunt-Lawrence pouch is required.

Reflux in Association With Esophageal Motor Disorders

Reflux esophagitis that persists after balloon dilation for achalasia despite medical therapy is an indication for early surgical intervention since esophagitis in the presence of a severe motility disorder progresses rapidly to stricture formation. The low outflow resistance of a Belsey Mark IV partial fundoplication is particularly suitable in these situations because the esophageal body has no propulsive activity. Once a stricture has developed under these conditions, esophageal resection and a colon interposition are usually necessary to reestablish alimentation.

REMEDIAL SURGERY FOR FAILED ANTIREFLUX REPAIRS

An antireflux procedure has failed if the patient is unable to swallow normally, experiences upper abdominal discomfort during and after meals, and has recurrence or persistence of reflux symptoms. Assessment of symptoms and selection of patients who need further surgery challenges the most experienced surgeon.[53-55] Functional assessment of patients who have recurrent, persistent, or new symptoms emerging after a primary repair is essential for identifying the cause of failure. A retrospective analysis of patients requiring reoperation showed that the most frequent cause of failure was placement of the wrap around the stomach.[39] Other causes include partial or complete breakdown of the wrap, herniation of the repair into the chest, and construction of a wrap that is too tight or too long. Attention to the technical details during construction of the primary procedure will avoid these failures in most instances. The importance of preoperative esophageal function tests is underscored by the fact that 10% of these patients had antireflux procedures for a misdiagnosed underlying esophageal motor disorder.

The preferred surgical approach in a patient who has a failed antireflux repair is a left thoracotomy using a peripheral circumferential incision in the diaphragm for simultaneous exposure of the upper abdomen and careful dissection of the previous repair from both the abdominal and thoracic sides of the diaphragm. Patients in whom heartburn and regurgitation recur but without dysphagia and who have good esophageal motility are most amenable to reoperation and can be expected to have an excellent outcome. If dysphagia is present, management is more difficult. Dysphagia occurring immediately after the repair usually indicates a technical failure, most commonly a misplaced fundoplication around the upper stomach, and can usually be corrected satisfactorily. When dysphagia is associated with poor motility and multiple previous repairs, esophageal resection and replacement should be seriously considered. Each redo surgery damages the esophagus further, jeopardizing the chance of preserving function. Blood supply is also reduced, and ischemic necrosis of the esophagus can occur after several mobilizations.

REFERENCES

1. Allison PR. Peptic ulcer of the esophagus. J Thorac Surg 15:308, 1946.
2. Allison PR. Reflux esophagitis, sliding hiatus hernia and the anatomy of repair. Surg Gynecol Obstet 92:419, 1951.
3. Allison PR. Hiatus hernia: A 20-year retrospective survey. Ann Surg 178:273, 1973.
4. Boerema I. Gastropexia anterior geniculata for sliding hiatus hernia and cardiospasm. J Int Coll Surg 29:533, 1958.
5. Nissen R. Gastropexy as the lone procedure in the surgical repair of hiatus hernia. Am J Surg 92:389, 1956.
6. Hill LD, Tobias JA. An effective operation for hiatal hernia: An eight-year appraisal. Ann Surg 166:681, 1967.
7. Baue AE, Belsey RHR. The treatment of sliding hiatus hernia and reflux esophagitis by the Mark IV technique. Surgery 62:396, 1967.
8. Nissen R. Eine einfache Operation zur Beeinflussung der Refluxoesophagitis. Schweiz Med Wochenschr 86:590, 1956.
9. Nissen R. Gastropexy and "fundoplication" in surgical treatment of hiatus hernia. Am J Dig Dis 6:954, 1961.
10. Negre JB. Hiatus hernia: Post-fundoplication symptoms: Do they restrict the success of Nissen fundoplication? Ann Surg 198:698, 1983.
11. DeMeester TR, Stein HJ. Gastroesophageal reflux disease. In Moody FG, Carey LC, Jones RS, et al., eds. The Surgical Treatment of Digestive Disease, 2nd ed. Chicago: Year Book, 1989, pp 65-108.
12. Costantini M, Crookes PF, Bremner RM, et al. Value of physiologic assessment of foregut symptoms in a surgical practice. Surgery 114:780, 1993.
13. DeMeester TR, Johnson LF, Joseph GJ, et al. Patterns of gastroesophageal reflux in health and disease. Ann Surg 184:459, 976.
14. Jamieson JR, Stein HJ, DeMeester TR, et al. Ambulatory 24-hour esophageal pH monitoring: Normal values, optimal thresholds, specificity, sensitivity, and reproducibility. Am J Gastroenterol 87:1102, 1992.
15. Wiener JG, Richter JE, Copper JB, et al The symptom index: A clinically important parameter of ambulatory 24-hour esophageal pH monitoring. Am J Gastroenterol 83:358, 1988.
16. Richter JE, Hewson EG, Sinclair JW, et al. Acid perfusion test and 24-hour esophageal pH monitoring with symptom index. Dig Dis Sci 36:565, 1991.
17. Bremner RM, Hoeft SF, Costantini M, et al. Pharyngeal swallowing: The major factor in clearance of esophageal reflux episodes. Ann Surg 218:364, 1993.
18. Zaninotto G, DeMeester TR, Schwizer W, et al. The lower esophageal sphincter in health and disease. Am J Surg 15S:104, 1988.
19. Bremner RM, DeMeester TR. Pre- and postoperative assessments in gastroesophageal reflux disease. In Scarpignato C, ed. Frontiers of Gastrointestinal Research, vol. 20. Clinical Investigation in Esophageal Disorders (in press).
20. Liebermann DA. Medical therapy for chronic reflux esophagitis: Long-term follow-up. Arch Intern Med 147:1717, 1987.

21. Brossard E, Mannier P, Ollyo JB, et al. Serious complications—stenosis, ulcer and Barrett's epithelium—developed in 21.5 % of adults with erosive reflux esophagitis. Gastroenterology 100:A36, 1991.
22. Lanspa SJ, Spechler SJ, DeMeester TR, et al. VA Cooperative Study Group No. 277. Incidence of stricture formation in patients with complicated gastroesophageal reflux disease (GERD). Gastroenterology 100:A107, 1991.
23. Spechler SJ, VA Cooperative Study Group No. 277. Comparison of medical and surgical therapy for complicated gastroesophageal reflux disease. New Engl J Med 326:786, 1992.
24. Fuchs KH, DeMeester TR. Cost-benefit analysis in the management of gastroesophageal reflux disease. In Siewert JR, Holscher AH, eds. Diseases of the Esophagus. New York: Springer-Verlag, 1987, pp 857-861.
25. DeMeester TR, Bonavina L, Iascone C. Chronic respiratory symptoms and occult gastroesophageal reflux. Ann Surg 211:337, 1990.
26. Bremner CG. The columnar-lined (Barrett's) esophagus. Surg Ann 9:103, 1977.
27. Bremner CG, Mason G. Bile in the oesophagus. Br J Surg 80:1374, 1993.
28. Gillen P, Keeling P, Byrne PJ, et al. Implication of duodenogastric reflux in the pathogenesis of Barrett's oesophagus. Br J Surg 75:540, 1988.
29. Attwood SEA, DeMeester TR, Bremner CG, et al. Alkaline gastroesophageal reflux: Implications in the development of complications in Barrett's columnar-lined lower esophagus. Surgery 106:764, 1989.
30. Stein HJ, Barlow AP, DeMeester TR, et al. Complications of gastroesophageal reflux disease: Role of the lower esophageal sphincter, esophageal acid and acid/alkaline exposure, and duodenogastric reflux. Ann Surg 216:35, 1992.
31. Stein HJ, Bremner RM, Jamieson J, et al. Effect of Nissen fundoplication on esophageal motor function. Arch Surg 127:788, 1992.
32. DeMeester TR, Bonavina L, Albertucci M. Nissen fundoplication for gastroesophageal reflux disease—evaluation of primary repair in 100 consecutive patients. Ann Surg 204:9, 1986.
33. Dallemagne B, Weerts JM, Jehaes C, et al. Laparoscopic Nissen fundoplication: Preliminary report. Surg Laparosc Endosc 1:138, 1991.
34. Schirmer BD, Dix J, Edge SB, et al. Laparoscopic cholecystectomy in the obese patient. Ann Surg 216:146, 1992.
35. Nathanson LK, Shimi S, Cuschieri A. Laparoscopic ligamentum teres (round ligament) cardiopexy. Br J Surg 78:947, 1991.
36. Bremner RM, DeMeester TR, Crookes PF, et al. The effect of symptoms and nonspecific motility abnormalities on surgical therapy for gastroesophageal reflux disease. J Thorac Cardiovasc Surg (in press).
37. Zaninotto G, DeMeester TR, Bremner CB, et al. Esophageal function in patients with reflux-induced strictures and its relevance to surgical treatment. Ann Thorac Surg 47:362, 1989.
38. Bremner RM, Crookes PF, Costantini M, et al. The relationship of esophageal length to hiatal hernia in gastroesophageal reflux disease (GERD). Gastroenterology 102:A45, 1992.
39. Collard JM, Kauer WKH, Peters JH, et al. Symptomatic, functional and anatomic assessment of failed antireflux procedures. Am J Surg (in press).
40. Lind JF, Duthie HL, Schlegal JR, et al. Motility of the gastric fundus. Am J Physiol 201:197,1961.
41. Richardson JD, Larson GM, Polk HC. Intrathoracic fundoplication for shortened esophagus: Treacherous solution to a challenging problem. Am J Surg 143:29, 1982.
42. Ollyo JB, Monnier P, Fontolliet C, et al. The natural history, prevalence and incidence of reflux esophagitis. Gullett 3(Suppl):3, 1993.
43. Johnson LF, Harmon JW. Experimental esophagitis in a rabbit model. J Clin Gastroenterol 8(Suppl):26, 1986.
44. Bremner RM, Crookes PF, DeMeester TR, et al. Concentration of refluxed acid and esophageal mucosal injury. Am J Surg 164:522, 1992.
45. Gotley DC, Ball DE, Ownen RW, et al. Evaluation and surgical correction of esophagitis after partial gastrectomy. Surgery 111:29, 1992.
46. DeMeester TR. Barrett's esophagus. Surgery 113:239, 1993.
47. Sarr MG, Hamilton SR, Marone GC, et al. Barrett's esophagus: Its prevalence and association with adenocarcinoma in patients with symptoms of gastroesophageal reflux. Am J Surg 149:187, 1985.

48. Zaninotta G, DeMeester TR, Bremner CG, et al. Esophageal function in patients with reflux-induced strictures and its relevance to surgical treatment. Ann Thorac Surg 47:362, 1989.
49. Bonavina L, DeMeester TR, McChesney L, et al. Drug-induced esophageal strictures. Ann Surg 206:173, 1987.
50. Pellegrini CA, DeMeester TR, Johnson LF, et al. Gastroesophageal reflux and pulmonary aspiration: Incidence, functional abnormality, and results of surgical therapy. Surgery 86:110, 1979.
51. Patti MG, Debas HT, Pellagrini CA. Clinical and functional characterization of high gastroesophageal reflux. Am J Surg 165:163, 1993.
52. McCallum RW, Polepalle S, Davenport K, et al. Role of antireflux surgery against achalasia in Barrett's esophagus. Gastroenterology 100:121, 1991.
53. Little AG, Ferguson MK, Skinner DB. Reoperation for failed antireflux operations. J Thorac Cardiovasc Surg 91:511, 1986.
54. Siewert JR, Isolauri J, Feussuer M. Reoperation following failed fundoplication. World J Surg 13:791, 1989.
55. Stirling MC, Orringer MB. Surgical treatment after the failed antireflux operation. J Thorac Cardiovasc Surg 92:667, 1986.

Chapter

10

Laparoscopic Nissen Fundoplication

Ronald A. Hinder, M.D., Ph.D. • Charles J. Filipi, M.D.

Gastroesophageal reflux disease is a common condition that can be easily controlled by self-medication. Most sufferers learn to modify their eating habits and use over-the-counter antacids to diminish symptoms. Forty-four percent of the U.S. population experiences heartburn at least once a month, and 18% of these regularly take some form of nonprescription medication for this problem. One tenth of the population experiences symptoms of gastroesophageal reflux at least once a week.[1] A large number of these patients will seek medical advice, making this the most common disease treated by gastroenterologists. Intermittent management with H_2 blockers or with the powerful acid suppressant omeprazole is effective in controlling symptoms in most patients.[2] However, there remain a significant number of patients who continue to have severe symptoms or who develop complications of the disease despite medical therapy. The complications include ulceration, stricture formation, Barrett's esophagus, and severe pulmonary symptoms. In these patients, antireflux surgery has been found to be of distinct benefit, allowing them to resume normal eating patterns and to enjoy a normal lifestyle without medication.[3] Surgeons who understand foregut physiology and are trained in the techniques of antireflux surgery are able to offer their patients an attractive alternative to lifelong symptoms or continuous medication. It is, however, the responsibility of the surgeon to ensure that patients are properly investigated prior to offering them surgical therapy so that appropriate therapy can be instituted.

SYMPTOMS

The most common symptom is heartburn, or pyrosis, of which more than half of patients with esophagitis complain.[4] It frequently occurs postprandially or at night. Occasionally it is reproduced by increasing intra-abdominal pressure by bending over or with exercise. Another common symptom is regurgitation, which is described as the effortless return of gastric contents into the pharynx or mouth. This should be differentiated from vomiting by the absence of nausea or forcible abdominal contractions. The sensation of dysphagia is frequently not accompanied by an esophageal stricture but may be produced by severe esophagitis or Barrett's esophagus. Some patients may have a problem initiating swallowing. The symptom of odynophagia is marked by painful swallowing that may occur with such complications as erosive esophagitis or a discrete ulcer. It is frequently associated with esophageal candidiasis, which may be secondary to a severe motor disorder of the esophageal body. Chest pain is a frequent symptom and should be differentiated from angina. This differentiation may require great clinical skill and a thorough cardiac investigation to be certain that the symptom is indeed esophageal in origin. Water brash as a result of excessive salivation is a well-recognized symptom. Reflux of acid into the lower esophagus may stimulate the production of saliva, which induces swallowing and aids in acid clearance.[5] Patients may complain of a feeling of something stuck in the throat, which is termed the globus sensation. Direct reflux of acid into the hypopharynx may lead to a sore throat and hoarseness. Occasionally aspiration may occur at night with nighttime cough, recurrent pneumonia, or unexplained fever.[6] This frequently occurs in the presence of systemic sclerosis, which is associated with poor esophageal body motility, preventing effective clearance of the refluxate. The onset of asthma in middle age is occasionally the result of gastroesophageal reflux disease. It is not always clear whether the symptoms are due to aspiration of esophageal contents into the trachea or to reflex bronchospasm resulting from vagal stimulation of the lower esophagus by the refluxate. Acid perfusion of the lower esophagus has been shown to result in reflex bronchial contraction.[7] Other symptoms that are often described in gastroesophageal reflux disease are abdominal bloating, early satiety, nausea, belching, and hiccoughs. The relationship of these symptoms to gastroesophageal reflux disease is obscure. It is possible that they may coexist as nonspecific dyspepsia rather than being directly related to gastroesophageal reflux disease. Rarely patients experience significant bleeding from ulcers in the diseased esophagus, but usually the bleeding is chronic and leads to iron deficiency anemia. It is important to exclude other lesions of the gastrointestinal tract before assuming reflux is the cause.

Relying on symptoms alone in the diagnosis of gastroesophageal reflux disease is dangerous and may lead to a misdiagnosis. It is essential that careful testing is carried out so that appropriate therapy can be instituted. Conditions such as systemic sclerosis, pill-induced stricture of the esophagus, duodenogastric reflux, or gastric conditions frequently masquerade as gastroesophageal reflux disease since the symptoms are similar. These patients will not be well served by Nissen fundoplication, and this accounts for many of the assumed failures of antireflux surgery. It is not the operation that has failed but rather the surgeon who has failed the patient in not obtaining the necessary physiologic information prior to embarking on surgical therapy.

DIAGNOSTIC AND PHYSIOLOGIC CONSIDERATIONS PRIOR TO ANTIREFLUX SURGERY

As other authors have stressed, the severity of gastroesophageal reflux disease cannot be assessed on the clinical history alone since other conditions may share the same symptoms and reflux patients may have severe disease with few symptoms. We underscore the importance of endoscopy with biopsies; a barium swallow, preferably with fluoroscopy; 24-hour esophageal pH studies; manometry of the esophageal body and lower esophageal sphincter; and occasionally gastric secretory or gastric emptying studies. Armed with this information surgeons can make the decision to operate on patients with a greater degree of certainty that gastroesophageal reflux will be effectively corrected. If esophageal body function is impaired, a partial fundoplication or "floppy" Nissen fundoplication must be considered. In those patients with gastric acid hypersecretion, particularly in the presence of peptic ulceration, a concomitant laparoscopic highly selective vagotomy may be indicated.

Recent reports show that the nature of the diet may not interfere with the results obtained with pH monitoring. Some argue that the diet should not be altered because the results would then not accurately reflect the patient's individual 24-hour pH profile and also because most reflux symptoms occur postprandially.[8,9] It has also been argued that smoking and alcohol should not be limited. The head of the bed should not be elevated, and patients are instructed to remain upright until retiring for the night. The testing period should exceed 18 hours.

Reasons for Increased Esophageal Exposure to Gastric Juice

The lower esophageal sphincter forms a barrier to acid reflux and should only open following a swallow. A defective sphincter is the cause of increased esophageal acid exposure in most patients with gastroesophageal reflux disease and the cause of a high rate of failed medical therapy.[10] Continual acid reflux eventually leads to esophageal injury and can result in permanent esophageal body dysmotility.[11]

The competence of the lower esophageal sphincter depends on the functional integrity of three factors: sphincter pressure, total sphincter length, and intra-abdominal length (i.e., that portion of the sphincter that will be exposed to increases in intra-abdominal pressure).[12-14] Although the most common cause of lower esophageal sphincter incompetence is inadequate pressure, the additional insult of having inadequate sphincter length, both the total or intra-abdominal component thereof, significantly increases the possibility of acid reflux.[10] The severity of esophagitis has been shown to be dependent on the number of defective components of the lower esophageal sphincter.[15]

The presence of a hiatal hernia appears to compromise sphincter function during dynamic stresses such as swallowing and abrupt increases in intra-abdominal pressure.[16] This is a reflection of the loss of intra-abdominal length in patients with hiatal hernia. Hiatal hernia also compromises esophageal acid clearance by impairing esophageal emptying.[17]

A second component central to the understanding of gastroesophageal reflux disease is acid clearance. Ineffective peristalsis in the esophageal body itself and as a consequence of esophageal injury due to acid reflux is an important factor in the development of the disease.[18] Progressive loss of lower esophageal sphincter function and esophageal body dysfunction not initiated by reflux disease may be related to neuromuscular disorders, metabolic disturbances, and especially collagen vascular diseases, of which scleroderma, mixed connective tissue disease, and dermatomyositis are the most common. Esophageal injury may result primarily from poor body function, especially in those with scleroderma. Furthermore, the finding of a short esophagus on manometry would be an indication for a transthoracic surgical approach, which allows for better mobilization of the esophagus (see Chapter 15).

Gastric acid hypersecretion may well be an important factor in gastroesophageal reflux disease, but its exact relationship is difficult to establish. In early studies in which varying criteria for reflux disease were used, gastric acid hypersecretion was shown to be prevalent in reflux patients.[19] The value of gastric acid analysis, however, appears to be in the evaluation of patients with high esophageal acid exposure and normal lower esophageal sphincter pressure. If these patients have gastric acid hypersecretion, they may be better served by a highly selective vagotomy combined with fundoplication.

LAPAROSCOPIC PROCEDURE

Indications

Most patients can be effectively treated with over-the-counter antacids, H_2 blockers, or omeprazole. However, a number of patients do not respond to medical therapy or develop complications such as stricture, ulceration, Barrett's esophagus, or pulmonary complications. Others may not wish to continue long-term medical therapy because of the inconvenience, cost, or fear of side effects of drugs such as omeprazole.

Surgery is strongly indicated in patients presenting with severe reflux esophagitis (grades 3 and 4). These patients are at high risk for developing further complications and require long-term therapy. Medical treatment fails in a high proportion of patients with severe reflux esophagitis, as has been demonstrated by Lieberman[20] and Spechler et al.[21] Mixed reflux episodes of acid or alkali are detected in many of these patients, making long-term acid blockade ineffective. Operative treatment is also advised in patients with low-grade reflux esophagitis (grades 1 and 2) with a mechanically defective sphincter. The latter predisposes to persistent reflux, as demonstrated by Zaninotto et al.[22] The response to long-term medical treatment (longer than a decade) is less than satisfactory under these conditions.[20]

Respiratory symptoms such as chronic laryngitis, pulmonary aspiration with recurrent pneumonia, and even asthma may respond to antireflux surgery. Only about 50% of these patients have a history of heartburn or show endoscopic evidence of reflux esophagitis.[23] The causal relationship between the pulmonary symptoms and gastroesophageal reflux can be confirmed by 24-hour pH monitoring. A positive 24-hour pH score with reflux-induced coughing, wheezing, or asthma attacks in addition to a mechanically incompetent sphincter represents a good indication for surgical intervention.

Patients without esophagitis should only be offered antireflux surgery if they have symptoms that severely affect their lifestyle. Patients with grade 0 to grade 2 reflux esophagitis who do not fulfill the preceding criteria on esophageal testing should be thoroughly investigated for other causes of their symptoms and are best treated medically initially. Patients with a large hiatal hernia presenting with severe dysphagia should be offered surgery regardless of whether reflux disease is present. Kaul et al.[24] have demonstrated that hiatal hernia may lead to dysphagia. The pathophysiologic basis is trapping of the herniated stomach by the diaphragmatic crura. The degree of dysphagia is directly proportional to the depth of diaphragmatic impression seen on contrast x-ray films. Patients with a paraesophageal hernia are seen occasionally. They usually have a normally positioned and well-functioning lower esophageal sphincter but may have symptoms of dysphagia, vomiting, gastric ulceration, or occult blood loss. These patients are well served by surgical therapy.

Barrett's esophagus is usually associated with a mechanically defective sphincter and evidence of acid or alkaline reflux warranting surgical therapy. It is not clear whether surgery will arrest the progression of Barrett's esophagus to malignancy. There are some reports of regression of Barrett's esophagus after antireflux surgery.[25,26]

Patients should be fully involved in the decision for surgical therapy since their cooperation is essential in the postoperative period. They should also be made aware of the risks of anesthesia and the surgical procedure.

Goals of Surgical Therapy

1. Reduce the hiatal hernia, which is present in approximately 50% of patients with gastroesophageal reflux disease
2. Fix the lower esophageal sphincter in the abdomen, allowing it to perform more satisfactorily under the positive intra-abdominal pressure
3. Narrow the crura to hold the lower esophageal sphincter and stomach in the abdomen and to act as a pinchcock on the lower esophagus
4. Lengthen the lower esophageal sphincter
5. Increase the lower esophageal sphincter resting pressure

These objectives must be met without producing undue obstruction to the forward passage of swallowed food.

Patient Preparation and Positioning

The laparoscopic procedure is carried out under general anesthesia with the patient in the lithotomy position. It is not necessary to place a urinary catheter in the bladder since this is an upper abdominal procedure. A nasogastric tube should be passed and the stomach aspirated of its contents. The lithotomy position allows the surgeon to stand between the legs of the patient and to comfortably address the upper abdomen without having to twist his body during the procedure. Assistants stand on the left and right of the patient. The operating table is placed in the steep reverse Trendelenburg position, allowing the stomach and other organs to fall away from the diaphragm so as to provide good access to the hiatus. This positioning also allows intra-abdominal fluid to drain from the hiatal area. Meticulous care is required to keep the blood loss to an absolute minimum.

Technique[27]

When a pneumoperitoneum has been established, two 10 mm ports are placed in the midline, the first 2 inches above the umbilicus and the other 1 inch below the xiphoid process (Fig. 10-1). The laparoscope is passed through the supraumbilical port. A third 10 mm port is placed in the left subcostal area in the midclavicular line. The upper midline and left subcostal ports are used by the surgeon in a two-handed approach to the esophageal hiatus. A fourth 10 mm port is placed in the right subcostal area to provide access for a liver retractor. A final 10 mm port is placed in the left lateral subcostal area to allow for downward traction of the stomach by the assistant and to elevate the esophagus off the posterior crura.

It is not usually necessary to detach the diaphragmatic connections of the left lobe of the liver. Hook electrocautery is used to elevate small amounts of tissue in the periesophageal area and to dissect the right crus of the diaphragm off the esophagus. This can best be achieved by first dividing the gastrohepatic omentum superior to

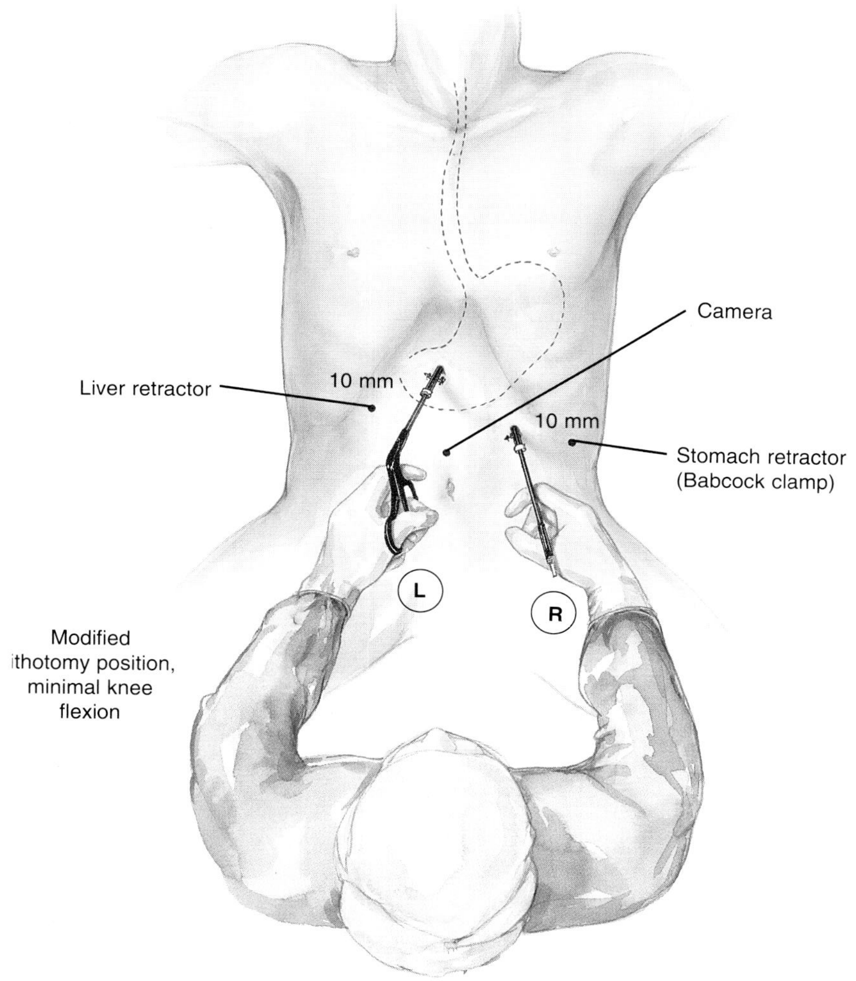

Fig. 10-1. Port positions for laparoscopic Nissen fundoplication.

the hepatic branches of the vagus nerve (Fig. 10-2). Care must be taken to identify and preserve an aberrant left hepatic artery in this area, which is found in 12% of cases. In most patients the esophagus can easily be identified to the left of the right crus and cleared of its connections to the hiatus (Fig. 10-3). The left, or anterior, vagus nerve is usually not identified and is left in contact with the esophagus. The left crus is then dissected off the esophagus. The esophagus is swept upward and to the left by using the side of a grasper passed through the left lateral port. This is an important maneuver that gives excellent access to the area behind the esophagus (Fig. 10-4). The right, or posterior, vagus nerve is identified and separated from the esophagus. It will be placed posterior to the crural repair and wrap. A window is created behind the esophagus in preparation for the fundoplication. Care must be taken to avoid damage to the pleura, esophagus, and stomach while dissecting in this area. The crura are approximated behind the esophagus using nonabsorbable sutures (Figs. 10-5 and 10-6). A size 58 to 60 F Maloney bougie is passed into the stomach by the anesthetist to ensure that the crura have not been approximated too closely and to calibrate the fundoplication. Attention is then focused on the greater curvature of the stomach where the short gastric vessels are divided for a distance of 10 to 15 cm from the angle of His (Fig. 10-7). This portion of the fundus of the stomach will be used for the

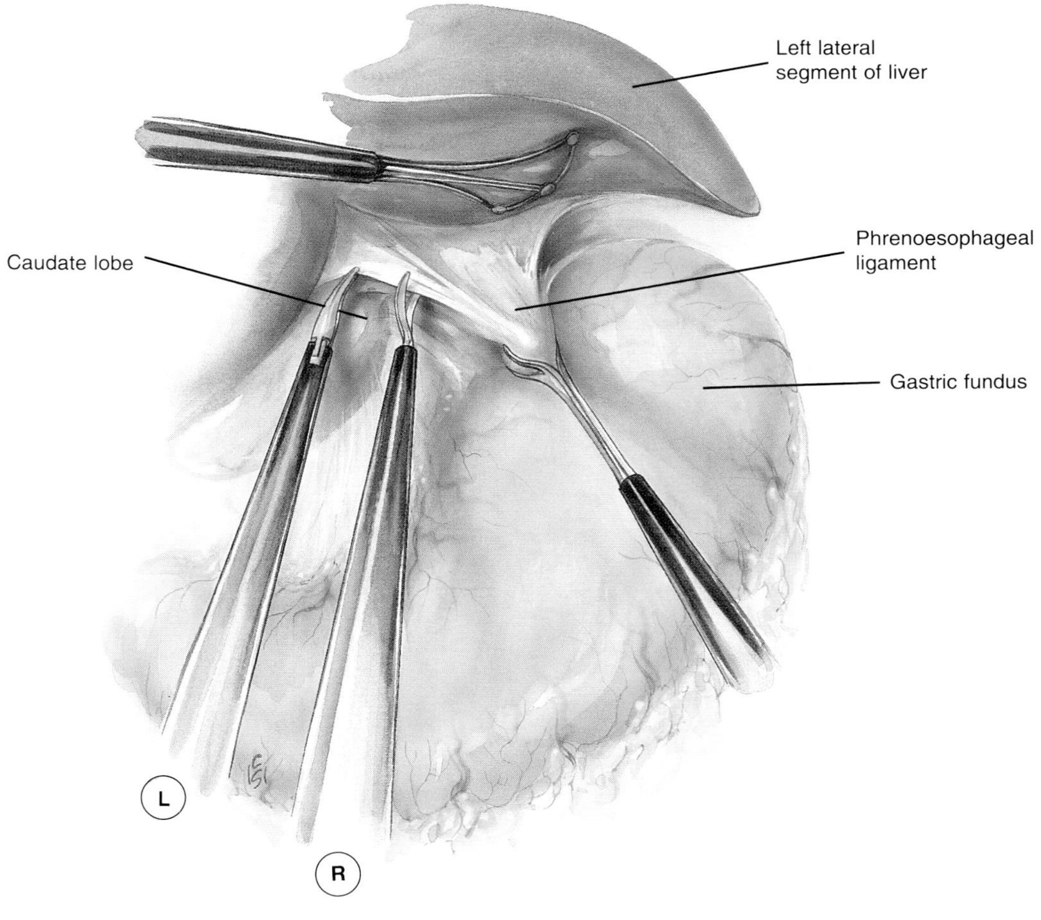

Fig. 10-2. Division of the gastrohepatic omentum.

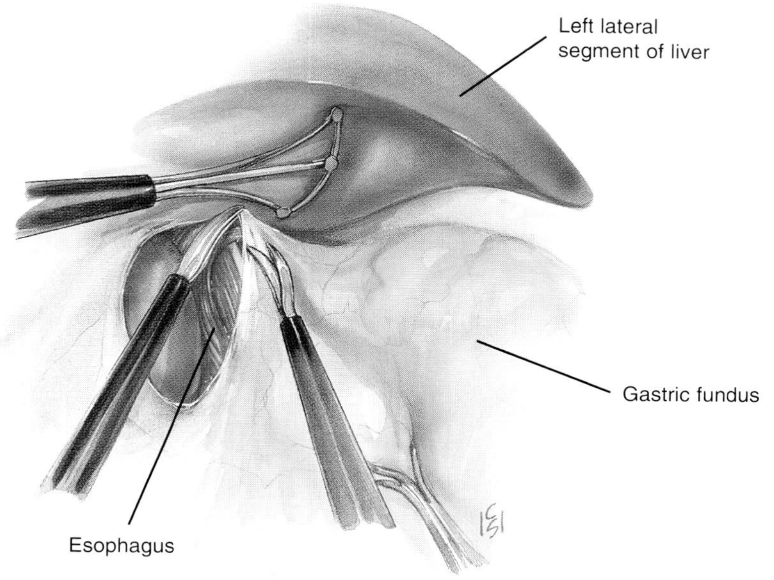

Fig. 10-3. Identification of the esophagus and right crus.

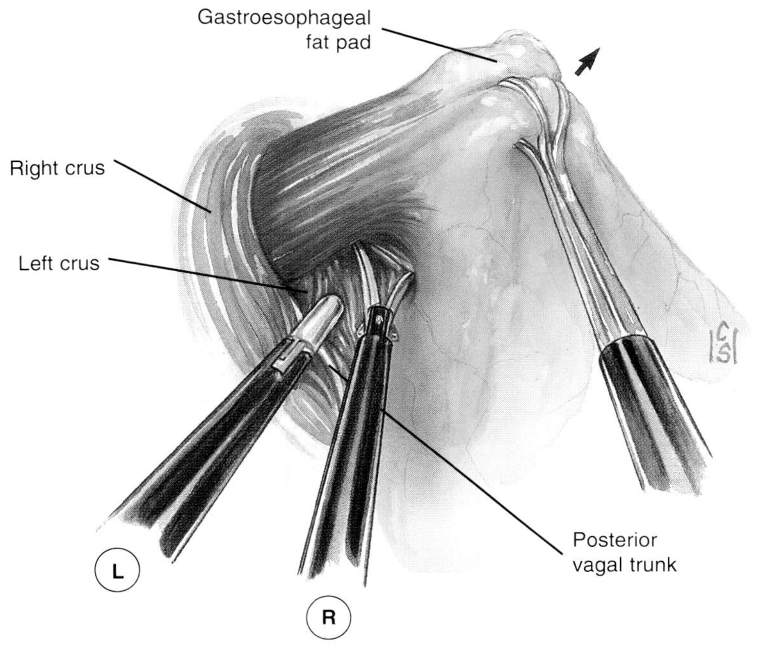

Fig. 10-4. Elevation of the esophagus off the crura and identification of the posterior vagus nerve.

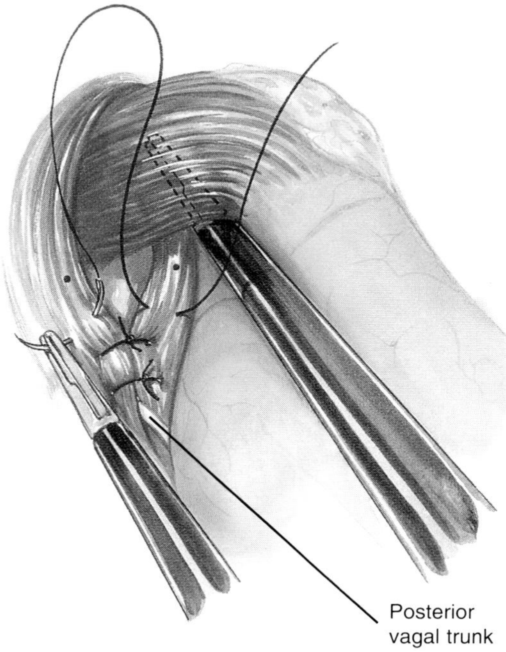

Fig. 10-5. Approximation of the crura.

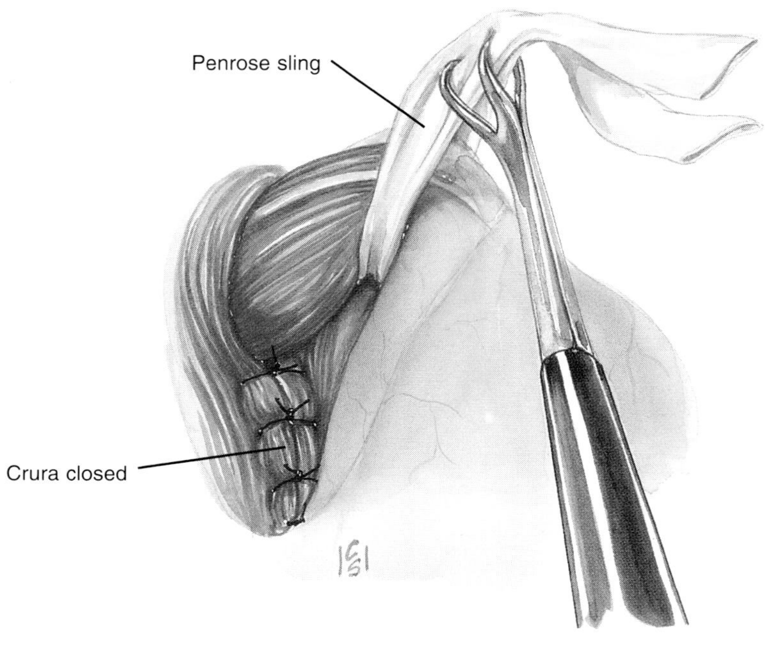

Fig. 10-6. A Penrose drain may be introduced to elevate the esophagus.

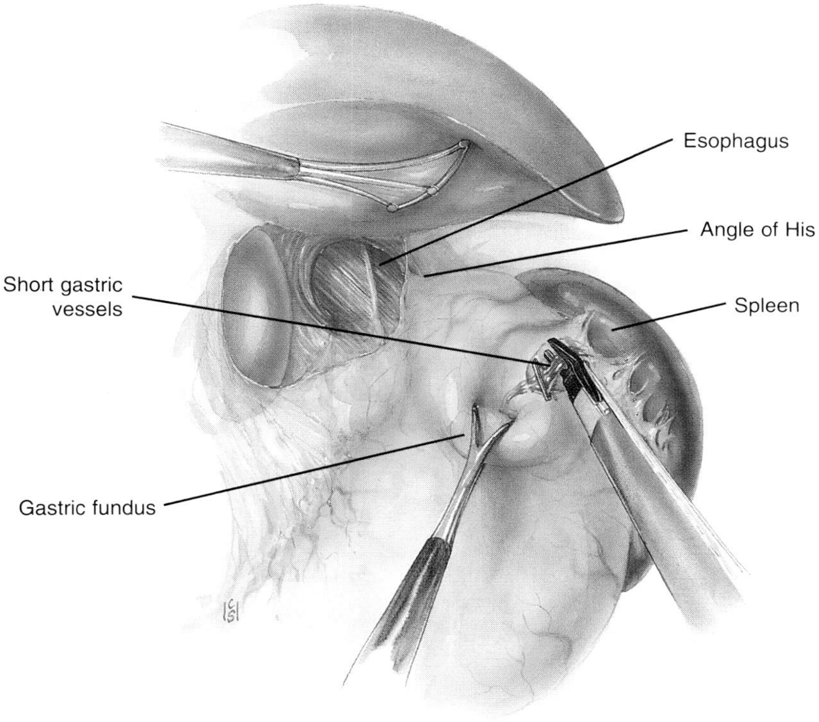

Fig. 10-7. Mobilization of the greater curvature and gastric fundus by dividing the short gastric vessels.

fundoplication. Care must be taken at this point to avoid damage to the spleen or stomach. The fundus of the stomach is brought around behind the esophagus and fixed with a horizontal U-stitch held by Teflon pledgets over the Maloney bougie within the esophagus (Figs. 10-8 to 10-11). The exact method of fixation of the fundoplication is the surgeon's choice.

Postoperative Care

No nasogastric tube is required and patients are encouraged to ambulate on the evening of surgery. The following day a Gastrografin swallow may be carried out to ensure that there is good passage of contrast material from the esophagus into the stomach and that there is no leakage at the surgical site. Patients are then allowed a liquid diet and are advanced to a soft diet on the following day. Many of the patients are discharged from the hospital on the second postoperative day. However, if there is any delay in advancing the diet or if additional postoperative concerns arise, we do not hesitate to keep the patient in the hospital.

Patients are encouraged to exercise frequently within the limits of their abdominal comfort and ability. They are instructed to eat cautiously and to avoid swallowing chunks of food such as solid meat or dry bread for the first 2 or 3 weeks after surgery since impaction in the lower esophagus occurs occasionally because of edema around the fundoplication. All medications are discontinued and a normal diet is resumed by the sixth postoperative week.

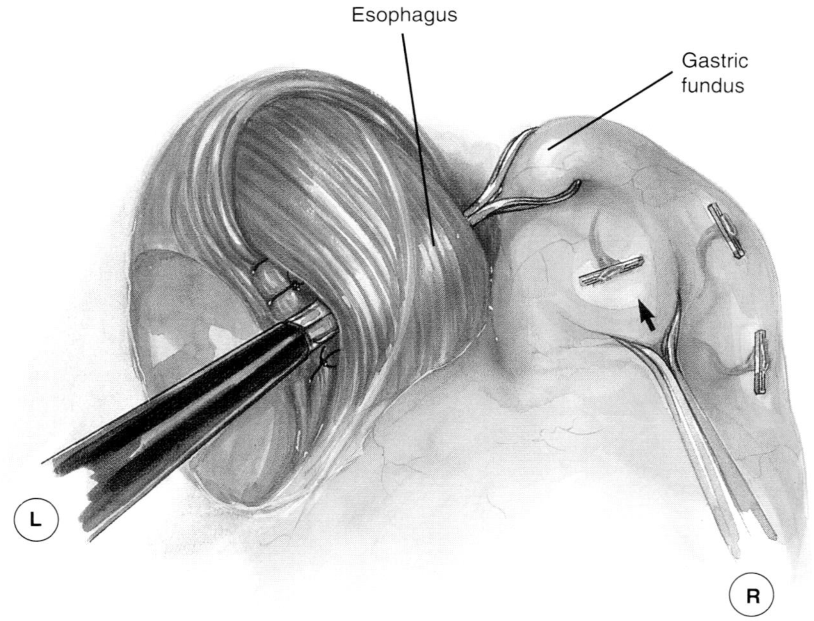

Fig. 10-8. Grasping of the fundus of the stomach.

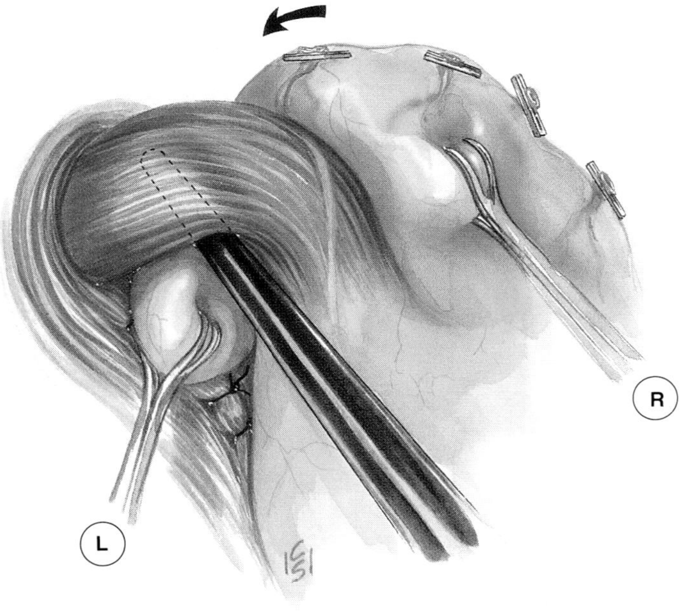

Fig. 10-9. The fundus is pulled behind the esophagus.

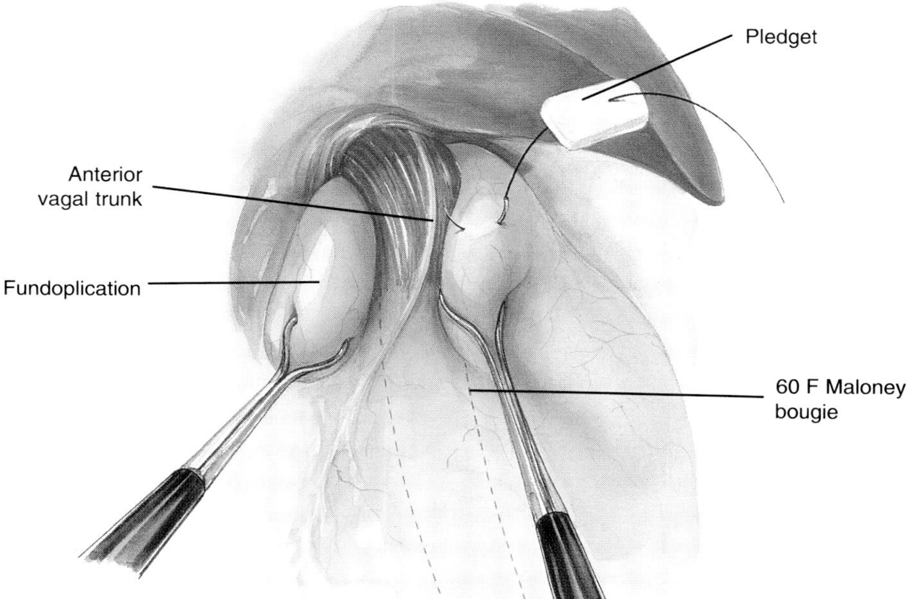

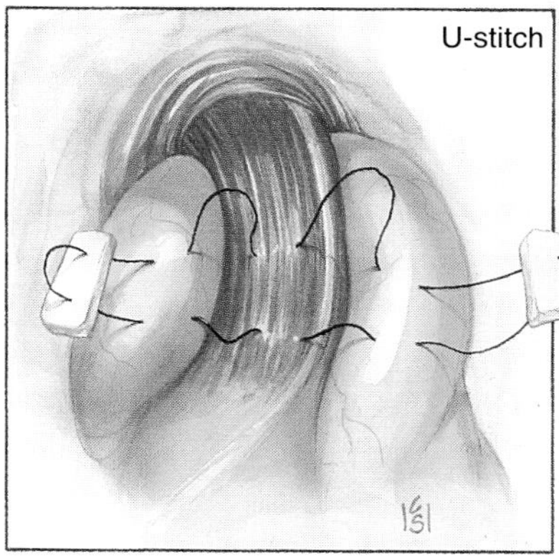

Fig. 10-10. Placement of U-stitch held with two Teflon pledgets. Size 58 to 60 F bougie in position in the esophagus.

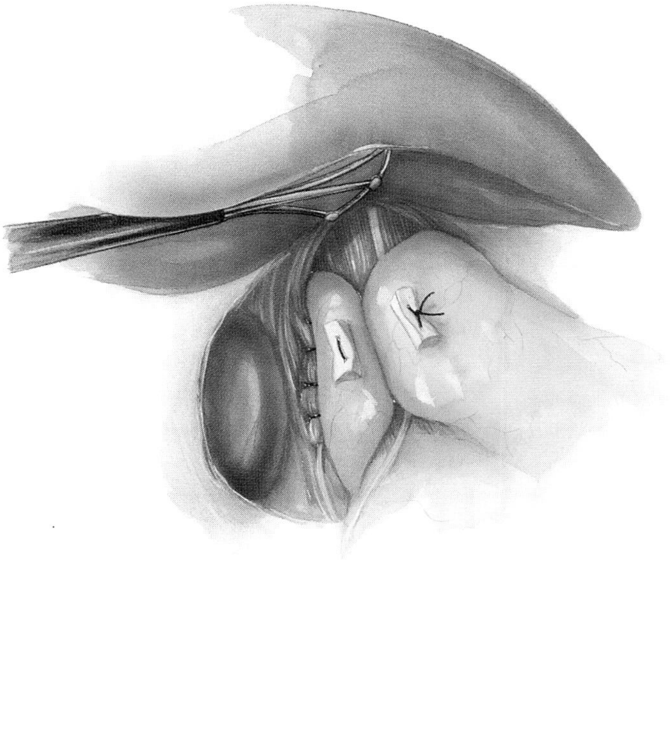

Fig. 10-11. Completed Nissen fundoplication.

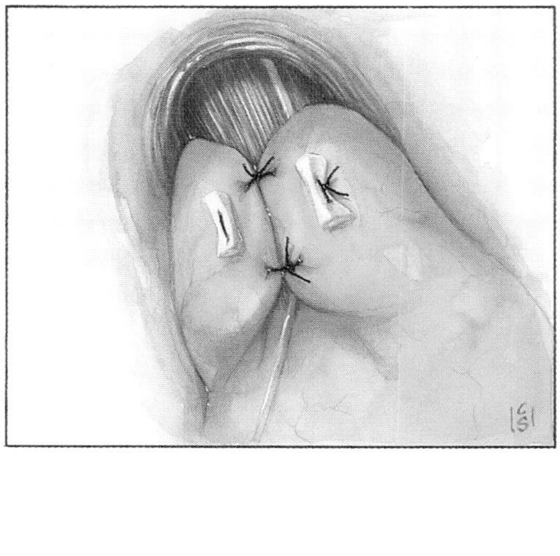

Results

In a collected series of 1141 patients followed for a period of 1 to 12 years after open fundoplication, good results were reported in 87%.[28] Seven percent had recurrence of reflux and 8% complained of dysphagia. Prolonged gas bloat was seen in 8%. The mortality rate in this combined series was 1%. Good results can be expected after Belsey, Hill, Nissen, or Angelchick procedures in 82% to 96% of patients. The recurrence of reflux in large series is less than 10% and the incidence of dysphagia is minimal. Patients are able to discontinue antacid medications and are able to eat a normal diet. The persistence of nausea, heartburn, regurgitation, dysphagia, chest pain, or epigastric pain after an antireflux procedure represents a poor outcome. The incidence of persistent dysphagia for longer than 30 days after surgery has been reported to be present in 0% to 21% of patients after Nissen fundoplication. By shortening the wrap to 1.5 cm this has been reduced to 3%.[28]

In some patients alkaline gastroesophageal reflux may be present. Fundoplication usually controls the esophageal reflux symptoms, but these patients may be left with severe duodenogastric reflux that causes significant abdominal symptoms and severe gastritis. A small proportion of these patients may have to be considered for subsequent surgical control of duodenogastric reflux by procedures such as the "duodenal switch."[29,30] Gastric ulceration has been reported after Nissen fundoplication. This may be caused by the dissection at the lesser curvature or by duodenogastric reflux.

In our first 150 patients treated by laparoscopic Nissen fundoplication, follow-up after 4 to 20 months has shown that 83% are symptom free and that 8% have mild dysphagia, 5% have some chest pain, 3% have occasional diarrhea, 2% have heartburn, and 2% have persistent asthma. One patient was found to have recurrence of gastroesophageal reflux. This patient had gastroenteritis in the early postoperative period with severe vomiting, which presumably disrupted the fundoplication. Another required reoperation for a stricture at the site of the fundoplication. These results are similar to those obtained after open fundoplication. The remaining patients have been satisfied with the results of the procedure. They had a shorter hospital stay and returned to work earlier and their symptoms have been controlled without the need for medication.

Blood loss is usually <50 ml and none of our patients have required intraoperative blood transfusion. The operative time required ranges from 1.5 to 3 hours. In 6 of our first 34 cases, conversion to an open procedure was precipitated by the inability to expose the anatomy to the surgeon's satisfaction, bleeding from a short gastric vessel, severe adhesions from previous operations, and perforation of the lower esophagus or stomach requiring immediate suturing. None of these led to untoward long-term complications. In only one patient in the following 130 cases was conversion to an open procedure required and this was because endoscopic access was limited by the presence of peritoneal adhesions from previous laparotomies. This indicates the lengthy "learning curve" of this procedure, but once mastered, the procedure can be safely completed by the laparoscopic route in almost all cases.

Complications

Early. Use of the laparoscopic technique has almost eliminated the need for nasogastric suction and allows for early ambulation followed by rapid discharge from the hospital. Patients with significant nausea or bloating occasionally may require a nasogastric tube. Because a large abdominal wound is avoided and the small bowel is disturbed less than during open surgery, laparoscopic Nissen fundoplication results in less ileus and a rapid return of bowel function. Forty percent of patients will have edema at the site of fundoplication that may obstruct the passage of solid food until the tissue swelling resolves. Whereas patients in the past have limited their food intake because of the prolonged ileus, this does not occur after laparoscopic surgery and may lead to symptoms of bloating and abdominal discomfort in the first weeks. The patient's focus is no longer on the abdominal wound but is now directed at intestinal symptoms. There is also a small incidence of diarrhea, chest pain, and early satiety. These symptoms usually disappear without the need for specific therapy.

Wound complications are rare after laparoscopic surgery. The occasional occurrence of infection constitutes no problem in these small wounds. In the early postoperative period an elevated temperature or white blood count should alert the surgeon to inadvertent bowel perforation at the time of surgery. Delayed perforation may potentially occur on the seventh or tenth day after surgery when the patient is at home. Other early complications include herniation at trocar sites in 1%, breakdown of the crural repair with herniation of the stomach into the chest in 1%, and the need for early esophageal dilatation in 3%.

Late. Most patients return to normal eating habits and can swallow normally and belch or vomit when necessary. As this procedure has only been performed for 3 years at the time of this writing, late complications beyond this length of follow-up are unknown. Because the procedure is carried out in exactly the same manner as open surgery, it is anticipated that the rate of late complications will be similar to that associated with open surgery.

CONCLUSION

Laparoscopic Nissen fundoplication is an excellent alternative to open fundoplication and offers the patient the same benefit via the minimal access route. As a final note, it is stressed that the procedure is technically demanding and should only be performed by a surgeon comfortable with advanced laparoscopic techniques.

REFERENCES

1. Thompson WG, Heaton KW. Heartburn and globus in apparently healthy people. J Can Med Assoc 126:46-48, 1982.
2. Klinkenberg-Knol EC, Jansen JM, Festen HP, Meuwissen SG, Lamers CB. Double-blind multicentre comparison of omeprazole and ranitidine in the treatment of reflux oesophagitis. Lancet 1:349-351, 1987.
3. DeMeester TR, Bonavina L, Albertucci M. Nissen fundoplication for gastroesophageal reflux disease. Evaluation of primary repair in 100 consecutive patients. Ann Surg 204:9-20, 1986.
4. Nebel OT, Fornes MF, Castell DO. Symptomatic gastroesophageal reflux: Incidence and precipitating factors. Dig Dis Sci 21:953-956, 1976.
5. Helm JF, Dodds WJ, Hogan WJ. Salivary response to esophageal acid in normal subjects and patients with reflux esophagitis. Gastroenterology 93:1393-1397, 1987.
6. Gonzalez ER, Castell DO. Respiratory complications of gastroesophageal reflux. Am Fam Physician 37:169-172, 1988.
7. Mansfield LE. Gastroesophageal reflux and respiratory disorders: A review. Ann Allergy 62:158-163, 1989.
8. DeCaestecker JS, Blackwell JN, Pryde A, Heading RC. Daytime gastroesophageal reflux is important in oesophagitis. Gut 28:519-526, 1987.

9. Shaker R, Helm JF, Dodd WJ, Hogan WJ. Revelations about ambulatory esophageal pH monitoring. Gastroenterology 94:421A, 1988.
10. Zaninotto G, DeMeester TR, Schwizer W, Johansson KE, Cheng SC. The lower esophageal sphincter in health and disease. Am J Surg 155:104-111, 1988.
11. Stein HJ, Eypasch EP, DeMeester TR, Smyrk TC, Attwood SE. Circadian esophageal motor function in patients with gastroesophageal reflux disease. Surgery 108:769-778, 1990.
12. DeMeester TR, Wernly JA, Bryant GH, Little AG, Skinner DB. Clinical and in vitro analysis as determinants of gastroesophageal competence: A study of the principles of antireflux surgery. Am J Surg 137:39-46, 1979.
13. O'Sullivan GC, DeMeester TR, Joelsson BE, Smith RB, Blough RR, Johnson LF, Skinner DB. The interaction of the lower esophageal sphincter pressure and length of sphincter in the abdomen as determinants of gastroesophageal competence. Am J Surg 143:40-47, 1982.
14. Bonavina L, Evander A, DeMeester TR, Walther B, Cheng SC, Palazo L, Concannon JL. Length of the distal esophageal sphincter and competency of the cardia. Am J Surg 151:25-34, 1986.
15. Rakic S, Stein HJ, DeMeester TR. Standard manometry of the esophageal body. What is normal? Unpublished data, 1990.
16. Sloan S, Rademaker AW, Kahrilas PJ. Determinants of gastroesophageal junction incompetence: Hiatal hernia, lower esophageal sphincter, or both? Ann Intern Med 117:977-982, 1992.
17. Sloan S, Kahrilas PJ. Impairment of esophageal emptying with hiatal hernia. Gastroenterology 100:596-605, 1991.
18. Joelsson BE, DeMeester TR, Skinner DB, LaFontaine E, Waters PF, O'Sullivan GC. The role of the esophageal body in the antireflux mechanism. Surgery 92:417-424, 1982.
19. Winkelstein A, Wolf BS, Som ML, Marshak RH. Peptic esophagitis with duodenal or gastric ulcer. JAMA 154:885-889, 1954.
20. Lieberman DA. Medical therapy for chronic reflux esophagitis: Long-term follow-up. Arch Intern Med 147:1717-1720, 1987.
21. Spechler SJ and the Department of Veterans Affairs Gastroesophageal Reflux Disease Study Group. Comparison of medical and surgical therapy for complicated gastroesophageal reflux disease in veterans. N Engl J Med 326:786-792, 1992.
22. Zaninotto G, DiMario F, Costantini M, Baffa R, Germana B, Dal Santo PL, Rugge M, Bolzan M, Naccarato R, Ancona E. Oesophagitis and pH of refluxate: An experimental and clinical study. Br J Surg 79:161-164, 1992.
23. Pellegrini CA, DeMeester TR, Johnson LF, Skinner DB. Gastroesophageal reflux and pulmonary aspiration: Incidence, functional abnormality, and results of surgical therapy. Surgery 86:110-119, 1979.
24. Kaul BK, DeMeester TR, Oka M, Ball CS, Stein HJ, Kim CB, Cheng SC. The cause of dysphagia in uncomplicated sliding hiatal hernia and its relief by hiatal herniorrhaphy: A roentgenographic, manometric, and clinical study. Ann Surg 211:406-410, 1990.
25. Williamson WA, Ellis FH, Gibb SP, Shahian DM, Aretz HT. Effect of antireflux operation on Barrett's mucosa. Ann Thorac Surg 49:537-542, 1990.
26. Brand DL, Ylvisaker JT, Gelfand M, Pope CE. Regression of columnar esophageal (Barrett's) epithelium after anti-reflux surgery. N Engl J Med 302:844-848, 1980.
27. Hinder RA, Filipi CJ. The technique of laparoscopic Nissen fundoplication. Surg Laparosc Endosc 2:265-272, 1992.
28. Stein HJ, DeMeester TR, Hinder RA. Outpatient physiologic testing and surgical management of foregut motility disorders. Curr Probl Surg 29:415-555, 1992.
29. DeMeester TR, Fuchs KH, Ball CS, Albertucci M, Smyrk TC, Marcus JN. Experimental and clinical results with proximal end-to-end duodenojejunostomy for pathologic duodenogastric reflux. Ann Surg 206:414-426, 1987.
30. Hinder RA. The duodenal switch—a new form of pancreatic-biliary diversion. Surg Clin North Am 72:487-500, 1992.

Chapter

11

Laparoscopic Partial Fundoplication

Lee L. Swanström, M.D. • John G. Hunter, M.D.

In 1956 Nissen first reported his technique of 360-degree plication of the gastric fundus around the lower esophagus.[1] After decades of careful clinical follow-up and prospective studies, Nissen fundoplication has become the operation of choice for preventing gastroesophageal reflux. The revolution in minimally invasive surgery has recently encompassed Nissen's procedure, leading to renewed interest on the part of surgeons and gastroenterologists in the laparoscopic treatment of gastroesophageal reflux disease. Early reports of good results coupled with a dramatic decrease in the length of the hospital stay and enthusiastic acceptance by the public have encouraged surgeons to learn this new technique.

As with most common diseases, gastroesophageal reflux has a broad spectrum of clinical presentations and cannot be adequately treated with a single operation.[2] In some circumstances a procedure other than Nissen fundoplication is warranted.

In patients with esophageal motility disorders, severely diminished contractility of the esophageal body, and extreme aerophagia or in those who have undergone cardiomyotomy for achalasia, the augmentation of the lower esophageal sphincter achieved with a Nissen fundoplication may potentially produce more adverse side effects or disability than is acceptable. In these clinical situations partial fundoplication has been advocated as the treatment of choice.[3] Because laparoscopic antireflux procedures mimic open antireflux procedures, the indications for partial fundoplication performed laparoscopically are the same as those for partial fundoplication through a laparotomy incision.

INDICATIONS

The classic indication for the use of partial fundoplication has been the treatment of gastroesophageal reflux disease in patients with esophageal motility disorders.[4] Esophageal dysmotility is a continuum ranging from weak esophageal body contractility (primary wave amplitudes of <30 mm Hg), uncoordinated peristalsis following swallowing, or true aperistalsis as seen in achalasia to end-stage connective tissue diseases (e.g., scleroderma) or occasionally advanced esophagitis from chronic gastroesophageal reflux disease. For such patients, increases in lower esophageal sphincter pressure via total fundoplication can create too much resistance to food passage for the weak esophageal pump mechanism and result in mild to profound dysphagia.[5]

Current Indications for Partial Fundoplication

Physiologic

1. Achalasia
2. Disordered motility
   a. Esophageal spasm
3. Decreased contractility
   a. Connective tissue diseases, scleroderma
   b. Long-standing gastroesophageal disease
4. Aerophagia

Anatomic

1. "Tubular" stomach
2. Gastric fibrosis (e.g., reoperative fundoplication)
3. Gastrosplenic adhesions

The most extreme example of an esophageal motility disorder is achalasia. This disorder is characterized by aperistalsis of the body of the esophagus and a hypertensive, nonrelaxing lower esophageal sphincter. The most effective albeit palliative treatment of this disease is division of the hypertensive lower esophageal sphincter (cardiomyotomy or Heller myotomy). Long-term relief of achalasia with this procedure has been shown to be superior to balloon dilatation.[6] Unfortunately, symptomatic gastroesophageal reflux following this procedure on average occurs in 12% of patients.[7] For this reason, some recommend that cardiomyotomy be accompanied by an antireflux procedure. As mentioned previously, Nissen fundoplication is probably contraindicated in this disease. On the other hand, partial fundoplications are well tolerated in this setting, causing little dysphagia and providing an effective defense against gastroesophageal reflux.[8,9]

Another subset of reflux patients are those whose disease is linked to profound aerophagia and abdominal bloating. Considering the difficulty or inability to belch following Nissen fundoplication, some have advised the use of partial fundoplication to avoid gas bloat in aerophagic patients.[3]

The most frequent indication for partial fundoplication is diminished esophageal body contractility not associated with a primary esophageal motor disorder (e.g., achalasia or diffuse esophageal spasm). Diminished contractility (esophageal body contraction amplitude <30 mm Hg) is often a result of severe gastroesophageal reflux and usually responds well to antireflux surgery. Unfortunately, it is difficult to identify preoperatively those in whom dysmotility will be relieved, and it is therefore risky to perform total fundoplication in these patients.

Although diminished esophageal contractility may be the most frequent indication for partial fundoplication in the United States, in Europe partial fundoplication has been advocated by some as the procedure of choice for all patients with gastroesophageal reflux disease to diminish the not-infrequent postoperative side effects of the 360-degree wrap. In fact, in several series of typical patients with gastroesophageal reflux, less postoperative dysphagia, gas bloat, and "slippage" were found when partial fundoplication was compared with total fundoplication.[10-12]

An additional element of theoretical appeal, especially when considering laparoscopic applications, is that less mobilization of the gastric fundus is required to perform a partial fundoplication than a total fundoplication. This may be important for the patient whose stomach is "tubular" as well as for patients with extremely short gastric vessels or gastrosplenic adhesions who may require extensive gastric mobilization for a 360-degree wrap.

TYPES OF REPAIRS

Several types of partial fundoplications have been described. All repairs, however, have certain physiologic features in common. Of primary importance is the fact that a portion of the lower esophagus above the gastroesophageal junction remains uncovered and is therefore exposed only to intra-abdominal pressure without any further augmentation of intragastric pressure. The percentage of unwrapped esophagus, however, is probably important in determining the strength of the antireflux barrier. By decreasing the amount of gastric fundic pressure on the dysfunctional lower esophageal sphincter zone, less augmentation of lower esophageal sphincter pressure is created as compared with Nissen fundoplication.[13,14] Although a lower resting pressure of the "neo-lower esophageal sphincter" is created by partial than by total fundoplication, care must to be taken not to make these partial wraps too long. Excessively long wraps could potentially increase the overall resistance to both reflux and swallowing as much as a typical short, floppy Nissen fundoplication.[15]

Partial fundoplications seem to create a different one-way valve configuration at the gastroesophageal junction as compared with Nissen fundoplication. These fundoplications may create a more physiologic flap valve than the Nissen nipple valve. This anatomic difference has been postulated to explain the diminished dysphagia and gas-bloat symptoms seen after partial fundoplication.[10] Whatever the reason, it has been demonstrated that partial fundoplication does indeed provide a competent lower esophageal sphincter and effectively prevents gastroesophageal reflux.

Numerous types of partial fundoplications have been described. These can be divided into the following three categories: a transthoracic partial wrap, a posterior gastric wrap, and an anterior gastric wrap. Each procedure has its advocates, with the individual bias depending on the surgeon's training and geographic location.

Transthoracic partial fundoplication is by far the most commonly performed type of partial fundoplication in the United States, perhaps because of the close association between thoracic and esophageal surgeons in this country. This repair is typified by the Belsey Mark IV procedure initially described in 1967 by Skinner and Belsey.[16] This repair is essentially an anterior partial wrap secured with U-stitches to the anterior two thirds of the esophagus. The fundoplication is accomplished via a left thoracotomy and the dissection and wrap are performed in the chest. After the repair the gastroesophageal junction is replaced in the abdomen and the esophageal hiatus is repaired by suture closure. Although studies of the Belsey repair have shown it to provide an adequate antireflux valve in mild reflux disease, few studies with large numbers of patients and long-term follow-up are available for direct comparison with transabdominal fundoplication.[17,18]

Transabdominal posterior partial fundoplication, as exemplified by the Toupet procedure, is commonly performed in Europe and appears to be extremely durable.[10,19] This procedure is not widely used in the United States because of the long history and general acceptance of the Belsey and Nissen fundoplication procedures. Toupet fundoplication was initially described in 1963 by Andrè Toupet as a posterior 180-degree gastric wrap securely fastened to the crura of the diaphragm and to either side of the esophagus with 12 to 16 interrupted sutures.[20] Fear that a 180-degree wrap would not be sufficient to prevent reflux in all cases led to a common modification of the Toupet procedure as a 270-degree wrap to increase augmentation of the hypotensive lower esophageal sphincter.[15] In a small randomized trial from Sweden comparing Toupet and Nissen fundoplications, the Toupet procedure proved to be durable over a 5-year follow-up and had a significantly lower incidence of postoperative side effects such as dysphagia, gas bloat, and wrap failure than Nissen fundoplication.[10] As expected, such clinical series also demonstrated that although this procedure provides adequate protection against reflux, less augmentation of the lower esophageal sphincter is obtained than with Nissen fundoplication. Because of such diminished lower esophageal sphincter augmentation, there remains some concern about the long-term efficacy of this procedure.

Anterior partial fundoplication was initially described more than three decades ago by Dor et al.[21] This 180-degree anterior wrap never achieved widespread acceptance despite its technical simplicity. The simplicity of the repair raises questions about its effectiveness as an antireflux procedure. The Dor procedure does not require extensive mobilization of the gastroesophageal junction or the posterior esophagus, leading to concern that a shortened (or absent) intra-abdominal esophagus may leave the wrap covering only the stomach and fail to provide adequate antireflux control. An additional concern about this repair is that it is difficult to construct an anterior wrap that is truly 180 degrees and thus in reality the Dor fundoplication will more likely span only 90 degrees of the esophagus. In 1984 Watson[22] described a modification of this procedure by pexing the gastroesophageal junction to the preaortic fascia in an attempt to provide a greater length of intra-abdominal esophagus. Unfortunately, this additional step made the procedure much more involved and therefore it lost some of the desirability of the simpler procedure described by Dor. No long-term comparative studies have been published comparing Dor fundoplication and its variations with more standard complete or partial fundoplications. The indications for anterior fundoplication remain somewhat limited. This procedure is commonly used only for perforations of the esophagus or to provide some reflux prevention after division of the lower esophageal sphincter in the setting of achalasia.[23]

Laparoscopic Procedure

Most gastrointestinal procedures can be performed with laparoscopic access, but few procedures, including cholecystectomy, are better suited for laparoscopic surgery than antireflux operations. Early results with laparoscopic antireflux procedures have confirmed their cost effectiveness, safety, efficacy, and desirability to patients. In skilled hands, with good prior training, the conversion and complication rates have been surprisingly low considering the complexity of the procedure. Nissen fundoplication was first performed laparoscopically by Cuschieri in 1989 and reported in

1992.[24] Since then, several significant series of laparoscopic fundoplications have been published.[25,26] In these reports the procedure most commonly performed was Nissen fundoplication, although Toupet and Hill repairs have been reported as well. Since laparoscopic fundoplication originated in Europe, early interest in partial fundoplication was characteristic of current clinical practices throughout Europe. The European lead has taken root in the United States and currently there is a great deal of interest both in laparoscopic fundoplication and in the appropriate applications of partial fundoplication.

Patient Preparation

All patients considered for laparoscopic fundoplication must undergo preoperative endoscopy to detect the presence of esophagitis and to perform a biopsy. Endoscopy is also helpful for assessing those patients with esophageal shortening and a stricture. Patients with esophageal shortening >5 cm should be considered for an alternative procedure such as Collis gastroplasty. Work in the animal laboratory has shown that a combined laparoscopic and thoracoscopic approach can be performed, but it is a complex procedure that may not be ready for clinical application. Patients with Barrett's esophagus who have severe dysplasia or frank carcinoma should not be considered candidates for fundoplication; instead esophageal resection is indicated.[27]

Preoperative esophageal motility studies and 24-hour ambulatory pH studies are necessary in all patients to ascertain the status of their esophageal function and to document the presence of acid reflux. A barium swallow, although not critical, is a helpful anatomic complement to upper endoscopy. A thorough medical evaluation is essential to evaluate the patient's ability to withstand general anesthesia and recover from a major operation. Patients with atypical symptoms or unusual physiologic findings should undergo further tests such as a gastric motility study, a gastric emptying study, or a HIDA scan to rule out other foregut motility disturbances that may produce symptoms similar to those of gastroesophageal reflux disease.

We have found that extensive preoperative counseling helps patients understand expected outcomes of the operation. Patients should be warned beforehand that transient dysphagia is not uncommon. Odynophagia is occasionally seen in the immediate postoperative period and such common side effects as bloating, flatulence, loose stools, and nausea frequently accompany fundoplications of any type.[12]

Patients are admitted the day of surgery, intravenous lines are placed, a single dose of preoperative antibiotic is given, and the patient voids before being taken to the operating room.

Toupet Fundoplication

Room setup and equipment for laparoscopic Toupet fundoplication are similar to that described for Nissen fundoplication.[23] Although some details are subject to the individual surgeon's preferences, it is essential that two video monitors be placed at the patient's head for viewing by both the surgeon and the assistant. We prefer to do all laparoscopic fundoplications with the patient in a low lithotomy position. The patient's thighs must be extended so that movements of the camera and instruments are not impeded. Allen stirrups or a modified "Y" table allows the legs to remain on the table but stretched outward (Fig. 11-1). When Allen stirrups are used in a low

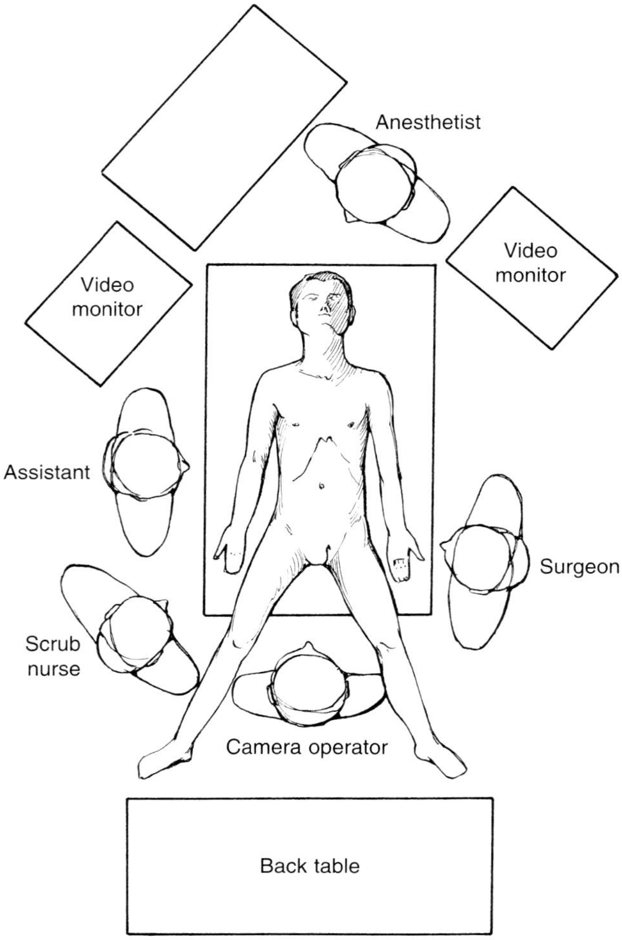

Fig. 11-1. Standard room setup and patient position.

lithotomy position, deep venous thrombosis may develop. We use pneumatic compression garments as a prophylactic measure. The surgeon can either stand between the patient's legs or to the patient's left according to his preference. A list of instruments we prefer for manipulation of the stomach and esophagus is listed below.

45- or 30-degree 10 mm telescope
5 mm atraumatic gastrointestinal graspers (Glassman)
10 mm atraumatic Babcock grasper
10 mm atraumatic liver retractor
5 mm fine curved dissecting forceps
Suction/irrigator
Curved 5 mm cautery scissors (mono- or bipolar)
Endoclip applier
2 axial grip 5 mm needle holders
3-10 mm trocars
2-5 mm trocars (valveless)
0 or 2-0 woven polyester or nylon suture on gastrointestinal curved needle

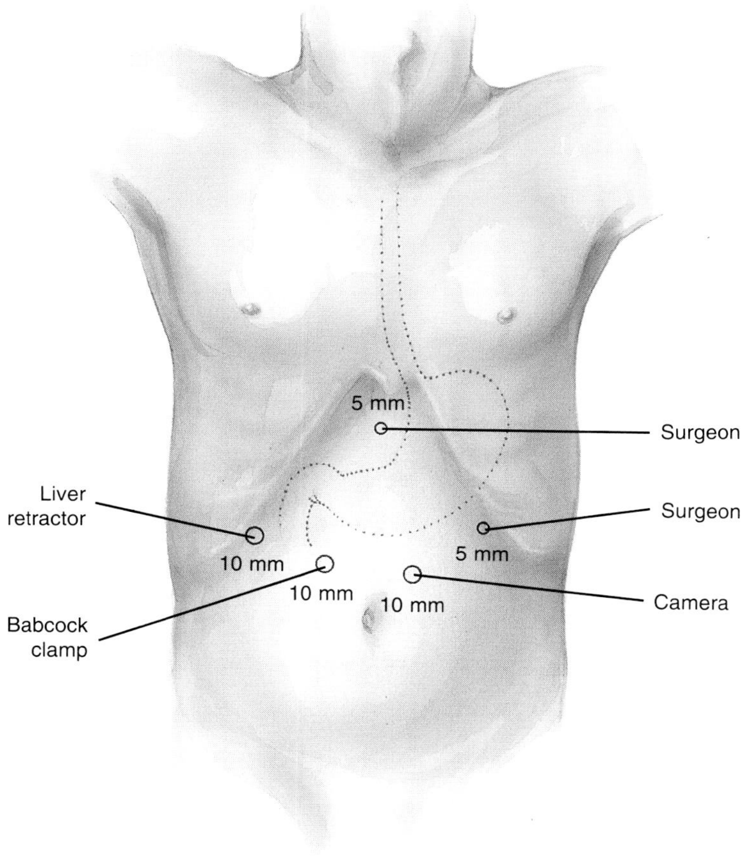

Fig. 11-2. Suggested trocar positions.

Insufflation of the abdomen is carried out in the standard manner using the Veress needle technique through the umbilicus. Insufflation to a maximum pressure of 16 mm Hg is performed slowly. A 10 mm port for the camera is placed to the left of the midline, approximately 15 cm below the estimated position of the gastro-esophageal junction. Additional ports are placed under direct vision, as illustrated in Fig. 11-2.

The left lobe of the liver is elevated with an atraumatic liver retractor from the right lateral port. An endoscopic Babcock clamp is introduced through the right paramedian port to apply downward traction on the proximal stomach. We have found that placement of a bougie at the beginning of the operation allows for rapid identification of the esophagus by instrument palpation. The primary surgeon uses the right upper quadrant 5 mm port and subxiphoid port to perform two-handed dissection, whereas the assistant on the patient's right retracts the liver and manipulates the stomach. It is frequently easier for the surgeon positioned between the patient's legs to operate through ports in the right epigastrium (left hand) and the left subcostal midclavicular region (right hand). The assistant on the patient's left retracts the stomach with a subcostal port in the left anterior axillary line.

After the liver is elevated, the thin gastrohepatic ligament is taken down with electrosurgical scissors, sparing the hepatic branch of the vagus nerve when possible. Caution must be exercised when dividing the gastrohepatic ligament since an aberrant left hepatic artery has been found in this region in approximately 4% of our patients. If the surgeon stays above the hepatic branch of the vagus nerve, this vessel is rarely seen. Division of the gastrohepatic ligament is continued until the right crus is identified. The right crus can then be dissected free and the phrenoesophageal ligament divided along the apex of the hiatus (Fig. 11-3). This typically provides a collar of tissue attached to the gastroesophageal junction that can be used as a safe and effective handle for manipulation. Dissection is then carried across the top of the

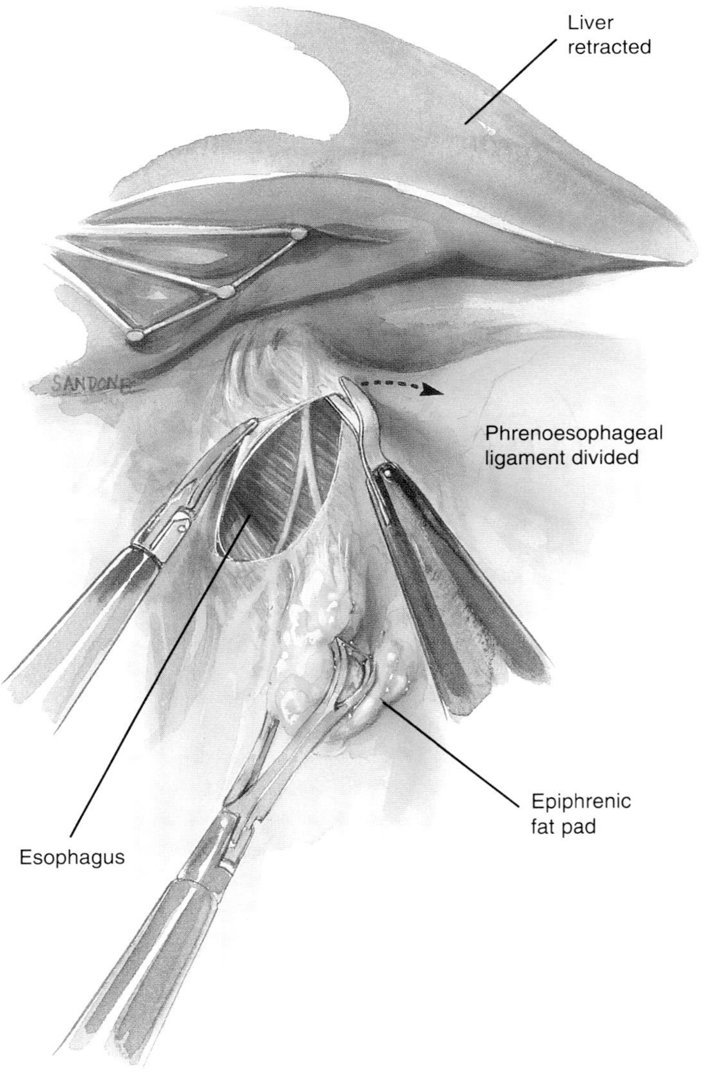

Fig. 11-3. Following division of the gastrohepatic ligament and identification of the right crus, the phrenoesophageal ligament can be taken down using electrocautery scissors.

hiatus to the left crus, which is exposed as much as possible from this angle. An acutely angled 30- to 50-degree laparoscope is essential to provide full visualization of the esophageal dissection and for mobilizing the gastrophrenic and gastrosplenic attachments.

Traction is placed on the fundus of the stomach, and attachments between the fundus of the stomach and the left diaphragm are carefully taken down, staying close to the fundus during dissection. The use of bipolar scissors provides an extra margin of safety during this maneuver and minimizes the possibility of inadvertently burning the stomach or esophagus. The superior pole of the spleen frequently adheres to the fundus of the stomach, and these adhesions should be taken down as well. We typically dissect the fundus down to the first short gastric vessels, and if these are tethering the stomach, they are routinely divided. Division of the short gastric vessels requires delicate dissection. The vessels are either tied in continuity or double hemoclipped and divided. For partial fundoplications, we have found that division of more than the first one or two short gastric vessels is rarely necessary; occasionally no division of any vessels is necessary.

Attention is then returned to the right side of the esophagus where the majority of the dissection is performed. The esophagus is freed circumferentially within the mediastinum for a variable distance, depending on the need to mobilize the mediastinal esophagus to bring it into the abdomen. In a moderately shortened esophagus the dissection can be carried far up into the mediastinum and in most cases adequate length can be obtained. If not, a Toupet fundoplication is contraindicated and alternative procedures such as Collis gastroplasty are indicated.

Dissection of the posterior portion of the esophagus and gastroesophageal junction is always performed under direct visualization (Fig. 11-4, *A*). The angled laparoscope turned at a 90-degree angle to the esophagus permits direct visualization of the posterior gastroesophageal junction. Dissection is continued until the left crus is exposed; it is cleared of all retroesophageal areolar tissue and a window is created into the left subphrenic space. At this point the mobilized gastric fundus can usually be seen, and the fundus can be grasped with a Babcock or atraumatic grasper and pulled beneath the esophagus (Fig. 11-4, *B*). The most redundant portion of the fundus should be found and securely grasped with an atraumatic clamp. The fundus can be used as a sling to retract the esophagus to the left upper quadrant and allow exposure of the hiatus posteriorly for fixation of the fundus to the crura of the diaphragm.

Occasionally the fundus of the stomach is not visible through the window created behind the esophagus. This happens most frequently in deep-chested men and those with a short esophagus. In these instances we have found it helpful to use a long, right-angled clamp (Jarit, Inc., New York, N.Y.) inserted percutaneously through the subxiphoid trocar site to reach behind the esophagus and elevate the esophagus anteriorly so that two hands can be used to feed the fundus into a grasper placed right to left through the window behind the gastroesophageal junction. The fundus that is pulled beneath the esophagus should be at least twice as long as the diameter of the esophagus and should hold its position to the right of the esophagus without retraction. If the fundus returns behind the esophagus when traction is released, additional dissection may be necessary, perhaps taking down additional short gastric vessels.

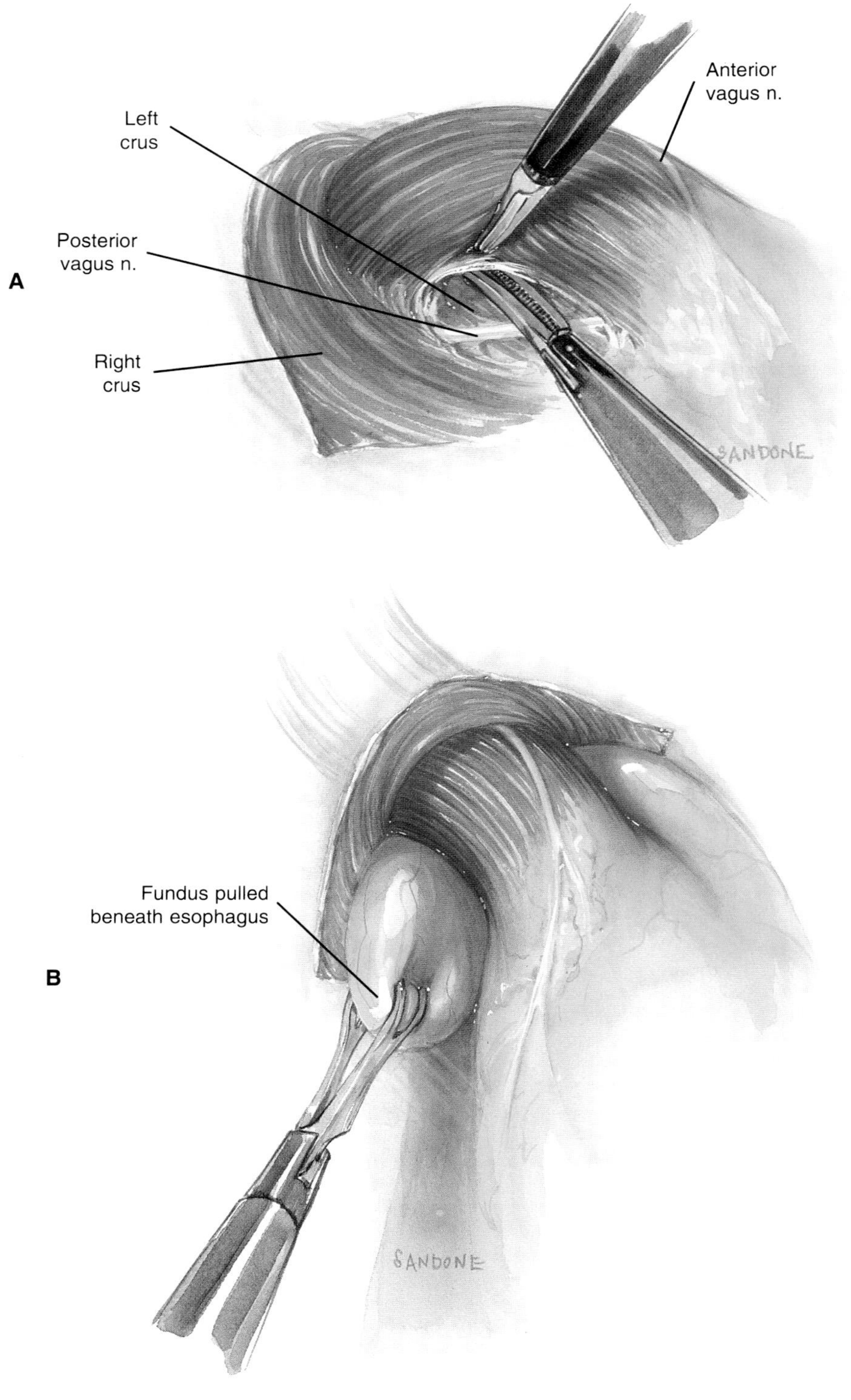

Fig. 11-4. A, Dissection of the posterior esophagus and gastroesophageal junction is performed under direct vision with an angled scope. **B,** The gastric fundus is grasped once a window has been created and brought to the right side of the esophagus.

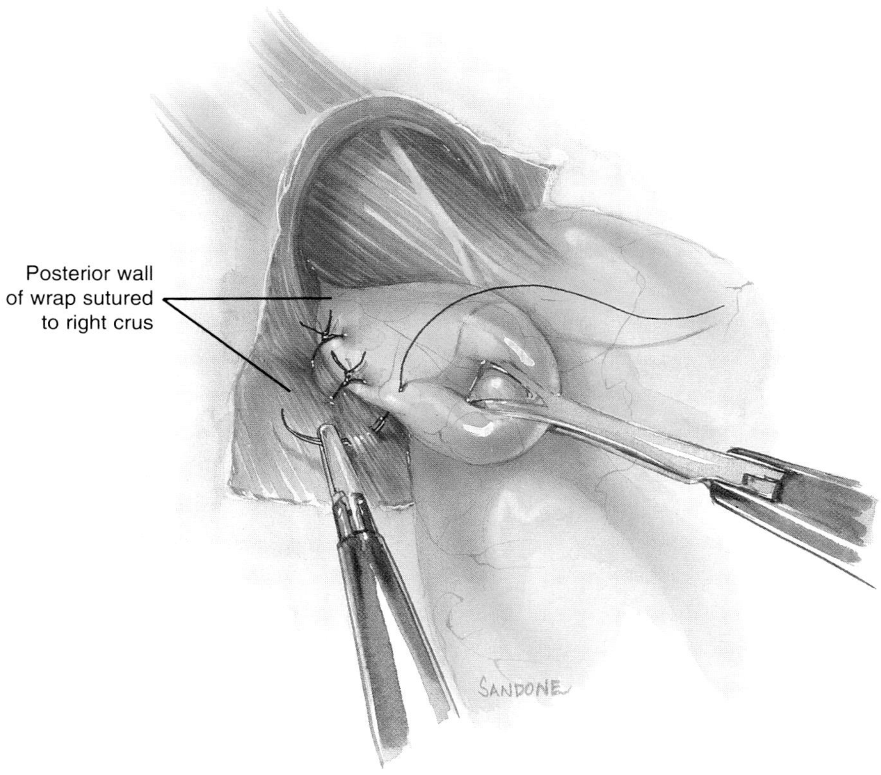

Fig. 11-5. The right side of the gastric wrap is used as a sling to expose the posterior wall of the wrap, which can then be sewn with interrupted sutures to the crura.

Using the fundic wrap as a sling and retracting toward the left upper quadrant exposes the right and left crura. Two or three posterior sutures can then be placed between the fundus and the left crus. The retraction is loosened to allow the fundus to come up against the right crus, and three additional sutures of 0 Ethibond or 2-0 Neurolon (Ethicon, Inc., Summerville, N.J.) attach the fundus to the right crus of the diaphragm (Fig. 11- 5). At this point a 56 F bougie is advanced into the stomach. This serves to distend the esophagus so that an accurate 270-degree wrap can be achieved. Often an additional suture is placed from the left crus to the left wrap to align the wrap with the esophagus (Fig. 11-6). Both sides of the esophageal wrap are then sewn to the lateral side walls of the esophagus with interrupted sutures tied intracorporeally (Fig. 11-7). Extracorporeal ties are not used for this portion of the procedure for fear of causing esophageal lacerations by the sawing action of long sutures that would be pulled through the friable esophageal wall. If the wrap is being performed as an adjunct to a Heller myotomy, the esophageal sutures are placed from the edge of the myotomy incision to the gastric wrap. This fixes the wrap in place and prevents reapproximation of the myotomy edges. After careful irrigation the liver is

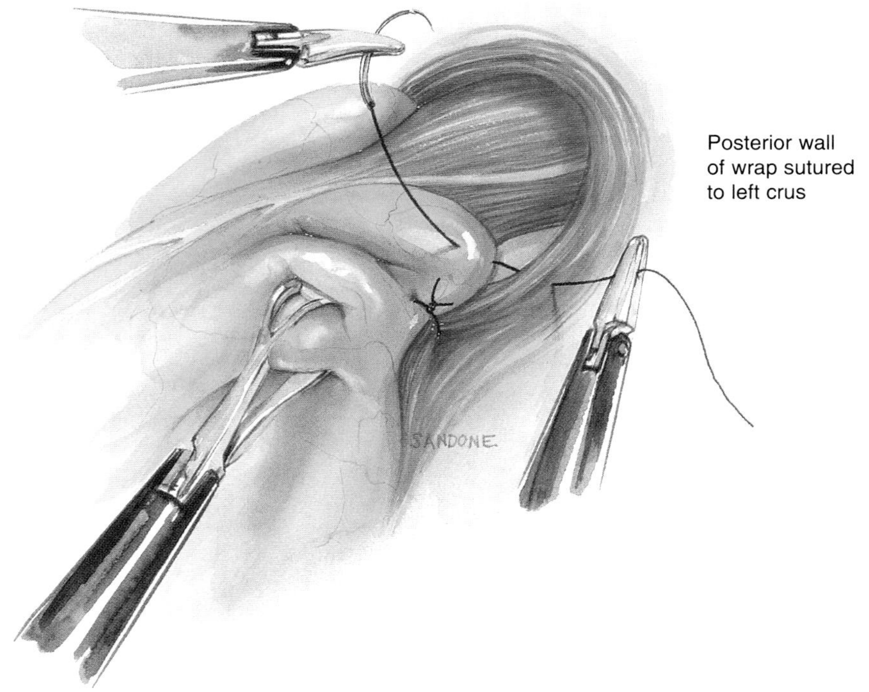

Fig. 11-6. Sutures are then placed from the left side of the gastric wrap to the left crus to pull this portion of the wrap up into the left lateral esophagus.

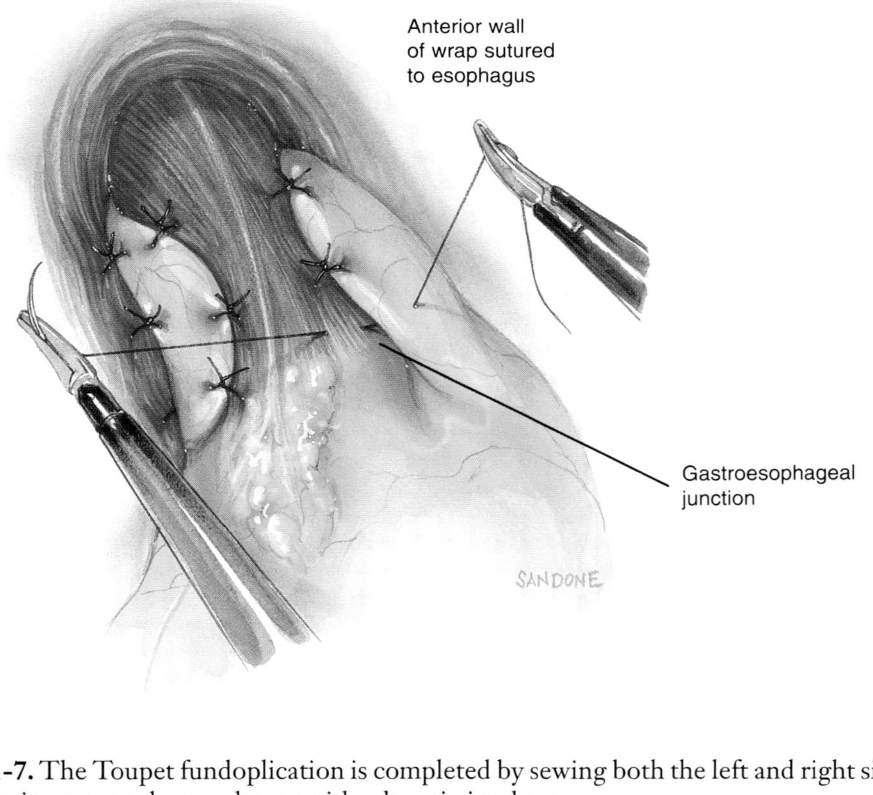

Fig. 11-7. The Toupet fundoplication is completed by sewing both the left and right sides of the gastric wrap to the esophagus with a bougie in place.

lowered, the instruments are withdrawn, and the procedure is terminated. Interrupted fascial sutures are placed to close all 10 mm trocar sites and the skin is closed in a standard fashion. Foley catheters and orogastric tubes are removed in the recovery room.

Patients are started on clear liquids when they are awake and nausea free. They are encouraged to ambulate and resume normal functions quickly. Aggressive antinausea measures are taken. Anesthetic agents that are known to cause nausea are avoided. Patients are premedicated with scopolamine patches and those who have a history of nausea or low tolerance for anesthetics are premedicated with antinausea medications. Simethicone is used liberally postoperatively since all patients seem to have some degree of gastrointestinal gas. Such postoperative bloating may be related to habitual aerophagia resulting from a physiologic attempt to clear refluxed acid from the esophagus. Patients are advanced to a full liquid diet as tolerated and discharged home on the first or second postoperative day with instructions to continue a full liquid diet and avoid carbonated beverages and extremes of hot or cold in their diet. This is usually adequate to get them through acute surgical edema and potential dysphagia or odynophagia. After 2 to 3 days a soft diet is begun, avoiding large pieces of meat, raw vegetables, breads, and large pills. Gradually patients are encouraged to resume a normal diet.

Cardiomyotomy and Dor Fundoplication

Since this procedure generally is performed following cardiomyotomy, the position of the patient and the trocar placement are the same as for cardiomyotomy and Toupet fundoplication (Figs. 11-1 and 11-2). Initial exposure is obtained by placing the patient in a reverse Trendelenburg position and introducing an atraumatic liver retractor from the right upper quadrant to elevate the left lobe of the liver. The gastrohepatic ligament is divided and the right crus is exposed. The phrenoesophageal ligament is divided to allow access to the mediastinum. Dissection is performed with bipolar scissors. An esophageal dilator is occasionally useful to help locate the esophagus and establish initial landmarks. Cardiomyotomy can then be performed under direct vision, as has been described elsewhere.[28]

In brief the cardiomyotomy divides the longitudinal and circular hypertonic smooth musculature for a distance of 7.5 cm, 6 cm above the gastroesophageal junction and 1.5 cm down the anterior gastric wall. Completion of the cardiomyotomy is ascertained by visualization with a gastroscope, confirming that all of the circumferential spastic fibers have been divided. The cardia and fundus of the stomach are freed from their diaphragmatic attachments. Extensive posterior esophageal and gastric dissection is not necessary with this procedure since the wrap is formed from the anterior gastric wall. The gastric cardia is grasped with a Babcock clamp and the greater curvature margin is brought up and over the esophagomyotomy site, as illustrated in Fig. 11-8. The anterior wrap is sutured to the right crus and to the side walls of the esophagus with interrupted sutures and tied intracorporeally. To prevent inadvertent suturing of both walls of the esophagus, a 42 to 52 F bougie should be inserted. The end result is illustrated in Fig. 11-9. The exposed esophageal mucosa is covered by the wrap, providing some security against microperforations and leakage

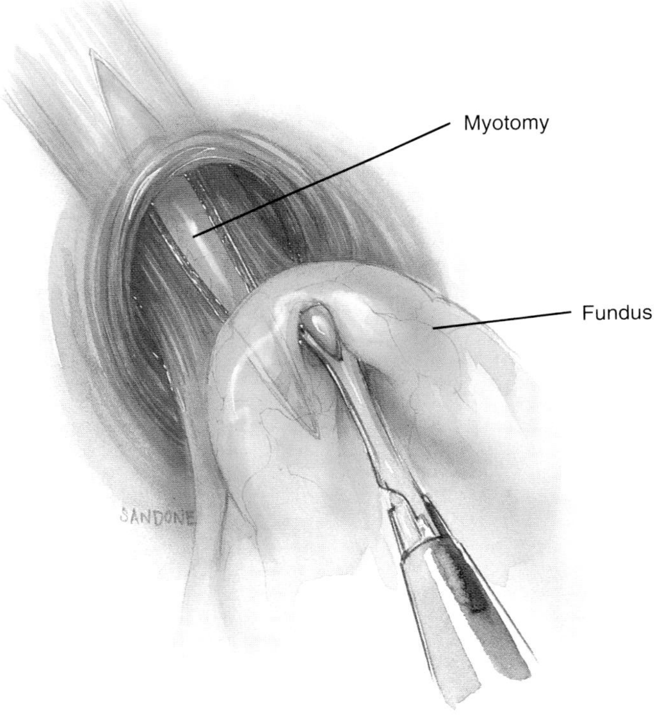

Fig. 11-8. The anterior wall of the gastric fundus is brought up and over the gastroesophageal junction from left to right covering the esophagomyotomy.

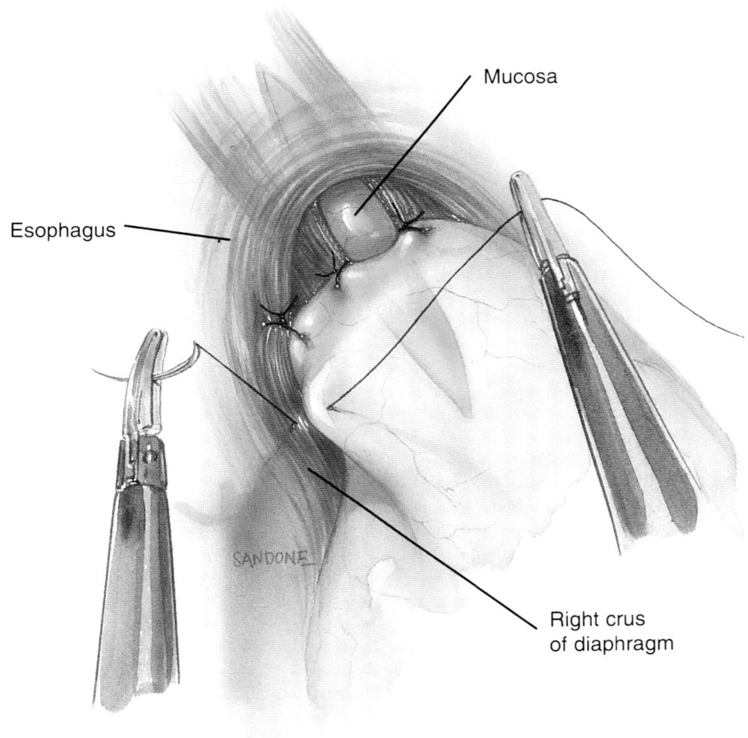

Fig. 11-9. Laparoscopic Dor fundoplication as an adjunct to the Heller procedure is completed.

from the myotomy and some additional assurance that reflux will not result from this procedure.

CLINICAL RESULTS

The literature demonstrates that open Belsey fundoplication produces good results in 82% to 89% of patients with mild disease.[16,17] Excellent results with Toupet fundoplication have been reported in 90% of patients.[3,10] Long-term results for laparoscopic fundoplication are not yet available since the first procedures were performed in 1990. Only small series with short follow-up have been published. The first published series of patients undergoing laparoscopic Nissen fundoplication was reported by Dallemagne et al.[29] in 1991. They described 12 cases performed with an average operating time of 188 minutes. Their initial experience was very encouraging. The conversion rate was 25%, the mortality rate was zero, and postoperative complications were seen in only one patient. Subsequent follow-up of a series now totaling 132 patients showed similar results.[25] Mortality was zero, morbidity was 7.5%, and good results were obtained in 94% of patients. The average operating time had decreased to 117 minutes and the conversion rate had decreased to 3.3%.

These early results show that the laparoscopic procedure is comparable to, if not better than, the open procedure. Other short-term reports have confirmed these early good results. To date, most studies have reported results of Nissen fundoplication. The only report discussing the use of laparoscopic partial fundoplication was a multicenter prospective, nonrandomized study with a 1-year follow-up.[26] This study included data from the University of Dundee, Scotland, University of California, Davis, University of Utah, and Legacy Hospital, Portland, Oregon. This study showed equal correction of reflux on postoperative pH monitoring with either total or partial fundoplication and a low incidence of dysphagia following Toupet fundoplication (0 of 36) as compared with Nissen fundoplication (9 of 80). Eight patients (10%) had persistent gas bloat following the Nissen procedure and one following the Toupet procedure (3%).

From October 1991 to September 1993 we performed laparoscopic Toupet fundoplication on 77 patients with a mean follow-up of 10 months. Short-term results are good, with 74 of 77 patients (97%) showing good to excellent control of preoperative reflux symptoms. The incidence of dysphagia is gratifyingly low: only 3 of 77 patients (3%) demonstrated persistent dysphagia after 6 weeks. Two of the three patients with dysphagia had significant esophageal motility disorders. These patients responded well to dilatation, and the third continues to have episodic solid food dysphagia despite dilatation. It should be noted that although postoperative pH monitoring showed reflux was eradicated in the majority of patients, five (6%) did have some residual esophageal reflux, although it was dramatically decreased. A major difference between the laparoscopic procedure and the open procedure is that the operating time is significantly longer for the laparoscopic Toupet procedure than for Nissen fundoplication, on average requiring 15% more operating time due to the difficulties of endoscopic suturing. Results of this experience are summarized in Table 11-1.

Although such results are encouraging, it is obvious that further follow-up will be necessary to ensure that the early excellent results with this procedure will hold up over the long term.

Table 11-1. Summary of results after laparoscopic fundoplication (October 1991 through September 1993)*

Esophageal motility disorders	21
With associated cardiomyotomy	9
Operative time (average)	138 min
Conversion to open procedure	0
Intraoperative complications	
Spleen injury	0
Bleeding >250 ml	0
Gastric perforation	1 (repaired laparoscopically)
Postoperative complications	
Death	0
Leaks	0
Wrap disruption	0
Wrap slippage	1
Recurrent reflux	2
Persistent dysphagia	3
Gas bloat	0
Continued reflux on postoperative 24-hr pH study	5
Average hospital stay	37 hr

*Toupet procedure in 77 patients and Dor procedure in one patient.

CONCLUSION

Gastroesophageal fundoplication is the procedure of choice for patients with gastroesophageal reflux disease in whom medical therapy has been unsuccessful and who can tolerate an operation. The introduction of laparoscopy has made it possible to treat patients effectively with a minimum of pain and disability and has made surgery a cost-effective alternative to prolonged medical therapy for a variety of diseases. In addition, minimally invasive surgery has provided an impetus for surgeons to reassess the surgical dogma of the past and jettison needless surgical practices that rely more on tradition than scientific validity. On the other hand, this new development has placed the burden of proof on surgeons to demonstrate that laparoscopic variations of the established open techniques are equally effective, safe if not safer than standard techniques, and hold up over the long run.

There is little doubt that patients of the 1990s who require antireflux surgery and who meet the eligibility criteria for a laparoscopic approach should undergo laparoscopic fundoplication. Patients with motility disorders of the esophagus should undergo partial fundoplication, most likely a modification of the Toupet procedure. The role that partial fundoplication may have in the treatment of patients with typical gastroesophageal reflux disease and no esophageal dysmotility remains to be demonstrated through prospective randomized trials and long-term follow-up.

REFERENCES

1. Nissen R. Gastropexy and fundoplication in surgical treatment of hiatal hernia. Am J Dig Dis 6:954-961, 1961.
2. DeMeester TR, Stein HJ. Surgical treatment of gastroesophageal reflux disease. In Castell DO, ed. The Esophagus. Boston: Little, Brown, 1992, pp 579-625.
3. Boutelier P, Jonsell G. An alternative fundoplicative maneuver for gastroesophageal reflux. Am J Surg 143:2260-2264, 1982.
4. Waters PF, DeMeester TR. Foregut motor disorders and their surgical management. Med Clin North Am 65:1235-1268, 1981.
5. Stein HJ, Bremner RM, Jamieson J. Effects of Nissen fundoplication on esophageal motor function. Arch Surg 127:788-791, 1992.
6. Csendes A, Braghetto I, Henriquez A, et al. Late results of a prospective randomized study comparing forceful dilatation and oesphagomyotomy in patients with achalasia. Gut 30:299-304, 1989.
7. DeMeester TR, Stein HJ. Surgery for esophageal motor disorders. In Castell DO, ed. The Esophagus. Boston: Little, Brown, 1992, pp 403-439.
8. Bjorck S, Dernevik L, Gatzinsky P, et al. Oesophagocardiomyotomy and antireflux procedures. Acta Chir Scand 148:525-529, 1982.
9. Peyton MD, Greenfield LD, Elkins RC. Combined myotomy and hiatal herniorrhaphy: A new approach. Am J Surg 128:786-790, 1974.
10. Thor KBA, Silander T. A long-term randomized prospective trial of the Nissen procedure vs a modified Toupet technique. Ann Surg 210:719-724, 1989.
11. Urschel J. Complications of antireflux surgery. Am J Surg 165:68-70, 1993.
12. Swanström L, Wayne R. Gastrointestinal side effects of laparoscopic fundoplication. Presented at the North Pacific Surgical Society Meeting, Vancouver, B.C., November 1993.
13. Stein HJ, DeMeester TR, Naspetti R. Three-dimensional imaging of the lower esophageal sphincter in gastroesophageal reflux disease. Ann Surg 214:374-384, 1991.
14. Jonsell G, Boutelier P. Gastroesophageal reflux. Evaluation of two fundoplicative methods by intraoperative esophageal manometry. Acta Chir Scand 493:47, 1979.
15. O'Sullivan GC, DeMeester TR, Joelsson BE, et al. Interaction of lower esophageal sphincter pressure and length of sphincter in the abdomen as determinants of gastroesophageal competence. Am J Surg 143:40-47, 1982.
16. Skinner DB, Belsey RH. Surgical management of esophageal reflux and hiatus hernia: Long-term results with 1030 patients. J Thorac Cardiovasc Surg 53:33-54, 1967.
17. Salama FD, Lammont G. Long-term results of the Belsey Mark IV anti-reflux operation in relation to the severity of esophagitis. J Thorac Cardiovasc Surg 100:517-519, 1990.
18. Heibert CA, O'Mara CS. The Belsey operation for hiatal hernia: A twenty-year experience. Am J Surg 137:532-535, 1979.
19. Boutelier P. Resultats d'une serie homogene de reflux gastrooesophagiens traites par valve tuberositaire retrooesophagienne fixee. Acta Chir 1:77, 1978.
20. Toupet A. Technique d' oesophago-gastroplastie avec phrenó-gastropexie appliquée dans la cure radicale des hernies hiatales et comme complément de l'operation d' Heller dans les cardiospasmes. Mem Acad Chir 89:394-399, 1963.
21. Dor J, Humbert P, Dor V, et al. L'intérêt de la technique de Nissen modifiée dans le prévention du reflux aprés cardiomyotomie extrazmuqueuse de Heller. Mem Acad Chir 88:877-884, 1962.
22. Watson A. A clinical and patholophysiological study of a simple and effective operation for correction of gastro-oesophageal reflux. Br J Surg 71:A991, 1984.
23. Cuschieri A. Hiatal hernia and reflux esophagitis. In Hunter J, Sackier J, eds. Minimally Invasive Surgery. New York: McGraw-Hill, 1993, pp 87-111.
24. Cuschieri A. Laparoscopic reduction, crural repair and fundoplication of large hiatal hernia. Am J Surg 163:420-430, 1992.
25. Weerts JM, Dallemagne B, Hamoir E, et al. Laparoscopic Nissen fundoplication: Detailed analysis of 132 patients. Surg Laparosc Endosc 3:357-364, 1993.
26. Cuschieri A, Hunter J, Wolfe B, et al. Multicenter prospective evaluation of laparoscopic antireflux surgery: Preliminary report. Surg Endosc 7:505-510, 1993.

27. DeMeester TR, Attwood SEA, Smyrk TC, et al. Surgical therapy in Barrett's esophagus. Ann Surg 212:528-542, 1990.
28. Pellegrini C, Wetter LA, Patti M, et al. Thoracoscopic esophagomyotomy: Initial experience with a new approach for the treatment of achalasia. Ann Surg 216:291-299, 1992.
29. Dallemagne B, Weerts JM, Jehaes C. Laparoscopic Nissen fundoplication: Preliminary report. Surg Laparosc Endosc 1:138-143, 1991.

Chapter

12

Laparoscopic Treatment of Gastroesophageal Reflux in Infants and Children

James B. Atkinson, M.D. • Keith E. Georgeson, M.D. • Sherif G.S. Emil, M.D., C.M.

Gastroesophageal reflux is a common finding in infants and children. Almost all newborn infants will have some demonstrable reflux, but this clears over time as the infant matures. Pathologic reflux, although less common, occurs with some frequency in infants and children. Neurologically impaired children may present with reflux symptoms such as failure to thrive or recurrent aspiration pneumonia. Signs of symptomatic reflux in children without central nervous system dysfunction include esophagitis, particularly if complicated by bleeding and stricture formation.

INDICATIONS

Minimally invasive techniques should theoretically decrease the morbidity of open surgical treatment. Advantages of this approach in the treatment of gastroesophageal reflux include decreased wound complications, fewer postoperative pulmonary problems, decreased adhesive bowel obstructions, improved cosmetic results, less severe postoperative pain, and shorter hospital stay. However, these advantages have not yet been documented and should not change the standard indications for the operative treatment of gastroesophageal reflux.

Standard indications for surgical treatment are divided into two categories depending on the central nervous system status of the patient. Children with central nervous system dysfunction usually require a gastrostomy for feeding access. These children should be evaluated for signs of gastroesophageal reflux such as pneumonia and frequent emesis and should undergo testing. Those with demonstrable reflux should have an antireflux procedure in addition to a gastrostomy. Children in this category who are symptomatic but have normal radiologic findings should undergo a 24-hour pH probe and gastric scintiscan. If reflux is found, these patients should also be considered candidates for fundoplication. Several recent reviews have addressed the particular challenges in this group of patients as well as outcome and long-term prognosis.[1-6]

Children without central nervous system impairment will usually present with failure to thrive, reactive airway disease, recurrent aspiration, stricture, bleeding, or a combination of these symptoms. Similar testing, possibly including endoscopic biopsy, will substantiate the diagnosis. Most children should then have a trial of medical therapy prior to being considered for surgical treatment.[7] The severity of the symptoms and resistance to medical therapy should be evaluated before proceeding with surgical treatment. As previously stated, the indications for proceeding with surgical treatment should be the same for open and minimally invasive techniques.

SELECTION OF PROCEDURE

Open Nissen fundoplication has been by far the most common procedure for treatment of gastroesophageal reflux in children and still constitutes one of the most common pediatric surgical procedures in North America. Several large case series have reported excellent success rates with this procedure.[2,5,8-10] Alternative open operations, abdominal as well as thoracic, have also been described, each having their enthusiastic proponents.[3,11-13] Almost all of the previously described methods for treatment of gastroesophageal reflux that have been used for open techniques can be accomplished with minimally invasive techniques. The Toupet partial fundoplication involves a 270-degree gastric wrap of the esophagus anchored to the crus of the diaphragm.[13] This procedure, which appears to produce excellent results, may be particularly amenable to laparoscopic techniques because it allows limited mobilization of the gastric fundus.[13,14]

Dallemagne et al.[15] in Belgium and Geagea[16] in Canada pioneered the laparoscopic Nissen fundoplication technique. Subsequently, several surgeons reported their preliminary experiences with different laparoscopic antireflux operations in adults and children.[17-20]

We consider Nissen fundoplication to be the open technique of choice and have developed an identical operation that uses minimally invasive technology. The 360-degree plication is the current standard for most surgeons. Any technique that is selected to be performed laparoscopically should include all of the essential steps performed in an open procedure. Compromises that are made as a result of impaired access or visibility will most certainly affect the quality and durability of the procedure and must be eliminated if the laparoscopic technique is to achieve widespread acceptance. We describe our experience and techniques with the Nissen fundoplication and encourage others to report on alternative operations such as the Toupet, Thal, Hill, or Belsey repair.

OPERATIVE PROCEDURE

Instrumentation

The standard instrumentation for any advanced laparoscopic procedure can be used. The instruments we use for laparoscopic Nissen fundoplication are as follows:

1	10 mm Hassan blunt trocar	1	Auto Suture clip applier
3	10 mm standard trocars	1	Endo Shears with cautery pole
1	5 mm standard port	2	needle holders
1	right-angle 10 mm instrument	1	knot pusher
1	Babcock forceps	1	30-degree 20 cm × 10 mm laparoscope

The 30-degree viewing laparoscope provides superior visibility for critical steps of the procedure such as esophageal mobilization and division of the short gastric vessels. It allows a "top down" view of the esophageal hiatus and improved depth perception. The standard 30 cm × 10 mm laparoscope may be used in most children weighing more than 10 kg. In children weighing less than 10 kg a modified 30-degree viewing scope 20 cm in length and 5 to 7 mm in diameter has proved to be superior.

Patient Positioning and Preparation

The surgeon, assistant surgeon, and camera operator must all have easy access to the operative ports. Larger children are placed in the lithotomy position and the surgeon works from the foot of the table. Smaller children can be positioned supine with the legs slightly abducted to allow positioning close to the foot of the table.

Because of the length of the procedure, careful attention to positioning, padding, and anesthetic monitoring is important to achieve successful results. Smaller children and those with chronic lung disease should have an arterial catheter inserted for monitoring of O_2 and CO_2 levels during abdominal insufflation.

Cannula and Port Placement

Port sites will vary in infants and children because of differences in abdominal cavity size (Fig. 12-1). Ideal placement in small infants is difficult to achieve because of the frequent overlapping of instruments and the camera.

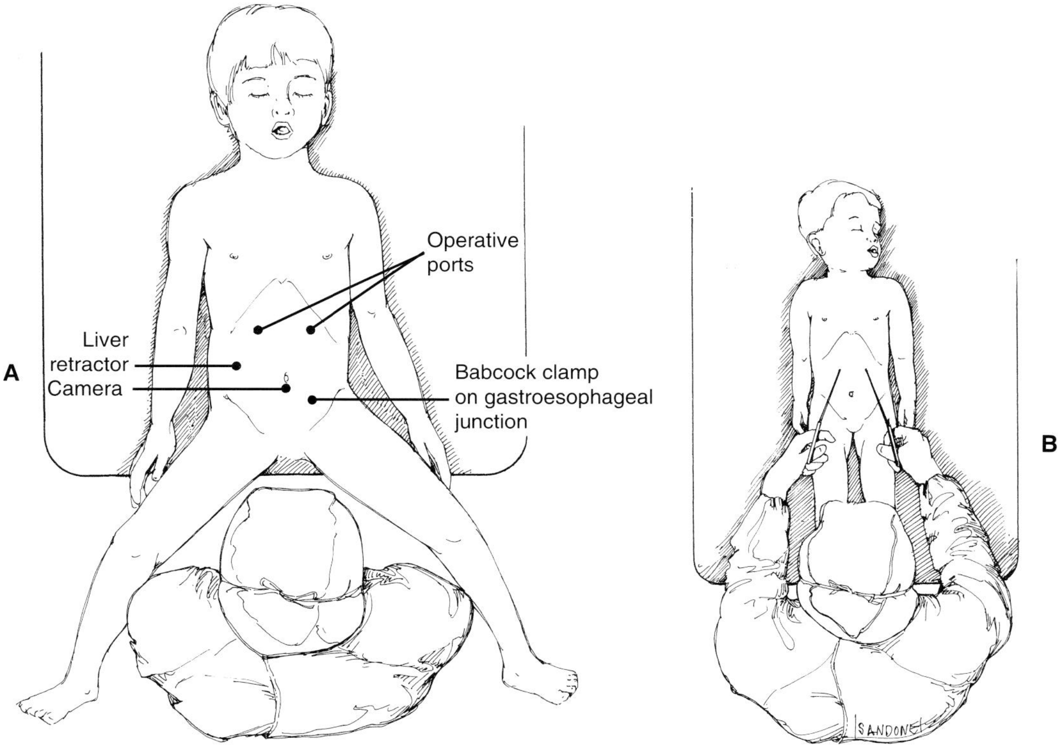

Fig. 12-1. A, Trocar positioning in the pediatric patient. Trocars must be placed lower to accommodate the smaller abdominal cavity. The surgeon is positioned at the foot of the table. Older children are placed in the lithotomy position with minimal elevation of the legs to allow the surgeon access between the legs. **B,** Children weighing less than 20 kg are placed in the supine position with the legs abducted.

An open technique for initial trocar placement is recommended. An infraumbilical location is selected and the skin, fascia, and peritoneum exposed and entered. A blunt 10 mm trocar is then introduced to insufflate the abdomen. Adequate visualization can usually be achieved with 10 cm H_2O insufflation pressure in small infants. Higher pressures of up to 15 cm H_2O may be used in older children. The laparoscope is inserted and the abdomen inspected for any abnormalities. Ports are placed in the epigastrium as the primary operative ports, the right flank for a liver retractor, and the left midabdomen for traction and elevation of the gastroesophageal hiatus. Exact port placement is adjusted according to the size and configuration of each patient.

Technique

A fan retractor inserted from the right flank port is used to elevate and retract the left lobe of the liver. A Babcock clamp is inserted via the left midabdominal port to grasp the stomach near the gastroesophageal junction and downward traction exerted. Scissors attached to cautery and blunt dissecting forceps are placed via the epigastric ports. Blunt and sharp dissection is used to divide the triangular ligament of the liver as needed. The peritoneum overlying the esophagus is sharply incised and the right and left borders of the esophagus delineated. The anterior vagus can be identified and preserved during these steps. Division of the hepatogastric ligament covering the caudate lobe of the liver facilitates identification of the right crus of the diaphragm. Once the right and left crura of the diaphragm are identified, further dissection will elevate the esophagus and create a posterior window for the fundoplication. A blunt instrument such as a Babcock clamp or right-angle clamp may then be passed around the esophagus and a Penrose drain inserted and clipped together. Passage of the clamp posterior to the esophagus is usually accomplished from right to left from the patient's perspective. The Penrose drain may then be used for traction and elevation during completion of the procedure.

The fundus of the stomach is exposed and the stomach and esophagus retracted to the patient's right side. The laxity of the fundus is assessed to determine the need for further mobilization. In most cases the mobility of the fundus is improved by dividing the uppermost short gastric vessels along the greater curvature. This is accomplished by grasping the gastrocolic omentum in this area and incising a clear area to enter the lesser sac. Individual short gastric vessels are then encircled, isolated, and doubly clipped using the automatic clip applier. This maneuver also provides exposure for further delineation of the diaphragmatic hiatus for repair.

Attention is then returned to the esophageal hiatus. The esophagus is retracted and several sutures are placed using a standard technique to close the esophageal hiatus after insertion of an appropriate-sized mercury dilator into the esophagus. Extracorporeal knot tying is used to secure the crural sutures.

The fundoplication is then completed by passing the mobilized fundus posterior to the esophagus using a Babcock clamp. The fundoplication is fixed with interrupted sutures to secure the stomach, esophagus, and fundus over a distance of 2 to 3 cm. Again the mercury dilator is placed into the esophagus and extracorporeal knot tying secures the wrap.

Gastrostomy Tube Placement

Many techniques for endoscopic and laparoscopic gastrostomy placement have been described.[21-27] We will discuss the two techniques used at our respective academic centers. At Children's Hospital Los Angeles we initially placed a percutaneous gastrostomy tube following decannulation and closure of the laparoscopic incisions. This dictated evacuation of the pneumoperitoneum and availability of additional endoscopic equipment. We have recently abandoned this method in favor of a simple procedure combining laparoscopic and extracorporeal techniques. A Babcock clamp introduced through the left upper quadrant port is used to select an ideal site on the greater curvature of the stomach. This site is grasped and exteriorized through the left upper quadrant laparoscopic incision by removal of the clamp and port together. A pursestring, Stamm-fashioned gastrostomy is then completed extracorporeally. The stomach with the gastrostomy tube attached is once again placed in the abdominal cavity. Finally, a separate stab incision is made in the left upper quadrant and the gastrostomy tube is grasped and exteriorized through the abdominal wall.

At The Children's Hospital of Alabama the following laparoscopic gastrostomy procedure has been developed and employed with great success. The liver is retracted from the anterior wall of the stomach. The dilator is removed from the esophagus and a nasogastric tube is passed into the stomach. CO_2 is infused into the stomach through the nasogastric tube using an auxiliary CO_2 pump. Pressures of up to 25 cm H_2O are used to insufflate the stomach. When deciding where to exteriorize the gastrostomy tube, allowance should be made for anterior displacement of the abdominal wall by the pneumoperitoneum. The pneumoperitoneum can be released momentarily to allow more accurate assessment of the appropriate site of exteriorization of the gastrostomy stoma. Care should be taken to place the stoma away from the costal margin.

Four Brown/Mueller T-fasteners (Flexiflo gastrostomy kit, Ross Laboratories, Columbus, Ohio) are introduced through the abdominal wall and into the anterior wall of the stomach, which is kept taut by the CO_2 insufflated through the nasogastric tube (Fig. 12-2). The anterior wall of the stomach can be stabilized with a laparoscopic

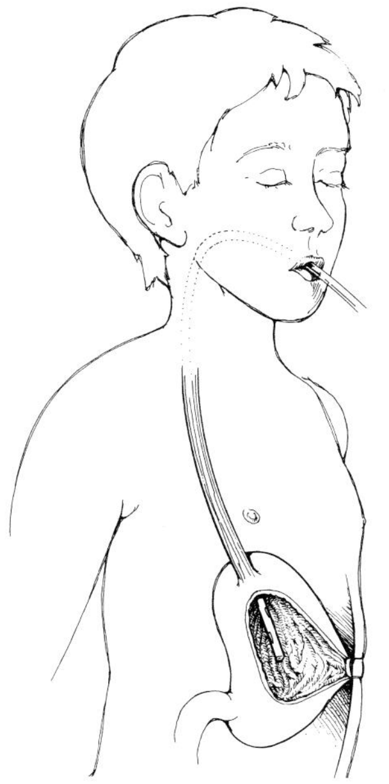

Fig. 12-2. The stomach is insufflated through a nasogastric tube. The gastrostomy site is selected after visualization through the laparoscope.

grasper if the T-fastener is deflected during an attempt to penetrate the gastric wall. The T-fasteners are placed so that they form a square or rectangle. Once the T-fasteners are in place, they are pulled upward, bringing the anterior wall of the stomach near the abdominal wall (Fig. 12-3). A needle is inserted through the abdominal wall beginning lateral or inferior to the T-fasteners and is angled through the abdominal wall so that it enters the peritoneal cavity in the middle of the four T-fasteners. The introducer is then passed into the stomach inside the four T-fasteners. A guidewire is inserted through the needle into the stomach (Fig. 12-4). After the introducer is removed, a dilator is inserted over the guidewire, and the abdominal wall and stomach are dilated appropriately to accept the Foley catheter selected for use as the gastrostomy tube (Fig. 12-5). A needle is passed through the tip of the Foley catheter, and a guidewire is passed in a retrograde direction through the needle and advanced through the catheter. The Foley catheter is then advanced over the guidewire through the abdominal wall into the stomach (Fig. 12-6). The lesser curvature of the stomach should be pulled snugly against the abdominal wall during this procedure. The guidewire is withdrawn and the Foley balloon is inflated. The T-fasteners are tied to each other over a bolster, and the gastrostomy tube is secured to the skin of the abdominal wall with a suture (Fig. 12-7).

Complications related to gastrostomy placement can be avoided with careful attention to details.[28-30] No attempt should be made to pass a T-fastener into the stomach without first insufflating CO_2 into the stomach. If a space is not created, there is a possibility that the T-fastener will go through both the anterior and posterior walls of the stomach. If a T-fastener is dropped outside the stomach, forceps can be used to retrieve it. It is also important not to dilate the opening in the stomach excessively. Too large a hole in the stomach may lead to leakage of gastric contents.

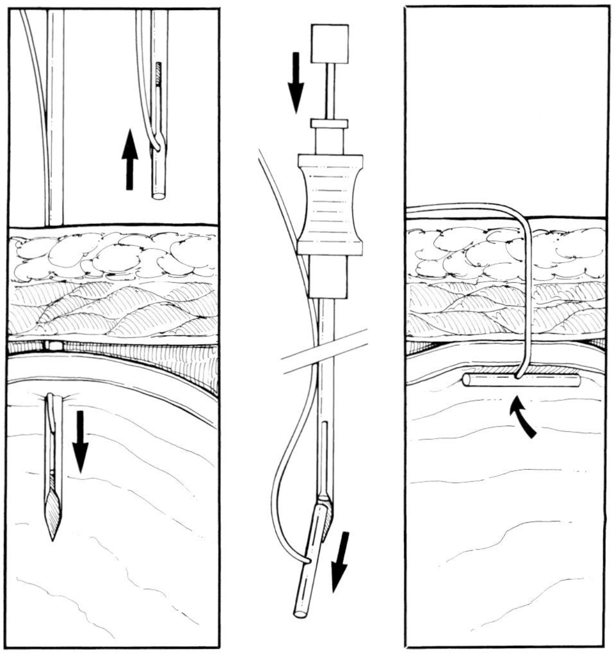

Fig. 12-3. The stomach is punctured with a needle and secured to the abdominal wall with T-fasteners.

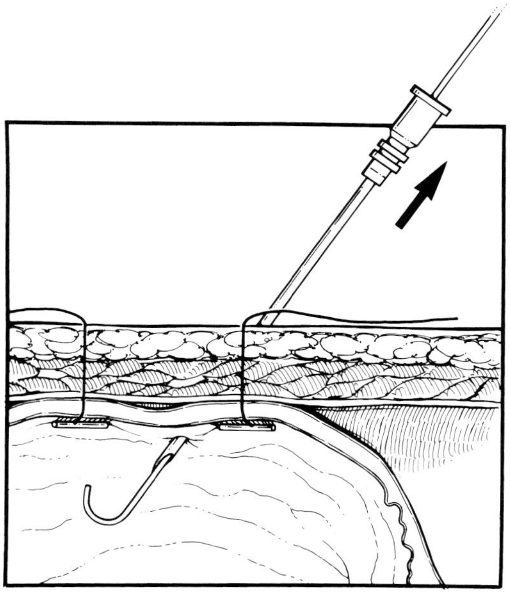

Fig. 12-4. Insertion of guidewire for placement of the gastrostomy tube.

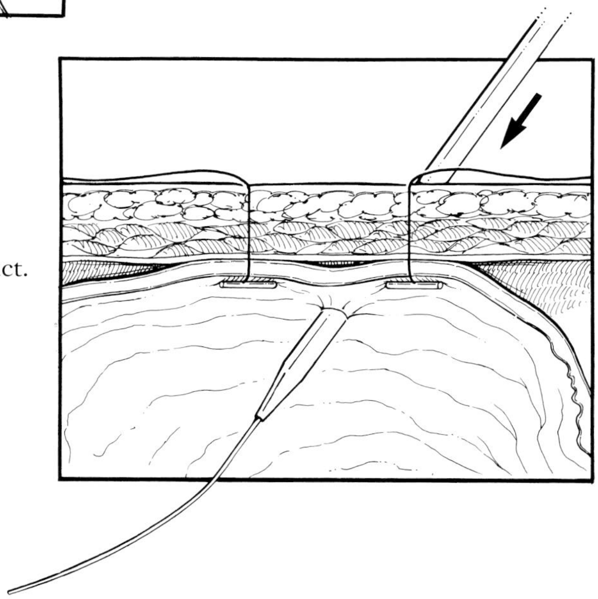

Fig. 12-5. Dilating the gastrostomy tract.

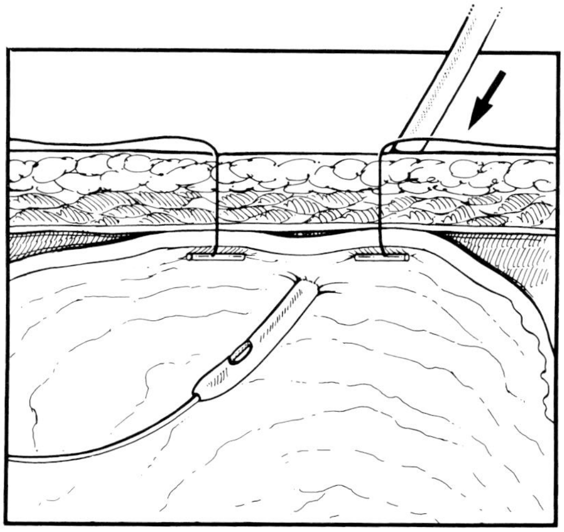

Fig. 12-6. Insertion of Foley catheter.

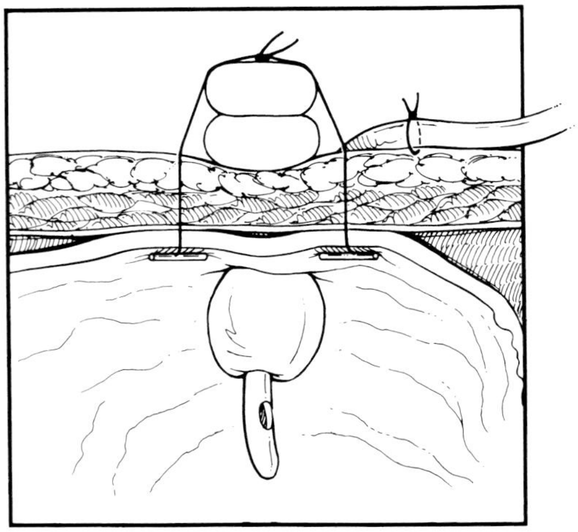

Fig. 12-7. Completed gastrostomy procedure.

Unique Laparoscopic Complications

Pneumothorax may occur during dissection of the esophageal hiatus. The pleura may be opened through the hiatus, allowing a tension pneumothorax to develop. Insertion of a chest tube is the treatment of choice and should be accomplished immediately if difficulty with ventilation is encountered. This complication can be prevented by avoiding dissection into the hiatus. Significant bleeding or insurmountable adhesion or exposure problems should be resolved by conversion to an open procedure without hesitation.

Postoperative Care

Most children may be extubated immediately at the conclusion of the procedure and returned to a routine-care hospital bed. Intravenous fluids and gastrostomy or nasogastric decompression are continued until the first postoperative day. Clear liquids and a gradually advancing diet are then permitted. Children may be discharged as soon as they are able to tolerate a full diet, usually within 48 to 72 hours. Occasionally a prolonged ileus may require a longer hospital stay. Postoperative analgesia may be accomplished with nonsteroidal anti-inflammatory or narcotic drugs depending on the individual needs of the patient.

Outpatient follow-up should include reevaluation at 6 weeks and 6 months for signs of reflux on upper gastrointestinal series and 24-hour pH probe. Long-term clinical and radiologic results of open procedures are well documented in the literature.* Careful documentation of efficacy is required when applying a new method to an established technique such as the Nissen fundoplication.

Clinical Experience

No randomized trials have been reported to date. The operative experience using laparoscopic fundoplication and gastrostomy at The Children's Hospital of Alabama

*See references 2, 3, 5, 6, 10, 11, 31, 32.

Table 12-1. Associated medical problems

	Open	Laparoscopic
Total patients	60	60
Seizures	30	31
Heart disease	5	2
Cystic fibrosis	2	3
Bronchopulmonary dysplasia	2	6
Tracheoesophageal fistula	2	1
Down's syndrome	2	1
Pierre Robin syndrome	2	1

Table 12-2. Preoperative symptoms

	Open	Laparoscopic
Total patients	60	60
Failure to thrive	58	51
Primary aspiration	23	22
Secondary aspiration	17	34
Retching	24	14
Pneumonia	9	24
Pain	1	14

Table 12-3. Postoperative complications

	Open	Laparoscopic
Total patients	60	60
Recurrent reflux	7	1
Gas bloat	3	2
Pneumonia	3	2
Retching	13	9
Perioperative death	1	1
Late death (>2 mo)	6	2

has been reviewed. Table 12-1 compares the associated illnesses of 60 consecutive patients undergoing open gastrostomy and fundoplication and the first 60 consecutive patients undergoing laparoscopic gastrostomy and fundoplication. Presenting symptoms are listed in Table 12-2. Table 12-3 compares the postoperative complications of the two procedures. Fig. 12-8 highlights the major advantages of laparoscopic fundoplication and gastrostomy over the open procedures.

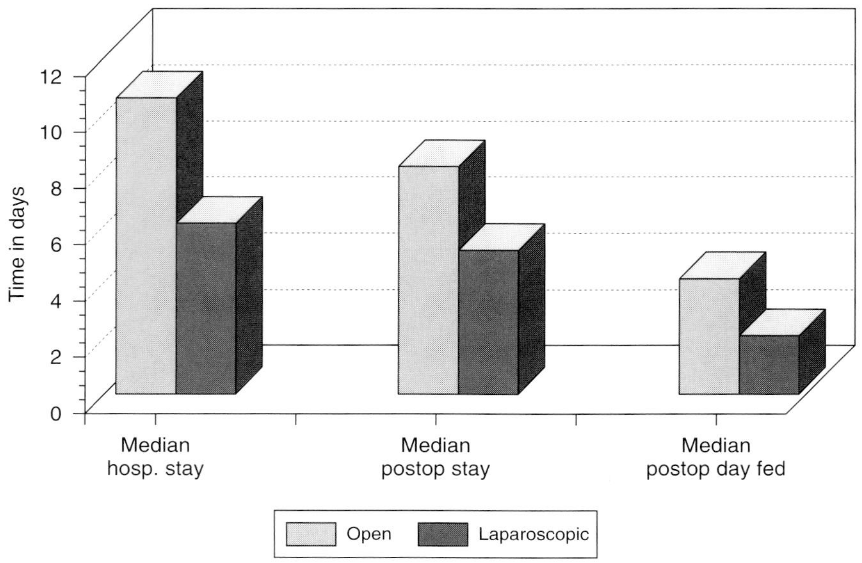

Fig. 12-8. Postoperative course following open and laparoscopic fundoplication/gastrostomy.

The most notable differences between the two groups were mean and median hospital stay. These findings suggest that laparoscopic fundoplication shortens the postoperative hospital stay and decreases the average cost. The cosmetic result is also superior in patients undergoing the laparoscopic procedure. Observation of other significant differences expected on a theoretical basis awaits long-term follow-up.

CONCLUSION

Minimally invasive techniques can be successfully applied to infants and children with gastroesophageal reflux. However, the advantages in terms of operative complications and long-term outcome remain to be proved. Careful adherence to the successful techniques of the open procedure should lead to an equally successful procedure accomplished using minimally invasive techniques. Caution is indicated in carefully evaluating the results of this technique prior to any expansion of the indications for surgical treatment of reflux in infants and children.

REFERENCES

1. Rice H, Seashore JH, Touloukian RJ. Evaluation of Nissen fundoplication in neurologically impaired children. J Pediatr Surg 26:697-701, 1991.
2. Stringel G, Delgado M, Guertin L, et al. Gastrostomy and Nissen fundoplication in neurologically impaired children. J Pediatr Surg 24:1044-1048, 1989.
3. Tuggle DW, Tunell WP, Hoezler DJ, et al. The efficacy of Thal fundoplication in the treatment of gastroesophageal reflux: The influence of central nervous system impairment. J Pediatr Surg 23:638-640, 1988.
4. Campbell JR, Gilchrist BF, Harrison MW. Pyloroplasty in association with Nissen fundoplication in children with neurologic disorders. J Pediatr Surg 24:375-377, 1989.
5. Vane DW, Harmel RP Jr, King DR, et al. The effectiveness of Nissen fundoplication in neurologically impaired children with gastroesophageal reflux. Surgery 98:662-667, 1985.

6. Martinez DA, Ginn-Pease ME, Caniano DA. Sequelae of antireflux surgery in profoundly disabled children. J Pediatr Surg 27:267-271, 1992.
7. Johnson DG. Current thinking on the role of surgery in gastroesophageal reflux. Pediatr Clin North Am 32:1165-1179, 1985.
8. Fonkalsrud EW, Foglia RP, Ament ME, et al. Operative treatment for the gastroesophageal reflux syndrome in children. J Pediatr Surg 24:525-529, 1989.
9. St. Cyr JA, Ferrara TB, Thompson TR, et al. Nissen fundoplication for gastroesophageal reflux in infants. J Thorac Cardiovasc Surg 92:661-666, 1986.
10. Turnage RH, Oldham KT, Otte JB, et al. Late results of fundoplication for gastroesophageal reflux in infants and children. Surgery 105:457-464, 1989.
11. Collard JM, De-Koninck XJ, Otte JB, et al. Intrathoracic Nissen fundoplication: Long-term clinical and pH-monitoring evaluation. Ann Thorac Surg 51:34-38, 1991.
12. Ferraris VA, Martinez L, Burrington JD. Modified fundoplication technique for correction of gastroesophageal reflux in children. Surg Gynecol Obstet 161:378-380, 1985.
13. Thor KBA, Silander T. A long-term randomized prospective trial of the Nissen procedure versus a modified Toupet technique. Ann Surg 210:719, 1989.
14. McKernan JB, Wolfe BM, MacFadyer BV Jr. Laparoscopic repair of duodenal ulcer and gastroesophageal reflux. Surg Clin North Am 72:1153-1167, 1992.
15. Dallemagne B, Weerts JM, Jehaes C, et al. Laparoscopic Nissen fundoplication: Preliminary report. Surg Laparosc Endosc 1:138-143, 1991.
16. Geagea T. Nissen fundoplication by laparoscopy. Union Med Can 120:417, 1991.
17. Cuschieri A, Shimi S, Nathanson LK. Laparoscopic reduction, crural repair, and fundoplication of large hiatal hernia. Am J Surg 163:425-430, 1992.
18. Cuschieri A, Nathanson LK, Shimi S. Laparoscopic ligamentum cardiopexy. Br J Surg 78:947-951, 1991.
19. Lobe TE, Schropp KP, Lunsford K. Laparoscopic Nissen fundoplication in childhood. J Pediatr Surg 28:358-361, 1993.
20. Cuschieri A. Laparoscopic antireflux surgery and repair of hiatal hernia. World J Surg 17:40-45, 1993.
21. Brown AS, Mueller PR, Ferrucci JT. Controlled percutaneous gastrosotomy: Nylon T-fastener for fixation of the anterior gastric wall. Radiology 158:543-545, 1986.
22. Edelman DS, Unger SW. Laparascopic gastrostomy. Surg Laparosc Endosc 1:251-253, 1991.
23. Cosgrove JM, Riou JP, Cooper B, et al. Percutaneous gastrostomy made simple. J Laparoendosc Surg 2:181-182, 1992.
24. Haggie JA. Laparoscopic tube gastrostomy. Ann R Coll Surg Engl 74:258-259, 1992.
25. Reiner DS, Leitman M, Ward RJ. Laparoscopic Stamm gastrostomy with gastropexy. Surg Laparosc Endosc 1:189-192, 1991.
26. Lathrop JC, Felix EJ, Lauber D. Laparoscopic Janeway gastrostomy utilizing an endoscopic stapling device. J Laparoendosc Surg 1:355-359, 1991.
27. Raaf JH, Manney M, Okafor E, et al. Laparoscopic placement of a percutaneous endoscopic gastrostomy (PEG) feeding tube. J Laparoendosc Surg 3:411-414, 1993.
28. Cave DR, Robinson WR, Brotschi EA. Nectrotizing fascitis following percutaneous endoscopic gastrostomy. Gastrointest Endosc 32:294-296, 1986.
29. Ditesheim JA, Sharp WR. Fatal and disastrous complications following percutaneous endoscopic gastrostomy. Am Surg 55:92-96, 1989.
30. Gallsgher MW, Tyson KRT, Ashcraft KW. Gastrostomy in pediatric patients: An analysis of complications and techniques. Surgery 74:536-539, 1973.
31. Blane CE, Turnage RH, Oldham KT, et al. Long-term radiographic follow-up of the Nissen fundoplication in children. Pediatr Radiol 19:523-526, 1989.
32. Dedinsky GK, Vane DW, Black T, et al. Complications and reoperation after Nissen fundoplication in childhood. Am J Surg 153:177-183, 1987.

Chapter

13

The Lessons of Failed Antireflux Repairs

Jeffrey H. Peters, M.D. • Tom R. DeMeester, M.D.

Of the benign esophageal diseases, management of gastroesophageal reflux disease can pose some of the most challenging diagnostic and therapeutic challenges. The surgical approach to gastroesophageal reflux requires four careful considerations: (1) documentation of gastroesophageal reflux as the cause of the patient's symptoms, (2) understanding the underlying cause of gastroesophageal reflux in the patient, (3) identifying those patients who should have a surgical antireflux procedure, and (4) meticulous performance of the appropriate antireflux procedure. Attention to these principles results in long-term success in more than 90% of patients. However, errors and mistakes are common and can result in the persistence or reappearance of symptoms following an antireflux procedure.

An antireflux procedure is considered a failure when the patient is unable to swallow normally, experiences upper abdominal discomfort during and after meals, or has recurrence or persistence of reflux symptoms. The assessment of these symptoms and the selection of patients for further surgery remains a challenge.[1-3] Functional assessment of patients who have recurrent, persistent, or new symptoms following a primary antireflux repair is critical in identifying the cause of failure. It also provides an opportunity to identify those operative principles that are crucial to performing a successful primary antireflux procedure.

PATIENT EVALUATION

Esophageal surgery is mechanistic surgery, that is, surgery performed to improve the function of the gastrointestinal system by altering the structure or arrangement of the system's moving parts. There are two requirements for successful mechanistic surgery: a precise preoperative diagnosis of the abnormality and surgical correction prior to the loss of organ function. Complete anatomic and functional evaluation of patients who have had failed antireflux surgery is the cornerstone of successful remedial surgery. Evaluation should include careful assessment of the patient's symptoms, video barium roentgenography, upper endoscopy, 24-hour esophageal pH monitoring, and assessment of esophageal motor function via stationary or ambulatory esophageal motility testing.

In some instances failure to perform esophageal function studies before surgery is the reason for the failed repair. This is exemplified by failed procedures in patients in whom a primary esophageal motor disorder was misdiagnosed or the strength of contractions in the esophageal body was inadequate to overcome the resistance of a complete fundoplication.

Twenty-four–hour esophageal pH monitoring is required to document the presence or absence of increased esophageal acid exposure, particularly before a remedial repair is undertaken. Failure to document increased esophageal acid exposure and determine its cause prior to surgery can lead to a poor outcome, which may require multiple procedures to correct. Endoscopy and biopsy are necessary to detect the presence of complications of gastroesophageal reflux disease such as esophagitis, stricture, and Barrett's esophagus. Patients with complications are more likely to have advanced disease and require careful attention to the choice of antireflux procedure. Endoscopic assessment can also aid in the evaluation of a failed antireflux repair. Video roentgenographic contrast studies using liquid barium, barium-impregnated hamburger, or radiopaque pills should be analyzed by replaying the study at various speeds. This technique is particularly useful for evaluating the rapid events of the pharyngeal phase of swallowing, the motility of the esophageal body, and structural abnormalities of the foregut.

SYMPTOMS RELATED TO A FAILED REPAIR

The most common symptoms of a failed antireflux procedure are recurrent or persistent heartburn and dysphagia. Fig. 13-1 shows the prevalence of these symptoms within 60 days of the primary repair. Symptoms of dysphagia will usually appear immediately after the initial antireflux repair, whereas heartburn has a delayed onset. This suggests that dysphagia is the result of a faulty repair or that an existing stenosis or a motor disorder of the esophageal body was not identified prior to surgery. In contrast, heartburn is usually a sign that the repair has broken down. Esophageal function studies will confirm that heartburn is related to abnormal acid exposure of the esophagus and will determine its cause. Increased acid exposure may result from a mechanically defective lower esophageal sphincter, ineffective esophageal motility, or a combination of the two. Esophageal function studies should also be used to in-

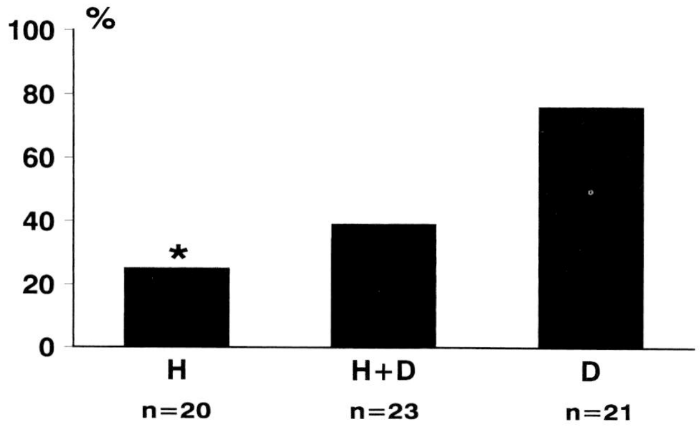

Fig. 13-1. Prevalence of patients with esophageal symptoms of heartburn alone *(H)* heartburn plus dysphagia *(H + D)*, and dysphagia alone *(D)* occurring within 60 days of a failed antireflux procedure. Four patients underwent two remedial operations. * = $p < 0.002$ vs. *D*.

vestigate dysphagia. Dysphagia may be associated with incomplete relaxation of the lower esophageal sphincter, ineffective esophageal motility, an anatomic stricture, or a combination of these.

Of the two symptoms, heartburn alone is more readily alleviated by remedial surgery than heartburn plus dysphagia or dysphagia alone. Remedial surgery has a 95% success rate in patients with heartburn alone, whereas 75% of patients with heartburn and 63% of those without heartburn who have dysphagia have a successful outcome. Esophageal resection and colon interposition may be necessary to alleviate symptoms of failed procedures in this latter group of patients.

REASONS FOR FAILURE OF PRIMARY ANTIREFLUX PROCEDURES

Technical errors account for the majority of failed antireflux repairs (Table 13-1). These include a misplaced fundoplication ("slipped" Nissen), breakdown of the repair, herniation of the repair into the chest, too long or too tight a fundoplication, and operative damage to the lower esophagus. An underlying primary motor disorder, an error in diagnosis, or an intact but ineffective repair is responsible for the remainder.

Misplaced Fundoplication

The most common technical error is placement of a Nissen fundoplication around the stomach instead of the lower esophagus. Historically this has been referred to as a "slipped" Nissen. A gastric wrap is most often misplaced because:

1. Poor exposure leads to insufficient dissection of the hiatal area, especially in obese patients.
2. The stomach is insufficiently reduced into the abdomen when the esophagus is shortened from long-standing disease. For example, the proximal stomach can assume a tubular shape after long-standing constriction by the diaphragmatic hiatus.

A short esophagus should be suspected if a hiatal hernia does not reduce during an upright barium swallow or the distance between the crura and the gastroesophageal junction is found to be in excess of 5 cm on endoscopic examination in patients with a stricture or severe disease. In these situations a thoracic approach is preferred to

Table 13-1. Reasons for failure of primary antireflux procedures

Finding	No.
Wrap around stomach	22
Delayed breakdown	17
Repair in chest	12
Too long or too tight Nissen fundoplication	5
Operative damage to lower esophagus	4
Unsuspected primary motor disorder	5
Ineffective but intact repair	5
	70

permit mobilization of the esophagus from the diaphragm to the aortic arch, to allow for the possibility of a lengthening procedure, and to ensure placement of a properly positioned fundoplication below the diaphragm without undue tension.

To position a wrap correctly the posterior lip of the wrap should be brought between the trunk of the right vagus nerve and the esophagus. If the repair cannot be placed below the diaphragm without undue tension, a Collis gastroplasty should be used to lengthen the esophagus.[4] Since it requires only 1.5 cm rather than 4 cm of intra-abdominal esophagus,[5] a short Nissen wrap may be effectively used in patients with a short esophagus. However, good esophageal contractility, which is often lost when the esophagus is shortened, is essential for a short Nissen wrap. Consequently, a Collis-Belsey procedure is usually necessary.

Delayed Partial or Complete Breakdown of the Repair

Breakdown of the fundoplication is the second most common cause of failure. Inadequate mobilization of the fundus is the most likely culprit and is suggested by intraoperative findings such as the lack of evidence of a crural dissection, removal of the esophageal fat pad, or division of the short gastric vessels. Excessive tension on the gastric wrap as a result of insufficient mobilization of the fundus or the incorporation of excessive fatty tissue may contribute to disruption of the wrap. Several technical maneuvers can prevent this from happening. Division of the short gastric vessels allows sufficient gastric fundus to construct the wrap without tension. Removal of the fat pad allows the serosa of the stomach to abut and heal to the esophageal wall.[5] Using permanent sutures with Teflon felt pledgets prevents them from tearing out of the gastric wall. Also, keeping a nasogastric tube in place for the first 24 to 48 hours after surgery prevents postoperative gastric distention from stressing the repair during the healing phase.

Herniation of the Repair Into the Chest

The third most common cause of failure is herniation of the repair into the chest because the repair is placed under too much tension, the crura are not adequately approximated, or the crural closure is disrupted. The sutures should incorporate the peritoneum covering the crura and not just the muscular tissue. The tendinous portion of the diaphragm at the apex of the right crus should be avoided. For these reasons the temptation not to close the crura during laparoscopic surgery should be avoided.

Too Tight or Too Long a Fundoplication

Other less common causes of failure are making the fundoplication too tight or too long and damaging the esophagus in the process. A wrap limited to 1 to 2 cm is just as effective an antireflux barrier as a longer wrap and reduces the potential for permanent dysphagia in the late postoperative course. Calibrating the diameter of the wrap with a 60 F intraluminal bougie prevents the fundoplication from being too tight and reduces the incidence of immediate postoperative dysphagia.[5] Gentleness in handling tissues is one of the cornerstones of esophageal surgery and prevents damage to the esophageal muscle that results in poor motility of that portion of the esophagus after surgery. This is particularly true of the laparoscopic approach.

Underlying Primary Motor Disorder

Patients who present with dysphagia and a severe motility disorder, weak or interrupted contractions, a stricture that cannot be dilated, or a history of multiple previous unsuccessful repairs and patients in whom fibrosis of the esophageal muscular layer is found intraoperatively have irreversible functional esophageal damage. An esophageal resection and colon interposition is, in our experience, the best way to restore alimentary function in these patients.[6]

Error in Diagnosis

An error in diagnosis is a preventable but relatively common reason for failure of an antireflux repair. Symptoms are an unreliable guide in diagnosing gastroesophageal reflux. Typical symptoms of functional foregut disorders include heartburn, regurgitation, dysphagia, postprandial fullness, epigastric pain, bloating, nausea, and vomiting. Ascribing the symptoms to a specific disease of the foregut in the absence of histologic findings and without further investigation can lead to an error in diagnosis.[1] This is because esophageal, gastric, duodenal, and nonforegut organs (i.e., lungs and heart) can cause symptoms of a similar nature, making it difficult to differentiate primary esophageal motor disorders, gastroesophageal reflux disease, and gastric, pulmonary, or cardiac disease. In addition, functional foregut disorders can present with atypical symptoms such as chest pain or chronic cough or occur concomitantly with cardiac or respiratory disease, further confusing the clinical picture. Consequently, objective methods are required to confirm the presence of a functional foregut abnormality and to distinguish it from other conditions.

Choice of Remedial Procedure

The preferred surgical approach in a patient who has had a failed antireflux procedure is an open thoracotomy. The diaphragm is divided via a peripheral circumferential incision to permit simultaneous exposure of the upper abdomen and dissection of the previous repair.

Four factors should be taken into account in choosing a remedial procedure: the patient's symptoms, the number of previous repairs, the results of esophageal functional tests, and the operative findings (Table 13-2). A 360-degree Nissen fundoplication should be performed in patients with positive 24-hour pH studies who complain primarily of heartburn and who have normal esophageal length and motility.[5] A Belsey partial fundoplication is performed in patients who complain of heartburn and have a positive 24-hour pH study, normal esophageal length, but abnormal esophageal motility (i.e., a contraction amplitude of <15 mm Hg) or patients who complain of dysphagia and have a normal 24-hour pH tracing but abnormal esophageal motility.[7] In these patients a gastroplasty can be added if the esophagus is shortened.[4] A myotomy of the esophageal body plus a Belsey procedure should be performed in patients who have >20% simultaneous waves and complete lower esophageal sphincter relaxation on swallowing. A myotomy of the sphincter plus a Belsey procedure is appropriate for patients whose initial wrap was properly placed around the sphincter but motility studies show incomplete relaxation of the lower esophageal sphincter on swallowing although esophageal peristalsis is adequate. An esophageal resection is often required for patients with dysphagia who have a history of two or more previous repairs with absent or severely depressed esophageal body contractility or a stenosis resistant to dilation.[6]

Table 13-2. Principles of procedure selection

Heartburn + positive 24-hr pH studies Normal motility and length	Nissen
Heartburn + positive 24-hr pH studies Abnormal motility, normal length *or* Dysphagia, abnormal motility	Belsey
Short esophagus	Collis-Belsey
>20% simultaneous waves *or* Incomplete lower esophageal motor relaxation	Belsey plus myotomy
Dysphagia, multiple previous repairs *or* Stricture resistant to dilation	Resection

Table 13-3. Procedures performed (70 reoperations in 65 patients)

Procedure	**No.**
Nissen	
Transabdominal	5
Transthoracic	29
Belsey	13
Collis-Belsey	4
Collis-Nissen	1
Colon interposition	13
Jejunal interposition	1
Other	4

CLINICAL RESULTS

We have recently analyzed 70 reoperations in 65 patients (Table 13-3). Fifty-six patients had an antireflux operation, and 14 patients underwent an esophageal resection and colon or jejunal interposition, one for a stricture that resisted dilation, two for severe mediastinal fibrosis and periesophagitis, two for immediate breakdown of the repairs and fistulization, and nine for a severe motility disorder, two of whom had a stricture. The patients were followed for a median of 15 months (range 2 to 96 months).

No deaths occurred. Postoperative complications are listed in Table 13-4. Altogether 23 complications developed in 19 of the 65 patients. Eight patients required reoperation for complications. One patient developed necrosis of the distal esophagus above the remedial Nissen fundoplication. The mediastinum and distal esophagus were extensively scarred from the initial antireflux repair and the ischemia was

Table 13-4. Complications of remedial surgery

Complication	Patients		%
Mortality		0	0
Morbidity	24/65		37
Incisional hernia*		4	
Pneumonia		3	
Wound infection		3	
Pancreatitis		2	
Empyema		1	
Bleeding*		1	
Perforated colonic diverticulum*		1	
Necrosis of distal stomach*		1	
Obstruction from internal hernia*		1	
Reoperation	8/65		11

*Required reoperation.

probably caused by the mobilization for the remedial repair. Esophageal resection and colon interposition were performed immediately.

Nineteen patients were operated on for heartburn alone and all had an antireflux procedure. One patient who developed recurrent symptoms 21 months after surgery underwent reoperation and was free of symptoms 13 months later. The success rate of an initial remedial antireflux procedure for the symptom of heartburn alone was 95%.

Twenty-two patients were operated on for heartburn plus dysphagia. Sixteen had an antireflux procedure and six underwent resection as the initial remedial procedure. Of the 16 patients who had an antireflux procedure, one required an esophagectomy and colon interposition for distal esophageal necrosis. Two patients developed recurrent symptoms of heartburn 24 and 36 months after surgery; one of them underwent a repeat Nissen fundoplication and is currently free of symptoms at 24 months and the other is currently receiving medical therapy. The success rate of an initial remedial antireflux procedure for the symptoms of heartburn plus dysphagia was 81%. Of the six patients who had initial resection, five were relieved of heartburn and dysphagia, one had persistent dysphagia after a jejunal interposition, one developed symptoms of duodenogastric reflux and had a bile diversion procedure, and another developed symptoms of gastric stasis and had a total gastrectomy. The latter two are currently free of symptoms.

Of the 19 patients operated on for dysphagia alone, 15 had an antireflux procedure and four had a resection. Four of the patients who had antireflux surgery had persistent dysphagia at 6, 10, 15, and 96 months, three after a remedial Belsey procedure and one after a Nissen procedure. The dysphagia was sufficiently severe in two to merit esophageal resection and colonic interposition, which has relieved their symptoms for 6 and 31 months. In the others, postoperative manometric findings in one were unremarkable and the other shows interrupted waves and weak contractions in the esophageal body. The success rate of an initial remedial antireflux procedure for the symptom of dysphagia alone was 67%. Of the four patients who

Table 13-5. Outcome of remedial surgery

Indication/Procedure	N	% Excellent/Good
Heartburn		
Antireflux procedure	19	95
Heartburn and dysphagia		
Antireflux procedure	16	81
Resection	6	83
Dysphagia		
Antireflux procedure	15	67
Resection	4	75

had an initial colon resection, one required resection of a stenosed cologastric anastomosis and all four are currently free of symptoms.

Of the 65 patients operated on for recurrent heartburn, dysphagia, chest pain, or immediate breakdown of the repair and fistulization, 17 had poor esophageal contractility. Of these, four had immediate resection (colon interposition in three and jejunal interposition in one) and 13 had a remedial antireflux operation followed by a poor result in five, two of whom required a resection with colon interposition to obtain symptomatic relief. The success rate of an initial remedial antireflux procedure in patients with poor contractility of the esophageal body was 61% (8/13 patients). In contrast, the success rate was 92% (37/40) in patients with good contractility ($p = 0.02$). Of the six patients with poor contractility who initially or eventually underwent an esophageal resection, five (83%) obtained symptomatic relief. The results after the initial and subsequent remedial procedures for the various esophageal symptoms are shown in Table 13-5. The overall combined good result rate was 94%. A good symptomatic and functional result was achieved in the patient who underwent reoperation for breakdown of the repair and pleural fistulization with sepsis. He was treated with resection and colon interposition. The three patients operated on for chest pain were aymptomatic following the remedial procedure.

CONCLUSION

Prevention is key to failed antireflux surgery. Detailed physiologic evaluation prior to surgery and attention to technical details during the operation will avoid failure in the vast majority of patients. There is no single remedial operation to correct a previously failed antireflux procedure. Rather, the operation must be tailored to each patient on the basis of the presenting symptoms, the number of previous repairs, the results of esophageal function tests, and the operative findings. In patients who present with heartburn and increased esophageal acid exposure secondary to a mechanically defective sphincter, a remedial antireflux procedure is generally sufficient. The choice of the procedure depends primarily on the motility study. If good lower esophageal sphincter relaxation and contraction amplitude of the esophageal body are present, a Nissen fundoplication can be used.[8] A transthoracic, transdiaphragmatic approach is helpful to free the esophagus and stomach from adjacent structures and allow takedown of the previous repair. If esophageal body contractility is poor, a Belsey partial fundoplication should be done to minimize outflow resistance. A gastroplasty can be added to a Belsey repair if the esophagus has shortened and the repair is under tension. Patients who present with nonobstructive dysphagia are best managed with a Belsey repair combined with a myotomy when a primary esophageal motor disorder or incomplete relaxation of the sphincter is present. If esophageal body function is adequate and the cause of dysphagia is too tight or too long of a fundoplication, an appropriate-sized Nissen fundoplication can be reconstructed.

REFERENCES

1. Little AG, Ferguson MK, Skinner DB. Reoperation for failed antireflux operations. J Thorac Cardiovasc Surg 91:511, 1986.
2. Siewert JR, Isolauri J, Feussuer M. Reoperation following failed fundoplication. World J Surg 13:791, 1989.
3. Stirling MC, Orringer MB. Surgical treatment after the failed antireflux operation. J Thorac Cardiovasc Surg 92:667, 1986.
4. Pearson FG, Cooper JD, Patterson GA, et al. Gastroplasty and fundoplication for complex reflux problems. Ann Surg 206:473, 1987.
5. DeMeester TR, Bonavina L, Albertucci M. Nissen fundoplication for gastroesophageal reflux disease. Evaluation of primary repair in 100 consecutive patients. Ann Surg 204:9, 1986.
6. DeMeester TR, Johansson K-E, Franze I, et al. Implications, surgical technique, and long-term functional results of colon interposition or bypass. Ann Surg 208:460, 1988.
7. DeMeester TR. Transthoracic antireflux procedures. In Nyhus LM, Baker RJ, eds. Mastery of Surgery. Boston: Little, Brown, 1984, pp 381-392.
8. DeMeester TR, Johnson LF, Kent AH. Evaluation of current operations for the prevention of gastroesophageal reflux. Ann Surg 180:511, 1974.

Part

IV

Peptic Ulcer Disease

Chapter

14

Pathophysiologic Basis of Peptic Ulcer Disease

Johannes Heimbucher, M.D. • Werner K.H. Kauer, M.D. • Jeffrey H. Peters, M.D.

HISTORY

Marinos first explored the pathophysiology of peptic ulcer disease nearly 2000 years ago in his studies of vagal anatomy. Galen continued Marinos' studies and speculated on the possible function of the nerves in control of the stomach.[1,2] The first scientific examinations on the secretory properties of the stomach were undertaken by René-Antoine Ferchault (1683-1757) in a pet buzzard. He found that the gastric liquid digested food, disproving the theory of putrefaction.[2,3] These studies provided a framework for experiments on digestion for many subsequent generations of physiologists. Chemical investigations were initiated in the first half of the nineteenth century after William Prout[4] (1785-1850) proved that gastric juice contained free hydrochloric acid. Prout's observations were confirmed by the classic observations of William Beaumont,[5] who studied gastric physiology in a patient with a gastric fistula. He demonstrated that the chemical activity of gastric secretion was responsible for the digestion of food. In 1910 Schwarz[6] more precisely elaborated the role of gastric juice in the development of gastric and duodenal ulcers.

The interactions between the vagus nerve, gastric juice, and stomach in the physiology of gastrointestinal function, however, were not well understood until the beginning of the twentieth century. The relationship between vagal innervation and gastric secretion was first elucidated by Ivan Petrovich Pavlov. He demonstrated in studies on dogs that the vagus nerves contain secretory fibers that are stimulated by eating, even if the food does not reach the stomach.[7] Subsequently, McCrea[8] in England recognized the vagi as the potential cause of disease. Lester Dragsted, chairman of the Department of Physiology and Pharmacology as well as associate professor of surgery at Northwestern University in Chicago, and his colleagues discovered that the vagal mechanisms responsible for gastric secretion play an important role in the determination of which physiologic events terminate and initiate gastric secretion to avoid the corrosive effects producing an ulcer.[9] Klein[10] and Berg[11] postulated that three factors were involved in ulcerogenesis: a specific ulcer gastritis, free hydrochloric acid in the stomach, and a secondary infection in the stomach or duodenum. Dragstedt was fascinated by this work and continued to investigate gastric physiology to better define the events surrounding peptic ulcer disease. He believed the key to understanding ulcerogenesis was acid secretion and that there were two stimuli of acid hypersecretion, neural and hormonal. After extensive experimental work on different dog models Dragstedt[12,13] finally formulated the mechanism of gastric acid secretion. Duodenal ulcers were of nervous origin and the pathologic stimuli that resulted in duodenal ulcers were transmitted by the vagi. Gastric ulcers were caused by abnormal hormonal stimuli secondary to prolonged antral contact with food and hypersecretion of gastrin.

Vagal physiology and anatomy was far from being completely understood, however. Previously unknown efferent vagus nerve fibers were discovered.[14] Similarly, reports documented the existence of a large number of different peptides and neurotransmitters with a yet undescribed function within the vagi.[15] The clinical implications of these cellular and biochemical studies are just beginning to be understood.

The understanding of the pathophysiology of peptic ulcer disease was revolutionized by the isolation of *Helicobacter pylori* from gastric biopsies by Marshall and Warren[16] in 1983. This was followed by a large number of publications concerning the role of the bacterium in several disorders of the upper gastrointestinal tract and changed the therapeutic approach to peptic ulcer disease.

The continuing high morbidity and mortality rates caused by the complications of peptic ulcers should lead to a resurgence of interest in surgery for peptic ulcer disease.[17] The central question is, Which patient will most benefit from which type of therapy? To answer this question, the physiology and pathophysiology of peptic ulcer disease must be further elucidated. The dictum "No acid, no ulcer" from the early 1900s is still commonly accepted as the explanation for the pathogenesis of both gastric and duodenal ulcers.[18,19] Unfortunately, neither this theory nor all other isolated pathogenic factors provide a definitive explanation for the various types of peptic ulcers. Peptic ulcer disease appears to be a multifactorial abnormality resulting from a variety of pathophysiologic mechanisms.

Normal Physiology

Normal gastric function includes three major components working in concert to aid in the digestion of food and protect gastric mucosa from injury. These include exocrine secretion of hydrogen ions, pepsinogen, mucus, and bicarbonate; gastric motor activity; and endocrine secretion of gastrin and somatostatin. Abnormalities of these normal physiologic mechanisms have been implicated in the development of peptic ulcer disease.

Acid Secretion

Acid-producing oxyntic cells are located in the cardia, fundus, and corpus. Normal acid secretion can be divided into three distinct phases: the cephalic phase controlled by vagal activity, a gastric phase mediated by intramural neural reflexes and gastric hormones such as gastrin, and an intestinal phase consisting of as yet poorly understood enteral hormones. Food stimulates acid secretion initially via the cephalic pathway. The simple smell or taste of food results in vagal stimulation with an increase in acid secretion and release of gastrin.[20] The gastric phase of acid secretion is induced both by distention of the stomach and the quality of the food. Gastric distention causes vagovagal and intramural reflexes that result in increased acid secretion.[21] Chyme in the intestine starts the intestinal phase of acid secretion by releasing a number of poorly understood intestinal hormones, including enteroxyntin, gastric inhibitory polypeptide, and somatostatin, that provide feedback loops modulating acid secretion. Absorbed amino acids provoke increased acid secretion. Acid in the stomach protects against bacterial colonization and converts pepsinogen into pepsin. Acid in the duodenum triggers the release of secretin, which induces pancreatic bicarbonate secretion.

The precise physiology of gastric acid inhibition is not well known. There is evidence of a cephalic phase of inhibition as well as neural and humoral inhibitory mechanisms located in the stomach, small intestine, and colon. Low gastric pH serves as a feedback mechanism, which stops gastrin release at pH <2. Fat in the duodenum is the most effective inhibitor of gastric acid secretion.

At the cellular level acid is produced by the parietal cell in response to stimulation of acetylcholine, histamine, and gastrin receptors. Via different intracellular pathways, all three receptor types activate the proton pump, the H^+K^+-ATPase resulting in the secretion of H^+(Fig. 14-1). The stomach secretes acid in an endogenous circadian rhythm. Acid secretion is greater in the evening than in the morning[22] (Fig. 14-2).

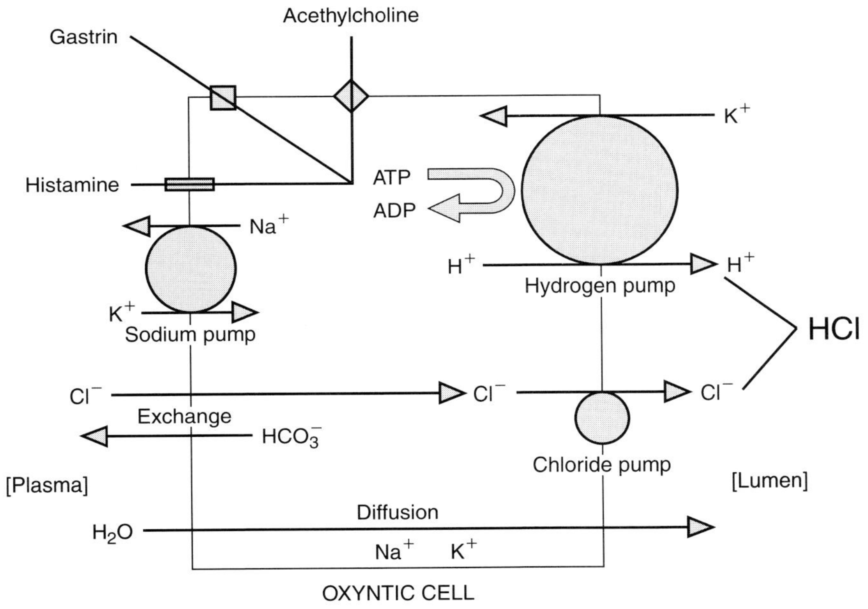

Fig. 14-1. Active and passive mechanisms of secretion in the oxyntic cell. The active transport is provided by Na^+K^+-ATPase and H^+K^+-ATPase pumps and the chloride pump that move substrates against electrochemical gradients. Passive secretion occurs by diffusion down the electrochemical gradient. The oxyntic cell has three different types of receptors for acetylcholine, gastrin, and histamine. Via different intracellular pathways, all three receptors activate the proton pump (H^+K^+-ATPase). The required energy is delivered by reduction of ATP to ADP.

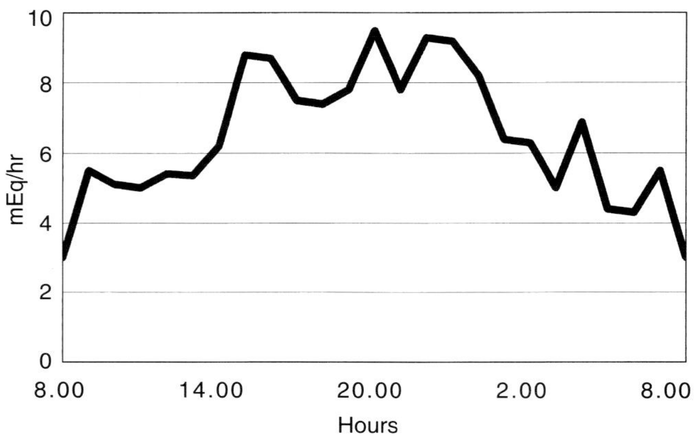

Fig. 14-2. Circadian gastric acid secretion. In the morning hours the acid secretion is at the lowest level. It increases during the afternoon with peak acid secretion occurring in the evening hours.

Mucosal Defense Mechanisms

Gastric mucosal defense is provided by mucous and bicarbonate secretion of the stomach, which serves to create a pH gradient from the acidic gastric lumen to the nearly neutral surface of the mucosa. Mucus is secreted by mucous cells present in all regions of the stomach in response to acetylcholine stimulation and contains protein, glycoproteins, and mucopolysaccharides. It protects the mucosa mechanically and preserves a constant moist milieu for mucosal cells. Gastric mucus also maintains an alkaline environment on the mucosal surface by trapping bicarbonate and acts to protect the normal gastric flora. Local bicarbonate secretion is stimulated by prostaglandins, glucagon, and secretin. Despite the fact that bicarbonate secretion is relatively small compared to acid secretion, its protective potential is maintained by the mucous gel at the mucosal cell surface. Moreover, gastric mucosal cells have a specialized apical surface membrane that resists the diffusion of acid back into the cell. Disruption of this specialized ability to resist acid back-diffusion has been shown to be a prominent mechanism in many types of gastric mucosal injury. Prostaglandins maintain the mucosal blood flow and stimulate the secretion of mucus and bicarbonate. Furthermore, other local factors such as the rapid renewal of mucosal cells and prompt repair after injury are important for mucosal defense. The extensive gastric blood flow quickly removes acid diffused across a compromised mucosa.

Motility and Gastric Emptying

Motility patterns of the stomach are complex. Contractile activities are regulated to produce at least four functions. First, receptive relaxation allows the storage of relatively large volumes with little increase in intragastric pressure. During ingestion of a meal the predominant action of the proximal stomach is one of accommodation. With swallowing, the muscle of the oral stomach relaxes so that the material being swallowed can enter the stomach without causing a significant change in intragastric pressure. This receptive relaxation is so efficient in the human stomach that it can accommodate 2 L of contents with a rise in intragastric pressure of $<$10 mm Hg. Receptive relaxation appears to be mediated by pathways of the vagus nerves.

Second, during digestion, gastric contractions mix the food with gastric secretions and break it down into small particles. The caudal region of the stomach exhibits phasic contractions that begin near the middle of the stomach and propagate toward the duodenum. Each primary contractile event in this region is a peristaltic contraction. In humans contractions occur at a rate of about three per minute, varying only in the depth and force of contraction according to the chemical and physical composition of the intraluminal contents. The peristaltic contraction of the caudal stomach causes fairly complex movements of the intragastric contents. Gastric emptying also occurs during these contractions. The amount, however, depends not only on the force of these contractions but also on the tone of the oral region of the stomach, on the contractile activity of the pylorus, and on the contractile activity of the duodenum.

Third, gastric contractions are coordinated with the pylorus and duodenum so that the gastric contents can be emptied in a regulated manner. Finally, during the interdigestive state, periodic contractions sweep remaining particles into the duodenum. Toward the end of this process, gastric contractions increase in force and depth so that they almost occlude the gastric lumen and tend to propel any remaining undigested particles into the duodenum, leaving the stomach relatively empty. After a burst of such contractions the entire motility pattern of the stomach changes to that characteristic of the fasted state until the next meal is ingested and the pattern begins again.

During the interdigestive period the activity of the stomach exhibits a specific integrated pattern called the migrating motility complex. The digestive burst is followed by a quiescent phase lasting approximately 1 to 2 hours in humans. Gastric contractions then appear and build rapidly to a 10- to 25-minute phase of intense contractions involving most of the stomach. This activity can be separated into three phases: phase I, quiescence; phase II, increasing activity; and phase III, intense contractions (Fig. 14-3). The entire period is referred to as migrating since the activity begins in the stomach and moves down the small bowel. The time between two consecutive phase III periods in many studies equals the time for the complex to reach the terminal ileum. Phase III contractions consist of a series of stripping waves that completely empty the stomach and small bowel. The migrating motility complex phases are probably determined by neural and hormonal influences. Phase I likely results from a lack of input, phase II seems to depend on vagal activity, and phase III depends on hormonal influences. Most studies have been able to correlate phase II activity with peaks in the plasma levels of motilin. Motilin is released during stimulation of the vagus, and it has been postulated that periodic discharges from the central nervous system regulate the migrating motility complex.

The stomach can be divided into two major functional subdivisions, proximal and distal. Proximal gastric muscle exhibits a tonic tone on relaxation during a meal, permitting a large meal to be accommodated with little change in intragastric volume. The distal functional unit includes the antrum and adjoining gastric body. Motor activity in the distal region is more phasic in nature and is organized to produce gas-

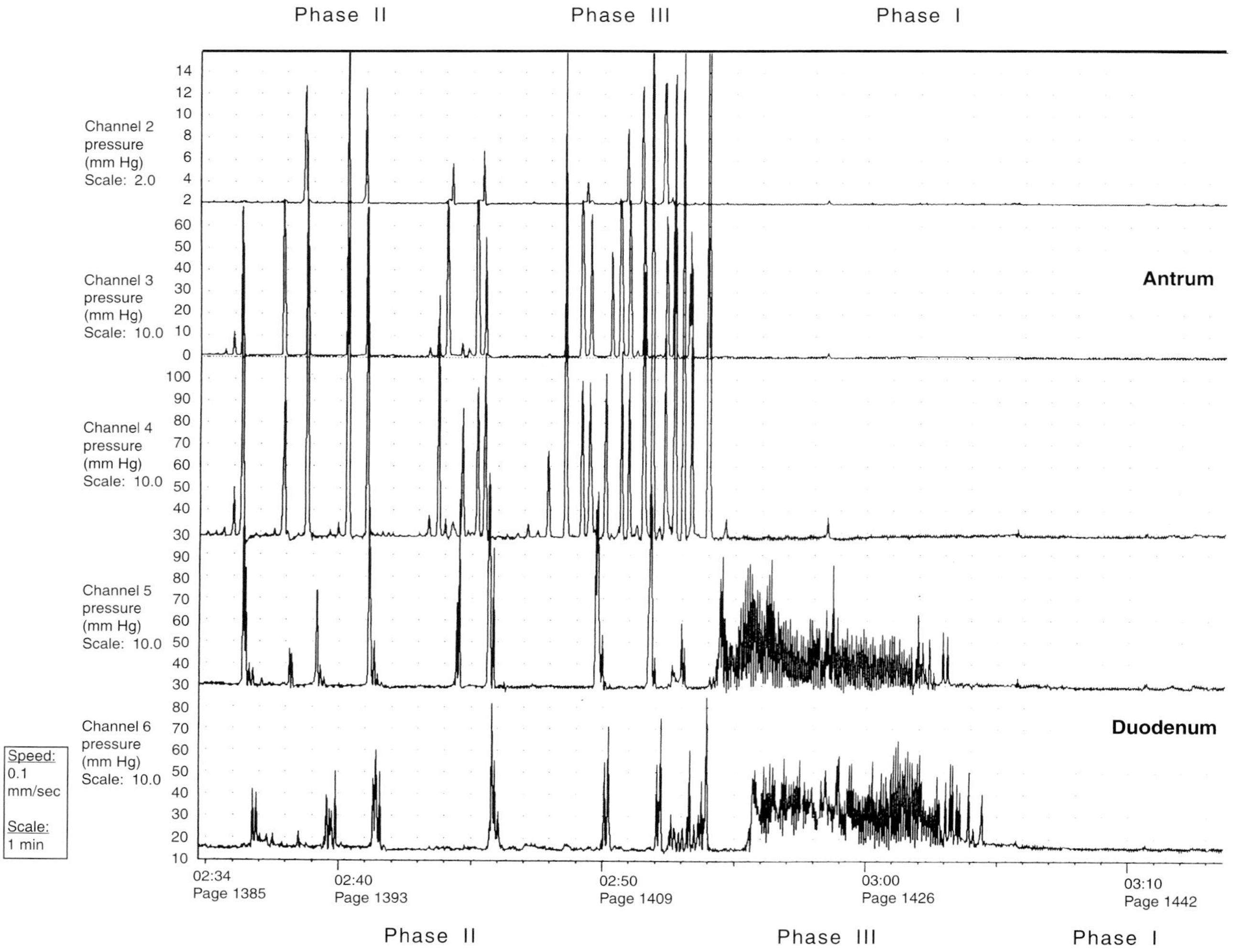

Fig. 14-3. Normal antroduodenal motility pattern during the fasting period. Three different phases of increasing activity produce the complete interdigestive motility cycle. The migration of phase III is generated in the stomach and moves down the duodenum. The duration of the complete cycle is normally 80 to 150 minutes.

tric emptying. Normal gastric function such as gastric emptying is influenced by contractions of both areas.

Smooth muscle cells of the stomach are arranged in three layers, an outer longitudinal layer, a middle circular layer, and an inner oblique layer. No layer completely envelops the entire stomach. The separation into three distinct layers is least obvious in the oral region. The stomach is richly innervated by both intrinsic and extrinsic nerves. The intrinsic nerves lie in various plexuses, the most prominent being the myenteric plexus. Axons from these nerves synapse with the muscle and glandular cells of the stomach.

Many neural and paracrine transmitters have been identified, including acetylcholine, adenosine 5'-triphosphate, enkephalins, norepinephrine, substance P, serotonin, and vasoactive intestinal polypeptide. Most of these substances originate within the enteric nerves, although the fact that vagotomy causes a loss of certain types of nerve endings suggests that the extrinsic nervous system accounts for some. Extrinsically the stomach is innervated by branches of the vagus nerve. Receptors have been identified that discharge in response to antral contractions, distention of the oral region of the stomach, and hot or cold temperatures. Vagal efferent fibers are of two types, cholinergic stimulatory and nonadrenergic inhibitory.

There is a marked difference in the intrinsic behavior of the smooth muscle cells of the two regions of the stomach. Cells of the oral region exhibit spontaneous tone and have no spontaneous fluctuations. Changes occur when nerves in the region are stimulated or certain chemicals are applied. Muscle cells of the distal region generate spontaneous fluctuations and in some respects resemble those seen in conducting tissue of the heart. Muscle cells from this region show an initial rapid depolarization and repolarization followed by a more prolonged depolarization or plateau phase and then repolarization. This entire complex has been called the gastric slow wave. Although action potentials are recorded from muscle cells from all areas of the distal stomach, their frequencies differ. The highest frequencies are recorded from cells of the midstomach near the greater curvature and are referred to as the gastric pacemaker. This gradient in frequency is not seen in the intact stomach. All areas influence each other, resulting in the expression of a single frequency.

Extrinsic nerves exert a major influence on gastric motility. The gastric effects of vagotomy have been studied for years and include decreased gastric contractions, decreased gastric distensibility (compliance), and decreased gastric emptying of solids and semisolids. Most chemicals and procedures that alter gastric motility through an action on the central nervous system act via the extrinsic nervous system.

In vivo all mechanisms are probably acting simultaneously in an integrated manner to produce the various patterns of contractions that occur. The primary unit of contractile activity, the smooth muscle cell, can contract on its own because of the intrinsic behavior of its action potential. In fact, however, this probably never occurs since muscle activity is modulated by at least two other factors, neurotransmitters released from nerve endings of the intrinsic and extrinsic nervous system and circulating and locally released chemicals.

PATHOPHYSIOLOGIC MECHANISMS

The pathophysiologic mechanisms involved in gastric and duodenal ulcers are different and will be discussed separately.

Gastric Ulcer

Four types of gastric ulcers have been described and have different implications for treatment (Fig. 14-4). Type I, the most common and typical gastric ulcer, is located in the proximal antrum, usually on the lesser curve near the incisura. Type II gastric ulcers are those that coexist with duodenal ulceration. Type III, or prepyloric gastric ulcers, behave similar to duodenal ulcers and typically are found in a prepyloric location or inside the pyloric channel.[18] Type IV gastric ulcers occur high in the gastric body near the gastroesophageal junction. Different disturbances of the gastric physiology are associated with each of the four types of gastric ulcers. The pathophysiology of types II and III is similar to duodenal ulceration.

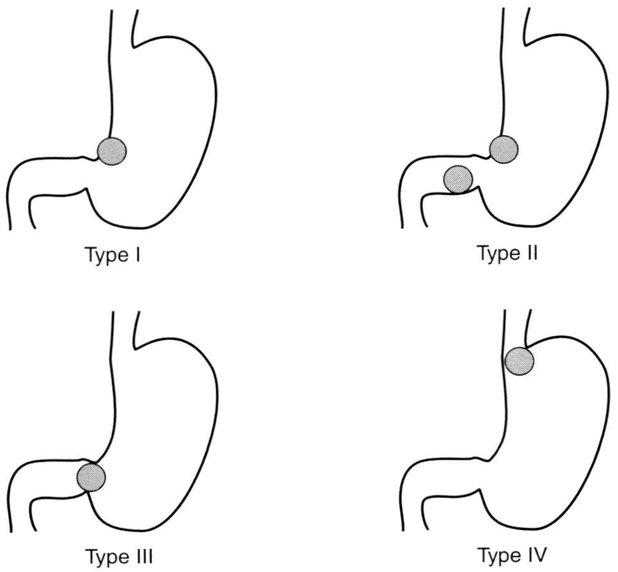

Fig. 14-4. According to their localization, gastric ulcers are classified into four types. Acid hypersecretion is present in types II and III, whereas the classic type I pattern shows normal or hyposecretion.

Acid Secretion. Most patients with gastric ulcers do not have gastric acid hypersecretion.[18] Patients with combined gastric and duodenal ulcer or ulcers in the prepyloric region (types II and III) exhibit findings similar to those with duodenal ulcers and may hypersecrete. Those with more classic lesser curve gastric ulcers have normal or diminished acid secretion. Davenport[23] first hypothesized that hydrogen ion back-diffusion through a damaged mucosal barrier was a cause of diminished acid in patients with classic gastric ulcer disease. Although a few cases of gastric ulcers have been reported in the presence of achlorhydria, it is believed that the presence of some acid-pepsin is required for ulcers to form. Thus it becomes clear that factors other than gastric acid must be involved in the pathophysiology of gastric ulcer in the vast majority of patients.

Impaired Mucosal Defense. Alterations in mucosal defense mechanisms may result from abnormalities of mucous or bicarbonate secretion or from the effects of exogenous agents. No definite defect of mucous composition or secretion has been demonstrated as yet. In contrast, the influence of several injurious agents on the mucosal barrier is well known.

DuPlessis[24] suggested that pathologic duodenogastric reflux may be involved in the development of gastritis, gastric ulcers, and posttraumatic stress ulceration. Bile salts act as detergents that disrupt the normal barrier function of the mucosa. Ritchie[25] has demonstrated that the combination of bile salts and gastric acid promotes severe gastric mucosal injury. Ethanol, cigarette smoking, and medications also weaken the mucosal barrier. Aspirin, corticosteroids, and nonsteroidal anti-inflammatory drugs are known to cause medication-induced injury. All inhibit cyclooxygenase, resulting in decreased mucosal prostaglandin synthesis and impaired mucosal defense. Damage is caused by back-diffusion of hydrogen ions, which produces histamine release, vasodilation, and finally bleeding. Chronic nonsteroidal anti-inflammatory drug use is associated with the development of mucosal ulceration in up to 20% of patients,

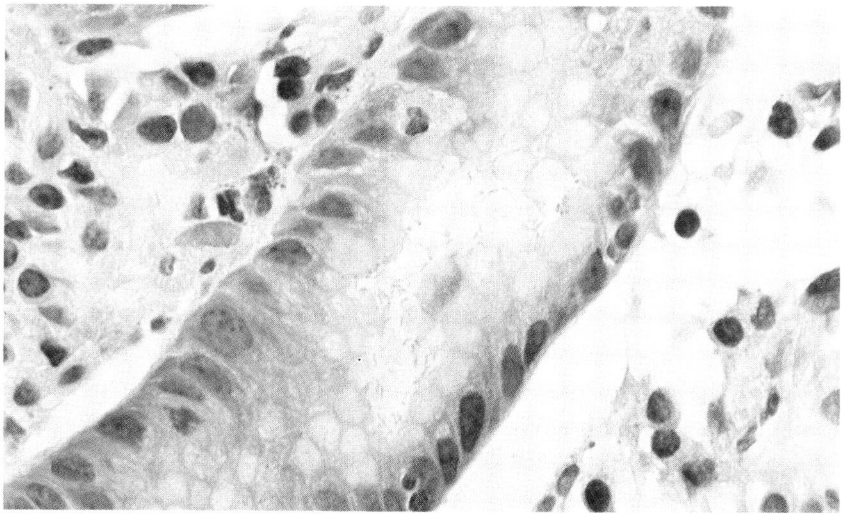

Fig. 14-5. Histologic section of mucous gland from the antrum shows large numbers of *Helicobacter pylori* in the lumen.

and they are more likely to experience serious complications such as hemorrhage or perforation than matched controls. Cigarette smoking is also known to impair healing and to promote recurrence of peptic ulcers. Hemorrhagic shock, decreased blood flow with mucosal ischemia, and endotoxemia probably act through similar mechanisms, allowing hydrogen ion back-diffusion. Combinations of these defense-impairing factors with hyperacidity and bile salts cause even more severe injury.[26]

Gastric Emptying and Antroduodenal Motility. Dragstedt[27] and Dragstedt and Woodward[28] first introduced the concept that delayed gastric emptying may be involved in the pathogenesis of gastric ulcers. Delay is caused by incomplete obstruction of the pyloroduodenal region or possibly antroduodenal dysmotility, with stasis causing reactive hypergastrinemia and acid hypersecretion. This theory would explain type II gastric ulcers. However, a large number of gastric ulcer patients have normal gastric emptying. Abnormal antroduodenal motility together with pyloric malfunction may also provide the mechanical basis for duodenogastric reflux. Increased duodenogastric reflux exposes the gastric mucosa to bile salts (particularly deoxycholate and taurocholate), lysolecithin, and pancreatic secretions.

Helicobacter pylori. *Helicobacter pylori* (Fig. 14-5) has been implicated as a major causative factor in the development of gastritis as well as the development of duodenal ulcers. Its association with gastric ulcers is less clear cut.[29] Although *Helicobacter pylori* infection does not appear to promote gastric ulcers in itself, the possibility of interactions with other pathogenetic factors must be considered. An interaction between *Helicobacter pylori* and other factors has not been confirmed. Studies have shown no significant difference in *Helicobacter pylori* prevalence in nonsteroidal anti-inflammatory drug users and nonusers, although there was a tendency toward lower infection rates in patients taking nonsteroidal anti-inflammatory drugs.[30] More severe mucosal inflammation, however, was found in *Helicobacter pylori*–positive gastric ulcer patients than in those without *Helicobacter pylori* infection.[31] The fact that gastric ulcers rarely occur in the large group of *Helicobacter pylori*–positive individuals but occur in 15% of nonsteroidal anti-inflammatory drug users suggests that *Helicobacter pylori* is of minor importance in the pathophysiology of gastric ulceration. Well-designed studies specifically addressing this problem are not currently available.

• • •

In summary, pathophysiologic events influencing the development of gastric ulcers in the presence of normal to decreased acid secretion include chemical or infectious damage of the mucosal defense resulting in chronic gastritis, mucosal barrier disruption, mucosal ischemia, and impaired mucous and bicarbonate secretion. These events are likely aggravated by the presence of gastric motility abnormalities manifested by delayed gastric emptying or pathologic duodenogastric reflux.

Duodenal Ulcer

Acid Secretion. Gastric acid hypersecretion resulting from an increased mass of acid-secreting mucosa or vagal hyperactivity is found in most patients with duodenal ulcers. Genetic determinants as well as acquired mechanisms that result in an increased release of gastrin and histamine are thought to be the basis for acid hypersecretion. Patterns of hypersecretion include increased peak secretion, prolonged response to stimuli, and elevated basal secretion. Increases in both basal and postprandial gastrin production may also influence the pattern of acid secretion. The prototype of this mechanism is Zollinger-Ellison syndrome. The fact that not all patients with Zollinger-Ellison syndrome develop a duodenal ulcer suggests that factors in addition to gastric acid hypersecretion are involved in the pathophysiology of duodenal ulcer.

Impaired Mucosal Defense. Microcirculatory ischemia, altered mucous secretion, and disturbed prostaglandin metabolism weaken mucosal resistance and seem to be an important element in ulcer formation. This is particularly true in patients without acid hypersecretion.[24] Disturbed prostaglandin metabolism results in diminished gastric and duodenal production of bicarbonate, leading to a high acid concentration in the duodenal bulb. The fact that recurrent ulcers commonly form at the same site suggests the possibility of locally impaired microcirculation and disturbed mucous secretion in the region. Cytokines and growth factors also contribute to mucosal defense, although their precise role is not yet clear.[25]

Gastric Emptying and Antroduodenal Motility. Rapid gastric emptying is present in many patients with duodenal ulcer disease. In this setting, gastric acid and pepsin are not sufficiently neutralized by gastric chyme and their premature entrance into the duodenum may result in duodenal hyperacidity and duodenal ulcer.[19] Other features of antroduodenal dysmotility such as increased postprandial retroperistalsis, reduction of pressure waves, atypical coordination, and decreased frequency and duration of phase III activity have been described by Kerrigan et al.[32] and Bortolotti et al.[33] in patients with active and healed duodenal ulcers. These motility factors may also lead to impaired acid clearance from the duodenal bulb and promotion of mucosal damage.

Helicobacter pylori. The recent discovery of *Helicobacter pylori* infection has significantly advanced our understanding of the physiopathology of peptic ulcer disease. *Helicobacter pylori* is a gram-negative, flagellated rod found in the antrum of more than 95% of patients with duodenal ulcer as well as in most patients with gastric ulcers that are not associated with nonsteroidal anti-inflammatory drugs.[34-36] The organism does not appear to invade the antral mucosa but does initiate an inflammatory response readily documented histologically in a high percentage of patients with duodenal ulcers. A clear-cut causal relationship such as for *Helicobacter pylori* and type B gastritis has not yet been demonstrated for *Helicobacter pylori* and duodenal ulcer disease. It is generally accepted that *Helicobacter pylori* plays an important role in the genesis of duodenal ulcer disease.

In addition to microbial gastroduodenitis, many other disease modifiers such as the acid-pepsin secretory potential, smoking, and genetic and environmental factors clearly play a role. The complex interplay of these factors might explain why only a small proportion of infected persons ever develop peptic ulcer disease, even though 50% to 75% of the asymptomatic general population is infected with *Helicobacter pylori*.[37] Thus we can reasonably deduce that *Helicobacter pylori* acts as a cofactor in the genesis of gastroduodenal ulcer disease.[38]

Helicobacter pylori infection is linked to hyperacidity, although it is not clear whether acid hypersecretion promotes the infection or is a consequence of it.[39] Fasting gastrin levels are generally normal in *Helicobacter pylori*–infected patients, although an exaggerated postprandial gastrin release appears to be linked to *Helicobacter pylori* and inflammation.[40,41] *Helicobacter pylori* infection seems to result in an interruption of the physiologic mechanisms responsible for gastrin–hydrochloric acid homeostasis.

• • •

In summary, pathophysiologic events influencing the development of duodenal ulcers include increased basal and stimulated acid secretion, decreased secretory inhibition, and increased secretion of tropic hormones. Motility disorders, rapid gastric emptying, mucosal defense alterations, and *Helicobacter pylori* infection act in concert with gastric acid to cause ulceration.

DIAGNOSTIC APPROACH TO PEPTIC ULCER DISEASE

The multifactorial nature of peptic ulcer disease makes a complete diagnostic approach essential. Radiographic or endoscopic verification of the location of the ulcer may suggest its possible pathogenesis, particularly in the case of gastric ulcers. Histologic examination is mandatory to identify the occasional neoplasm presenting as an ulcer.

The presence of *Helicobacter pylori* infection should be established. The *Campylobacter*-like organism urease test and histologic examination are commonly used for this purpose. Gastric analysis of secretion by aspiration of gastric juice and calculation of basal and maximal acid output is widely used to analyze the patient's secretory status.[42] The clinical value of gastric acid analysis is, however, limited by the short study period and the overlap in secretion rates of healthy persons and patients with gastroduodenal ulcer diseases.[43] Therapeutic decisions can be made only in the event of markedly increased acid secretion, such as patients with Zollinger-Ellison syndrome or antral hyperplasia. Ambulatory 24-hour pH monitoring may allow more sensitive discrimination between the normal and pathologic state. Typical 24-hour pH patterns have been described for different ulcer types and may also suggest delayed gastric emptying and duodenogastric reflux[44] (Fig. 14-6). If the clinical presentation and

A

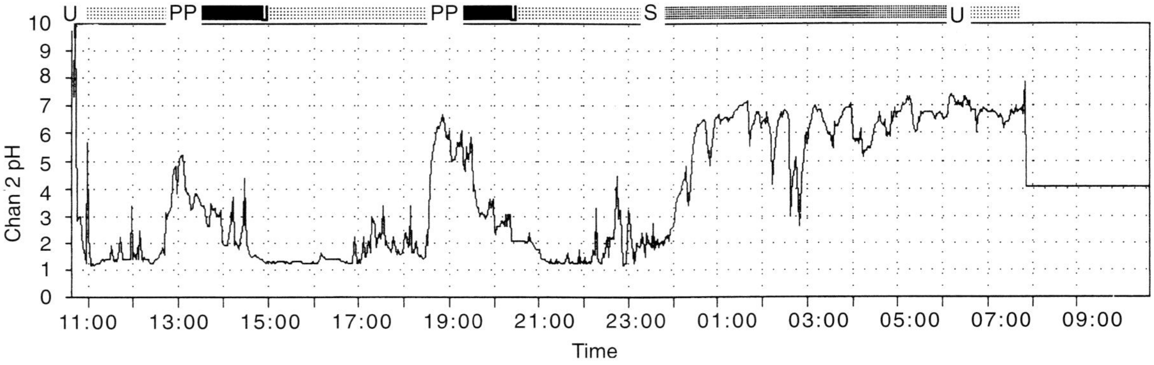

B

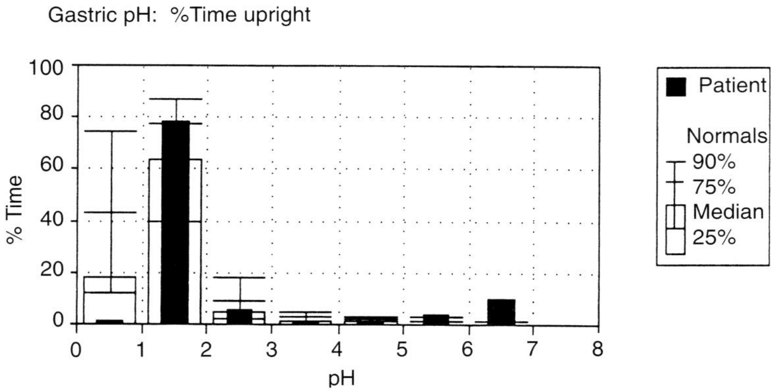

Range	Min	Max	Patient
0-1	0.0	93.5	0.9
1-2	4.8	98.9	78.7
2-3	0.0	50.0	5.5
3-4	0.0	6.5	0.5
4-5	0.0	5.5	0.5
5-6	0.0	3.6	3.7
6-7	0.0	13.7	10.1
7-8	0.0	3.7	0.1

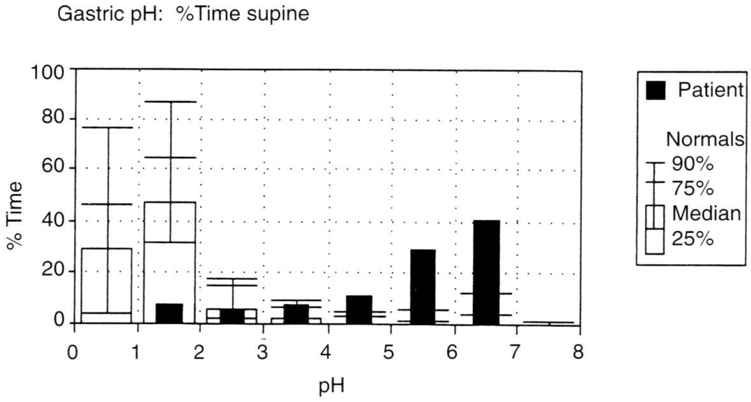

Range	Min	Max	Patient
0-1	0.0	89.9	0.0
1-2	10.1	97.9	6.8
2-3	0.0	20.5	5.6
3- 4	0.0	10.3	7.2
4-5	0.0	5.7	11.2
5-6	0.0	6.3	28.6
6-7	0.0	32.7	40.3
7-8	0.0	36.6	0.2

Fig. 14-6. Gastric 24-hour pH metry with computerized analysis. **A,** The original tracing with postprandial, upright, and supine phases marked. Note the normal alkalinization during the postprandial phases and the pathologic alkalinization during the supine time, starting at 0:300 A.M. **B,** The computerized analysis shows the % time spent in each pH interval for the upright and the supine periods. The white bars indicate the median of normal and the lines the 75th and 95th percentile of normal. The black bars indicate the patient's result. There is a right shift of pH in both periods, but it is more evident in the supine phase.

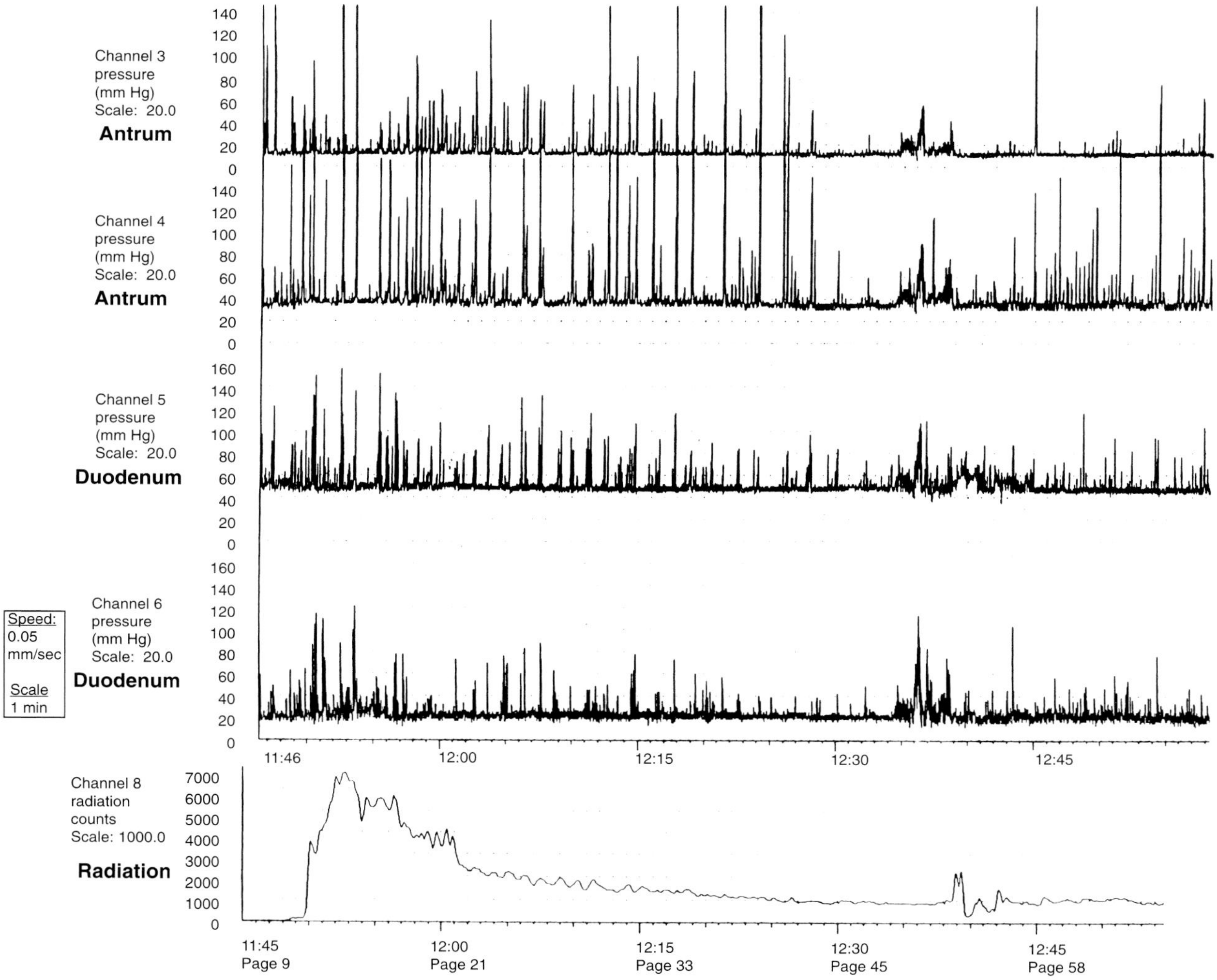

Fig. 14-7. Postprandial antroduodenal motility study with simultaneous scintigraphic gastric emptying study, both performed in ambulatory patients with internal electronic probes. The test meal (scrambled egg labeled with 1 mCi technetium 99m) provokes the conversion of the motility to a fed pattern (compare with Fig. 14-3 showing the fasting pattern), which exhibits strong antral and duodenal contractions. One hour after the meal less than 20% of the initial activity is left in the stomach. The spasmlike contractions between 12:35 and 12:40 P.M. are followed by a short increase of radiation, indicating a chyme movement in the orad direction.

the gastric pH pattern imply a gastric motility disorder, a gastric emptying scan should be performed. Antroduodenal motility studies may provide additional information, especially in a simultaneous setup with the gastric emptying scan (Fig. 14-7). However, the interpretation of those studies is not yet standardized. Detection of pathologic duodenogastric reflux is also possible with the recently introduced bile probe that can detect the presence of bilirubin via a fiberoptic probe in the stomach (Fig. 14-8).

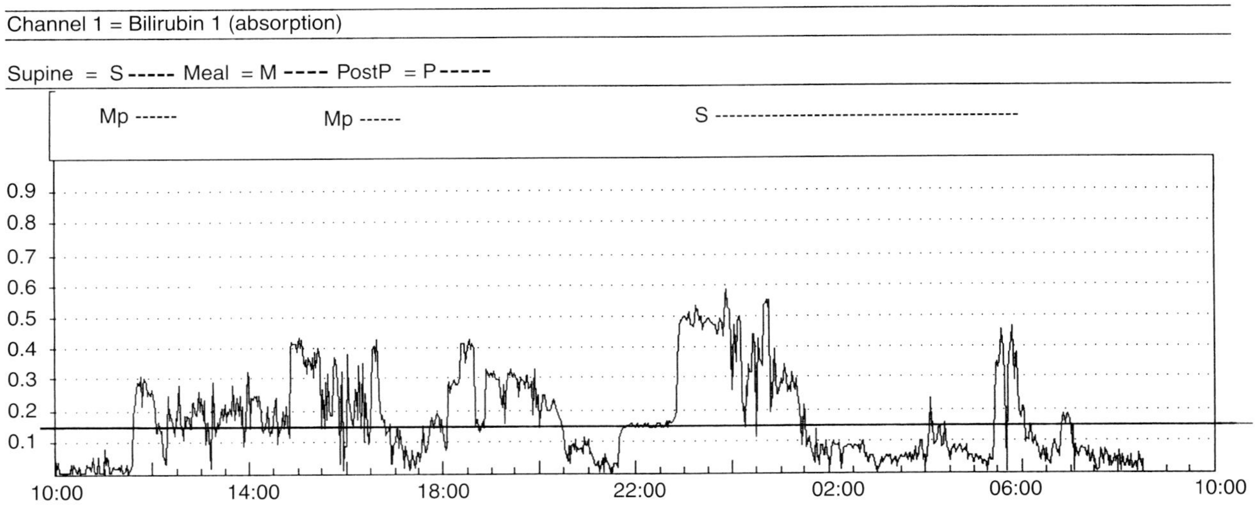

Fig. 14-8. Intragastric measurement of bilirubin with fiberoptic bile probe (absorption above 0.14). Meals and supine times are indicated. The example shows increased bile exposure of the mucosa during the upright period and during the first 3 hours of the supine period.

MEDICAL TREATMENT

Ideally the treatment of peptic ulcer disease should be individualized according to the underlying pathophysiologic cause. Relapse rates after short-term therapy with H_2 blockers are as high as 90%. Complications such as bleeding, stenosis, or perforations occur in 3% to 6% of patients within the first 6 weeks of therapy.[17] Continuous H_2-blocker therapy decreases the recurrence rate, but 20% of patients still have a recurrence within 18 months.[45,46] Proton pump blocker therapy improves these results, but long-term use remains controversial. Unless *Helicobacter pylori* infection is addressed, ulcers rapidly recur when therapy is stopped, reflecting the noncurative nature of antisecretory therapy. For this reason medical therapy should not only focus on acid reduction but also address the *Helicobacter pylori* infection. Eradication of the infection is most effective with so-called triple therapy that includes colloidal bismuth subcitrate, tetracycline, and metronidazole in concert with antisecretory agents. More recently a combination of omeprazole and amoxicillin has been found to be effective, although not in all cases. Ulcer recurrence drops to 6% to 10% 1 year after eradication of *Helicobacter pylori*. Recrudescence rates are largely unknown but will play a role in long-term efficacy.[47,48]

REFERENCES

1. Galen L. On the Usefulness of the Parts of the Body. (Translated by MT May.) New York: Cornell University Press, 1968, p 32.
2. Garrison F. History of Medicine, 4th ed. Philadelphia: WB Saunders, 1929.
3. Holmes FL. Claude Bernard and Animal Chemistry. Cambridge, Mass.: Harvard University Press, 1974, pp 140-159.
4. Prout W. On the nature of the acid and saline matters usually existing in the stomach of animals. Philos Trans R Soc Lond 1:45-49, 1824.

5. Beaumont W. Experiments and observations on the gastric juice and the physiology of digestion. Plattsburg, N.Y.: FP Allen, 1883.
6. Schwarz C. Über penetrierende Magen- und Jejunalgeschwüre. Beitr Klin Chir 67:96-128, 1910.
7. Babkin BP. Pavlov, a Biography. Chicago: The University of Chicago Press, 1949, pp 217-269.
8. McCrea ED. The nerves of the stomach and their relation to surgery. Br J Surg 13:612-648, 1925.
9. Dragstedt LR, Oberhelman HH, Smith CA. Experimental hyperfunction of the gastric antrum with ulcer formation. Ann Surg 134:332-345, 1951.
10. Klein E. Left vagus section and partial gastrectomy for duodenal ulcer. Ann Surg 90:65-68, 1929.
11. Berg A. The mortality and late results of subtotal gastrectomy for the radical cure of gastric and duodenal ulcer. Ann Surg 92:340-346, 1930.
12. Dragstedt LR. Contributions to the physiology of the stomach: Gastric juice in the duodenum and gastric ulcers. JAMA 68:330-333, 1917.
13. Dragstedt LR. Vagotomy for gastroduodenal ulcer. Ann Surg 122:973-989, 1945.
14. Donahue P, Yoshida J, Polley E, et al. Preganglionic vagus nerve fibers also enter the greater curvature of the stomach in rats and ferrets. Gastroenterology 94:1292-1299, 1988.
15. Uvnas-Moberg K, Jarhult J, Alino S. Neurogenic control of release of gastrin and somatostatin. Scand J Gastroenterol 19 (Suppl 89):131-136, 1984.
16. Marshall B, Warren JR. Unidentified curved bacillus on gastric epithelium in active chronic gastritis. Lancet 1:1273-1275, 1983.
17. Andersen D, Amdrup E, Hostrup H, et al. Surgery of cimetidine? Comparison of two plans of treatment: Operation or cimetidine given as a low maintenance dose. World J Surg 7:378-384, 1983.
18. Johnson HD. Gastric ulcer: Classification, blood group characteristics, secretion patterns and pathogenesis. Ann Surg 162:996-1004, 1964.
19. Malagelada JR, Longstreth GF, Deering TB, et al. Gastric secretion and emptying after ordinary meals in duodenal ulcer. Gastroenterology 73:989-994, 1977.
20. Richardson CT, Walsh JH, Hicks MI, et al. Studies in the mechanisms of food stimulated gastric acid secretion in normal human subjects. J Clin Invest 58:623-629, 1976.
21. Grossman MI. Secretion of acid and pepsin in response to the distension of vagally innervated fundic gland area in dogs. Gastroenterology 41:718, 1962.
22. Moore JG, Englert E. Circadian rhythm of gastric acid secretion in man. Nature 226:1261-1262, 1970.
23. Davenport HW. Destruction of the gastric mucosal barrier by detergents and urea. Gastroenterology 54:175-181, 1968.
24. DuPlessis DJ. Pathogenesis of gastric ulceration. Lancet 1:974, 1965.
25. Ritchie WP. Alkaline reflux gastritis: Late results on controlled clinical trial of diagnosis and treatment. Ann Surg 203:537-544, 1986.
26. Ritchie WP. Acute gastric mucosal damage produced by bile salts, acid, and ischemia. Gastroenterology 68:699-705, 1975.
27. Dragstedt LR. Pathogenesis of gastroduodenal ulcer. Arch Surg 44:438-451, 1942.
28. Dragstedt LR, Woodward ER. Gastric stasis a cause of gastric ulcers. Scand J Gastroenterol [Suppl] 6:243-252, 1970.
29. Isenberg J, McQuaid KR, Laine L, et al. Diseases of the stomach and duodenum: *Helicobacter pylori*, peptic ulcer disease, and gastritis. In Yamaha T, ed. Textbook of Gastroenterology. Philadelphia: JB Lippincott, 1991, p 1241.
30. Graham DY, Lidsky MD, Cox AM, et al. Long-term nonsteroidal anti-inflammatory drug use and *Helicobacter pylori* infection. Gastroenterology 100:1653-1657, 1991.
31. Laine L, Marin Sorensen M, Weinstein WM. *Helicobacter pylori* (HP) prevalence and mucosal injury in gastric ulcers: Relationship to chronic nonsteroidal anti-inflammatory drugs ingestion. Gastroenterology 100:A103, 1991.
32. Kerrigan DD, Read NW, Houghton LA, et al. Disturbed gastroduodenal motility in patients with active and healed duodenal ulceration. Gastroenterology 100:892-900, 1991.
33. Bortolotti M, Pinotti R, Sarti P, et al. Interdigestive gastroduodenal motility in patients with active and inactive duodenal ulcer disease. Digestion 44:95-100, 1989.
34. Börsch GMA, Graham DY. *Helicobacter pylori*. In Collen MJ, Benjamin SB, eds. Handbook of Experimental Pharmacology, vol 99. Pharmacology of Peptic Ulcer Disease. Berlin: Springer Verlag, 1991, pp 107-147.
35. Graham DY. *Campylobacter pylori* and peptic ulcer disease. Gastroenterology 96:615-625, 1989.

36. Tytgat GNJ, Axon ATR, Dixon MF, et al. *Helicobacter pylori*, causal agent in peptic ulcer disease? In Working Party Report of the World Congresses of Gastroenterology. Oxford: Blackwell Scientific, 1990, pp 36-45.
37. Dooley CP, Fitzgibbons P, Cohen H, et al. Prevalence and distribution of *Campylobacter pylori* in an asymptomatic population. Gastroenterology 94:A102, 1988.
38. Isenberg JI, Selloing JA, Hogan DL, et al. Impaired proximal duodenal mucosal bicarbonate secretion in patients with duodenal ulcer. N Engl J Med 316:374-379, 1987.
39. Graham DY, Opekum A, Lew GM, et al. Ablation of exaggerated meal-stimulated gastrin release in duodenal ulcer patients after clearance of *Helicobacter* (*Campylobacter*) *pylori* infection. Am J Gastroenterol 95:394-398, 1990.
40. Levi S, Beardshell K, Haddad G, et al. *Campylobacter pylori* and duodenal ulcers, the gastrin link. Lancet 1:1167-1168, 1989.
41. Graham DY, Opekum A, Lew GM, et al. *Helicobacter pylori*–associated exaggerated gastrin release in duodenal ulcer patients. Gastroenterology 100:1571-1575, 1991.
42. Wormsley KG, Grossmann MI. Maximal histalog test in control subjects and patients with peptic ulcer. Gut 6:427-435, 1965.
43. Fuchs KH, Selch A, Freys SM, et al. Gastric acid secretion and gastric pH measurement in peptic ulcer disease. Probl Gen Surg 9:138-151, 1992.
44. Fuchs KH, Heimbucher J, DeMeester TR, et al. The role of 24-hour gastric pH monitoring in gastroduodenal ulcer disease. Paper presented at Digestive Disease Week, San Francisco, May 9-15, 1992.
45. Murray WR, Cooper G, Laferla G, et al. Maintenance ranitidine treatment after hemorrhage from a duodenal ulcer. A 3-year study. Scand J Gastroenterol 23:183-187, 1988.
46. Hentschel E, Brandstätter G, Judmaier G, et al. Dreijährige Langzeittherapie des rezidivierenden Ulcus duodeni mit 400 mg Cimetidin nocte. Wien Med Wochenschr 9:184-187, 1987.
47. Brunner G, Creutzfeld W, Harke U, et al. Therapy with omeprazole in patients with peptic ulcerations resistant to extended high-dose ranitidine treatment. Digestion 39:80-90, 1988.
48. Bayerdörfer E, Mannes GA, Sommer A, et al. Long-term follow-up after eradication of *Helicobacter pylori* with a combination of omeprazole and amoxicillin. Scand J Gastroenterol 28 [Suppl 196]:19-25, 1993.
49. Dragstedt LR. Section of the vagus nerves to the stomach in the treatment of peptic ulcer. Ann Surg 126:687-708, 1947.
50. Burge HW, Hutchinson JSF, Longland CJ, et al. Selective nerve section in the prevention of postvagotomy diarrhea. Lancet 1:577-581, 1964.
51. Sawyers JL, Herrington JL, Burney DP. Proximal gastric vagotomy compared with vagotomy and antrectomy and selective gastric vagotomy and pyloroplasty. Ann Surg 186:510-517, 1977.
52. Johnston D, Humphrey CS, Smith RB, et al. Should the gastric antrum be vagally denervated if it is well drained and in the acid stream? Br J Surg 58:725-729, 1977.
53. Johnston D. Operative mortality and postoperative morbidity of highly selective vagotomy. Br Med J 4:545-547, 1975.
54. Taylor TV, Gunn AA, MacLeod DAD, et al. Morbidity and mortality after anterior lesser curve seromyotomy and posterior truncal vagotomy for duodenal ulcer. Br J Surg 72:950-951, 1985.
55. Oostvogel HJM, Van Vroonhoven TJMV. Anterior seromyotomy and posterior truncal vagotomy. Technic and early results of a randomized trial. Neth J Surg 37:69-74, 1985.

Chapter

15

Minimally Invasive Approaches to Ulcer Therapy

Namir Katkhouda, M.D. • Jean Mouiel, M.D.

The pathogenesis of duodenal ulcer, a multifactorial disease, is very complex. Schwartz's aphorism coined at the beginning of the century, "No acid, no ulcer," is being replaced with Graham's dictum, "No *Helicobacter pylori*, no ulcer."[1] Although no study has demonstrated an immediate cause-and-effect relationship, *Helicobacter pylori* is always seen in association with antral gastritis and is commonly associated with duodenal ulcer. All studies point to a strong association between this organism and ulcer disease.[1-4]

The ideal treatment for chronic duodenal ulcer continues to elude us. Therapy with proton pump blockers is controversial and has not been approved for long-term use. Triple antibiotic therapy, proposed more recently to eradicate *Helicobacter pylori*, contains bismuth, which may have a cicatrizational effect on gastric mucosa. Recent studies show reinfection rates of between 6% and 10% 1 year after the initial treatment.[3-5] Nor do we know the prevalence of *Helicobacter pylori* in the general population as compared with ulcer patients. Thus the treatment of ulcers remains to be standardized. Medical treatment produces side effects. Carcinoid tumors have been demonstrated in the rat after long-term administration of proton pump blockers, and pseudomembranous colitis may be related to triple antibiotic therapy.

Taylor et al.[6] from Great Britain have shown that despite improvements in medical therapy the mortality rate associated with peptic ulcer disease has been stable or increasing slightly, with an incidence of 4500 cases a year. A comparison of surgical and medical treatment is necessary to put the issue into perspective. Since its introduction in Leeds in 1970 by David Johnson, highly selective vagotomy has been considered the treatment of choice for elective ulcer surgery.[7]

Bilateral truncal vagotomy and antrectomy for ulcer disease has the lowest recurrence rate (1.2%), but the associated mortality and morbidity are higher. We believe gastric resection should not be performed for a benign disease such as duodenal ulcers. Highly selective vagotomy offered the promise of an improved technique for ulcer therapy without the side effects of truncal vagotomy. The recurrence rate in the hands of expert surgeons was low, 2% to 10% at 5 to 10 years. Hoffman et al.[8] reported recurrence rates of almost 20% to 40%. The success of this operation is directly related to the skill of the performing surgeon. Johnson warned that recurrence rates would be unacceptably high if this operation were performed by the occasional ulcer surgeon.

Our operation of choice is posterior truncal vagotomy and anterior seromyotomy because it offers the same benefits as bilateral truncal vagotomy without its side effects. The procedure is not as tedious as highly selective vagotomy, making the results less dependent on surgical virtuosity. It was first described by Taylor et al.[9] in 1982 and was performed laparoscopically for the first time in Nice in 1989. Historically, it was among the first advanced laparoscopic procedures.[10-13]

The principles of the operation are based on the anatomic studies of Latarjet, which showed that the secretory vagal nerves originating from the anterior and posterior gastric nerves course through the superficial seromuscular layer of the stomach before penetrating the gastric wall beyond the vascular pedicles. Division of the seromuscular layer, sparing the inner mucosa, interrupts these secretory branches. It has been established experimentally that seromyotomy should be performed precisely 1.5 cm from and parallel to the lesser curvature. In his original technique described in 1979, Taylor[14] advocated incision of the seromuscular layer of both the anterior and posterior aspects of the stomach beginning at the angle of His and coursing to the incisura angularis. This, in effect, corresponds to a fundic denervation. In 1982 he proposed replacing the posterior seromyotomy with posterior truncal vagotomy, as Hill and Barker[15] had advocated in 1978 for a modified highly selective vagotomy. Complete division of the posterior vagus nerve ensures total denervation of the posterior vagal territory with no secondary effects on the pancreas or digestive tract, as shown by Burge et al.[16] This means that there is no postoperative diarrhea and that antropyloric motility is preserved.[6,17]

Because anterior seromyotomy preserves the antropyloric branches of Latarjet's nerve, adequate motility of the antropyloric pump is maintained and pyloric spasm is prevented. This ensures normal physiologic emptying of the stomach and obviates the need for associated drainage procedures. Experimentally, Daniel and Sarna[18] showed that preservation of the antropyloric branches of Latarjet's nerve in the dog ensured adequate gastric emptying through vagovagal arcs. The results of the operation are the same as for open surgery.[6,9,19,20]

Indications and Patient Selection

In general, preoperative evaluation of patients with chronic duodenal ulcer disease is similar to that for laparoscopic cholecystectomy. In the elective setting, surgical intervention for duodenal ulcer disease is indicated in:

1. Patients in whom the disease is resistant to medical treatment despite medical therapy for at least 2 years and/or two or more documented recurrences after thorough medical treatment
2. Patients who cannot be followed regularly because of geographic or socioeconomic reasons or who cannot afford medication
3. Patients with complications such as perforation or hemorrhage

Taylor's Operative Procedure

Preoperative Preparation

As in elective open surgery, preoperative evaluation of the patient's general medical status, operative risk factors, and endoscopic and secretory investigation of the peptic ulcer diathesis are important. Endoscopy documents the ulcer typically seen as a linear defect without associated stenosis or hemorrhage. Secretory tests include measurement of basal acid output and peak acid output after stimulation with pentagastrin. These tests are necessary to evaluate the degree of acid hypersecretion in patients who are intractable to medical treatment. They are also useful for documenting a postoperative reduction of acid output. The serum gastrin level should always be assessed to exclude gastrinoma.

General Considerations and Patient Positioning

As in traditional open surgery, general anesthesia and endotracheal intubation are used. The techniques for establishing and maintaining pneumoperitoneum, performing aspiration and lavage, and using electrocautery are the same as for other forms of laparoscopic surgery. We will discuss only the details specific to laparoscopic vagotomy.

The patient is positioned in much the same way as for open cholecystectomy. The trunk is elevated 15 degrees. Since lateral (left or right) tilting (also 15 degrees) of the patient is necessary, a pillow roll or a bolster (10 cm) should be available for this purpose. The operating surgeon stands between the legs of the patient; the scrub nurse and first assistant are on the left and the second assistant (camera assistant) is on the right of the patient. The video endoscopic system with irrigation/suction is placed on the left, and a second monitor is placed on the right. Electrocautery Systems (Valleylab, Boulder, Colo.) complete the operating room units.

Instrumentation

In addition to standard laparoscopic instruments, we recommend the following:

An L-shaped hook coagulator/dissector with a canal for evacuation of smoke (Karl Storz, Tuttlingen, Germany)
Clip appliers (Ethicon Endo-Surgery, Cincinnati, Ohio)
2 needle holders (Karl Storz)
Absorbable monofilament sutures with 2 cm straight needles (Ethicon)
Endoloops with preformed Roeder knot (Ethibinder)
Application systems for laser coagulation and fibrin sealant spray (Karl Storz)

Port Placement (Fig. 15-1)

Once the pneumoperitoneum has been established, the first trocar to be inserted is the video laparoscopic 11 mm port introduced approximately one third of the distance between the umbilicus and the xiphoid process. Four other 10 to 12 mm trocars are then inserted under visual control. These 10 mm ports allow the position of the scope to be changed if necessary. Port sites are closed at the end of the operation, including fascial closure for the 10 and 11 mm trocars.

Exploration and Hemostasis

The abdominal cavity is explored as soon as the video laparoscope is inserted. The surgeon should be certain that the operation is feasible and that the liver can be retracted so that the operative area is visible. Associated lesions amenable to laparo-

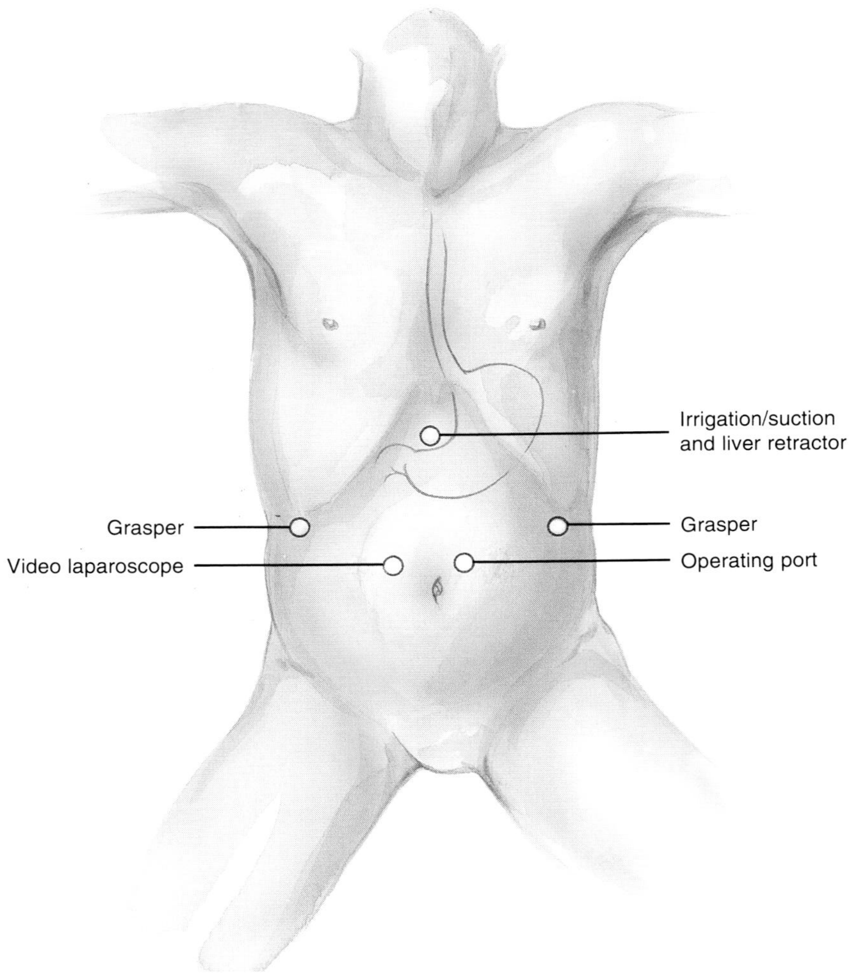

Fig. 15-1. Trocar placement.

scopic surgery are noted (adhesions, appendicitis, cholecystitis, and biliary cysts). Should problems arise, conversion to open surgery is indicated. This situation was not encountered in our practice. The patient should be informed of this possibility beforehand.

A variety of methods may be used to ensure hemostasis:

1. The hook coagulator is used with monopolar current to coagulate small-caliber vessels safely. Electrical scissors are used for most of the dissection.
2. The Nd:YAG laser, if available, coagulates superficial surfaces by contact fiber.
3. Titanium clips are used for gastric vessels.
4. Suture ligation with a 15 cm long 3-0 monofilament suture ensures hemostasis.

All types of knots (flat, double, and Roeder) may be used. The Endoloop is required only occasionally in this operation. Running sutures may also be used. The

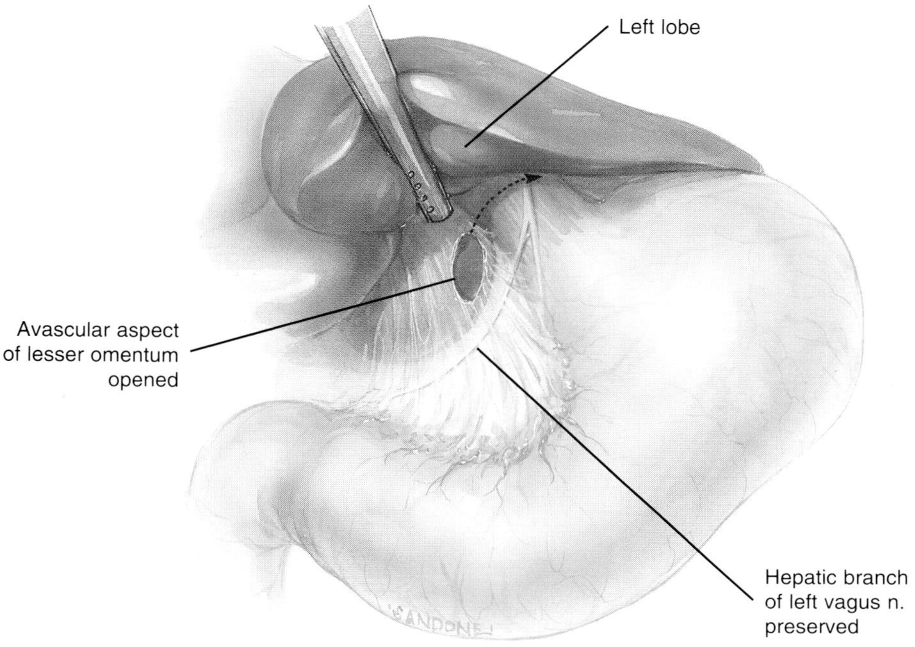

Fig. 15-2. Lateral approach to the hiatus.

suture may be stopped with a knot secured by a clip (Laprotic, Ethicon) if knot tying represents a difficulty.

Hiatal Dissection (Fig. 15-2)

The left lobe of the liver is retracted with the subxiphoid probe. The lesser sac is entered through an opening in the pars flaccida. This avascular area is always recognizable even in obese patients. Areolar tissues are carried to the hook coagulator/dissector with two angulated graspers. Dissection is continued until the muscular portion of the right crus is reached. If left gastric veins are encountered, they may be divided between clips as necessary. Although it is not proved that division will result in clinically significant postoperative complications, injury of the hepatic branch of the vagus nerve should be avoided if possible.

Posterior Truncal Vagotomy (Fig. 15-3)

The two major landmarks for posterior truncal vagotomy are the *caudate lobe* and the *right crus*. They should be grasped with the right-sided forceps and held to the right while the coagulator/dissector hook is used to open the pre-esophageal peritoneum. The abdominal esophagus is retracted to the left, allowing visualization of the areolar tissue. The posterior vagus nerve, easily recognized by its white color, can then be identified. With gentle traction on the nerve, adhesions are coagulated and divided and the nerve transsected between two clips. A segment of the nerve is retrieved for histologic verification.

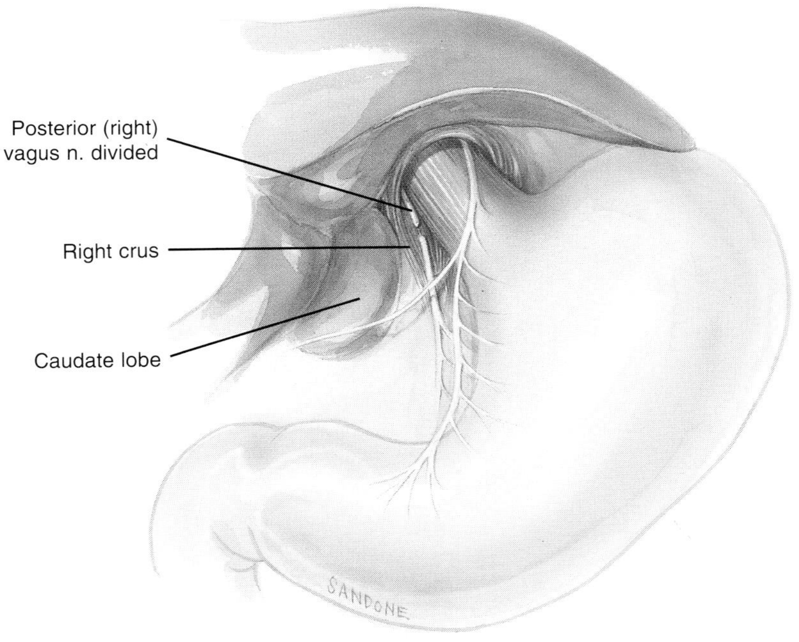

Fig. 15-3. Posterior truncal vagotomy (important landmarks).

Anterior Seromyotomy (Fig. 15-4)

The anterior aspect of the stomach is spread between two grasping forceps. Starting at the esophagogastric junction, the line of incision is outlined by light electrocoagulation parallel to and 1.5 cm from the lesser curvature. The line stops 5 to 7 cm from the pylorus at the level of the crow's-foot. The two most distal branches of the nerve are left intact to be sure that the antropyloric innervation is preserved. Seromyotomy is then performed with the hook coagulator using monopolar current, blending coagulation, and cutting at average intensity. The hook successively incises the serosal layer, the oblique muscle layer, and the circular muscle layer. The two borders are then grasped and gently spread apart, breaking the remaining deep circular fibers. Electrocautery completes the division when necessary.

Once the last muscular fibers have been divided, the mucosa can easily be identified by its typical blue color as it "pops" out of the incision. The sumucosal layer should not be incised as the mucosa is strongly adherent to this layer. Because of the magnification afforded by laparoscopy, the surgeon can easily verify that no holes have been made inadvertently. We have had no cases of perforation. Two or three short vessels may be encountered during the incision. They should be divided before starting the seromyotomy as described by Taylor after dissection with the hook coagulator/dissector and lifted off the seromuscular layer. It is of utmost importance that the incision be anatomically accurate and hemostasis ensured. On completion, the seromyotomy appears as a 7 to 8 mm trench in the gastric wall. Air is injected through the nasogastric tube to make sure that there are no leaks. Methylene blue can also be injected for the same purpose. The seromyotomy is closed with an overlap-

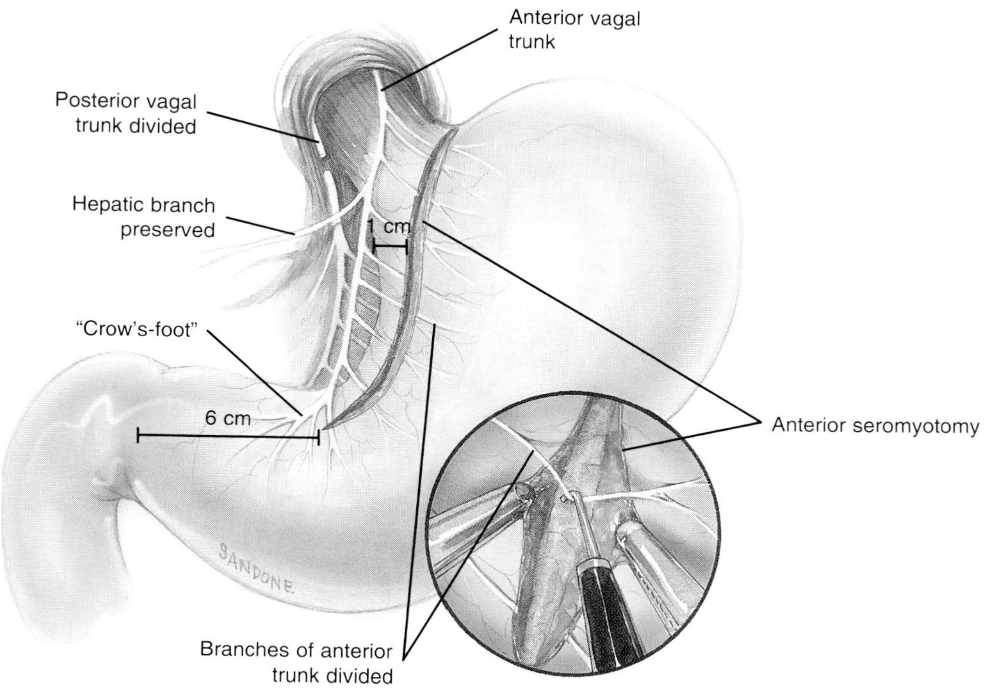

Fig. 15-4. Anterior lesser curve seromyotomy.

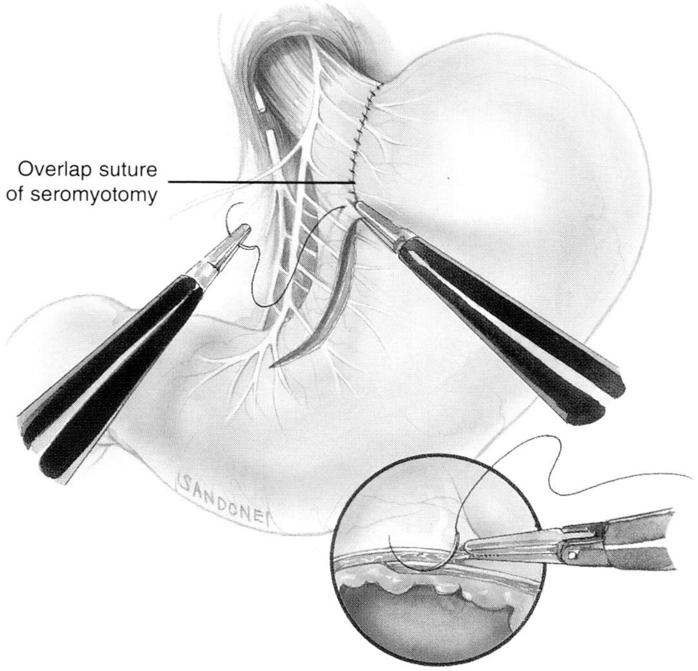

Fig. 15-5. Suture for seromyotomy.

ping running suture (Fig. 15-5) knotted at both ends. This will prevent postoperative adhesion, allow perfect hemostasis, and prevent nerve regeneration by disturbing the architecture of the gastric layers. The abdomen is closed without drainage.

Postoperative Care

The postoperative course is usually uneventful, as is typical of laparoscopic procedures. Postoperative pain is minimized by the fact that the surgical wounds are very small and infiltrated with local anesthetics, making systemic analgesia unnecessary. The minimally invasive nature of the procedure makes early ambulation possible. Patients may resume light, soft meals within 24 hours and are discharged from the hospital 2 days after surgery or earlier in some cases. Our ultimate goal is to be able to perform laparoscopic vagotomies in 1 hour on an outpatient basis.

TREATMENT OF COMPLICATIONS OF PEPTIC ULCER DISEASE

Peritonitis From a Perforated Anterior Duodenal Ulcer (Fig. 15-6)

Suspected intraperitoneal perforation of a chronic duodenal ulcer is a good indication for laparoscopic repair. Duodenal perforations should be treated laparoscopically if

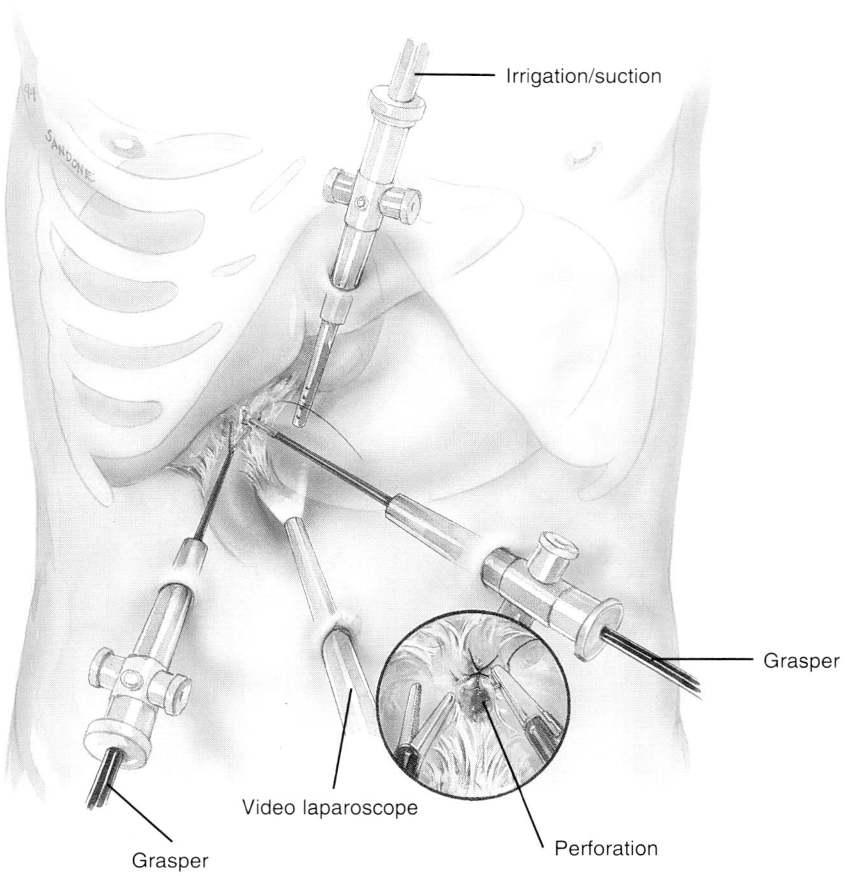

Fig. 15-6. Management of duodenal ulcer perforation.

detected within 12 hours and the patient has not eaten. It should not be performed in patients in septic shock. This procedure is therefore reserved for "chemical peritonitis." Age is not a contraindication. Our oldest patient was 77 years of age. Occasionally numerous inflammatory adhesions will have to be taken down since they seal the ulcer. The gallbladder commonly adheres firmly to the perforation and must be carefully removed to gain access to the duodenum. The first step is to irrigate the abdomen and ensure that all quadrants are rinsed and aspirated with isotonic saline solution and antibiotics. We think that this an important step in the management of perforated ulcers. Details of the laparoscopic technique to repair perforated duodenal ulcers are discussed in Chapter 21.

Gastric Outlet Obstruction by Intractable Chronic Duodenal Ulcer (Fig. 15-7)

This is a frequent complication of chronic duodenal ulcer disease, which we treat by bilateral truncal vagotomy and stapled gastrojejunostomy. Posterior truncal vagotomy is performed as described above. Anterior (left) truncal vagotomy is performed using five trocars, as shown in Fig. 15-7. An electrical scissors and grasper are used to free the phrenoesophageal membrane on the anterior aspect of the lower esophagus. The

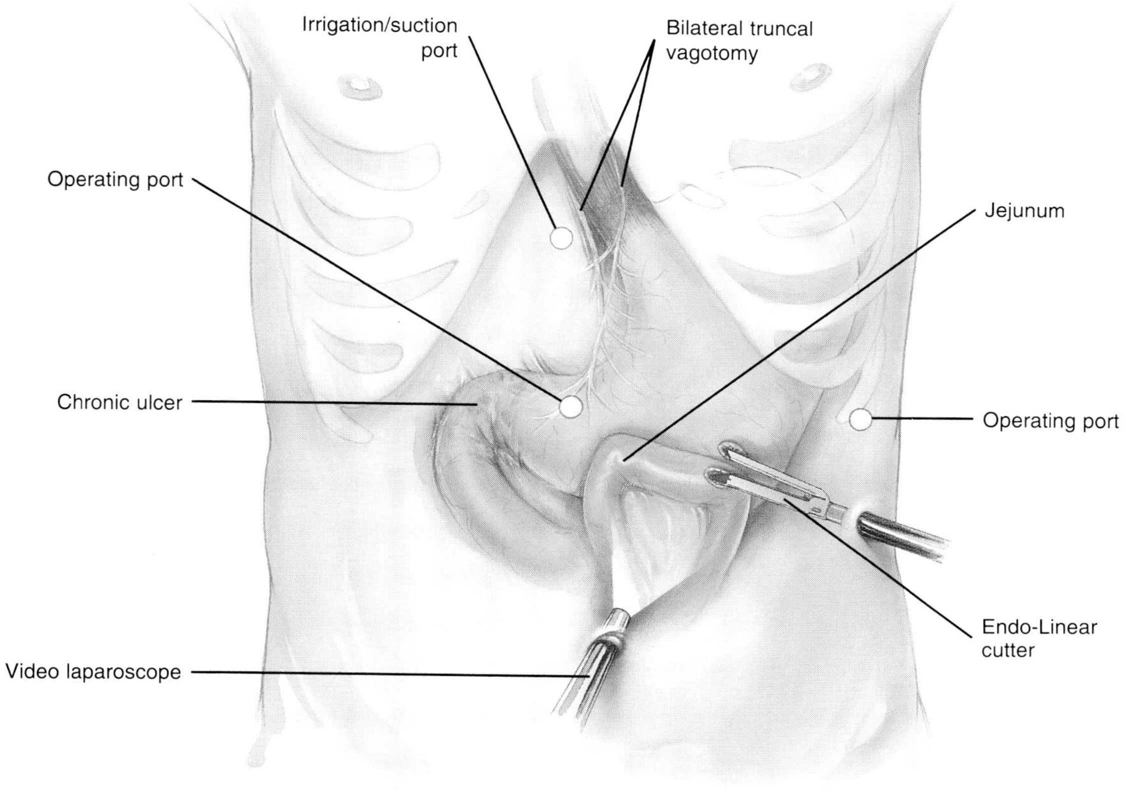

Fig. 15-7. Bilateral truncal vagotomy and gastrojejunostomy.

trunk of the left vagus nerve and its numerous branches must be identified since they usually divide in a plexiform manner in the abdomen. The esophagus should be cleared of any nerve fibers on both the anterior and posterior aspects to search for any aberrant nerves of Grassi. A complete dissection will skeletonize several centimeters of the lower esophagus. Specimens should be sent for histologic assessment.

The gastrojejunostomy must be performed on the greater curvature of the lowest part of the antrum as close to the pylorus as possible. The second loop of jejunum is identified and approximated to the body of the stomach. A hernia stapler can be used to approximate the ends of the stomach and the jejunum. A Babcock clamp can also be used for this purpose. Two incisions are made in both the stomach and the small bowel to allow the Endo-Linear cutter 65 (Ethicon Endo-Surgery) to be introduced. The instrument is closed and rolled to ensure that the anastomosis will be fired in a good position. The interior aspect of the anastomosis is checked for bleeding and inappropriate stapling. The stapler is fired again to close the incisions used to introduce the instruments. To ensure that the second staple line has left no stenosis, we recommend checking the diameter of the afferent loop of the jejunum with a large bougie before firing the Endo-Linear cutter. If stenosis is likely to occur, the incisions should be closed with a running suture technique.

We have used this approach for management of gastric outlet obstruction secondary to peptic ulcer disease or inoperable pancreatic cancer with good clinical results. However, long-term follow-up is necessary to assess the function and physiologic effects of this laparoscopic approach.

LAPAROSCOPIC BILATERAL TRUNCAL VAGOTOMY AND ANTRECTOMY FOR TREATMENT OF COMPLICATIONS OF BENIGN GASTRIC ULCERS (Fig. 15-8)

Gastric ulcers may be complicated by perforation, usually in the posterior aspect, and bleeding. However, before treatment is begun, a meticulous search for malignancy must be made and excluded by the histologic examination of at least 12 biopsy specimens obtained during flexible endoscopy.

Gastric ulcers do not respond well to medical treatment, and surgical intervention is frequently indicated. Historically, bilateral truncal vagotomy and antrectomy have been used to treat intractable duodenal ulcers after multiple recurrences. This operation can also be used to resect distal gastric ulcers by extending the antrectomy to a hemigastrectomy using a laparoscopic approach. Since bilateral truncal vagotomy was described earlier in this chapter, we will limit this discussion to distal gastrectomy.

The procedure begins by opening the gastrocolic ligament under the right epiploic vessel using electric scissors. Clips are used to secure all vessels and prevent hemorrhage. The dissection is carried toward the duodenum and the stomach retracted with a Babcock clamp. This permits dissection of the posterior aspect of the duodenum and placement of a tape to be held by one grasper. The tape assists in transsection of the duodenum using an Endo-Linear cutter 60 with blue staples. Division of the duodenum permits the retraction of the specimen via two Babcock clamps and the ligation of of the right gastric artery and the distal branches of the left gastric artery. The right gastroepiploic artery is then ligated and the posterior aspect of the stomach freed from the pancreas.

Two enterotomies are performed on the posterior aspect of the stomach and on the second jejunal loop to allow the introduction of the Endo-Linear cutter 60 for

A

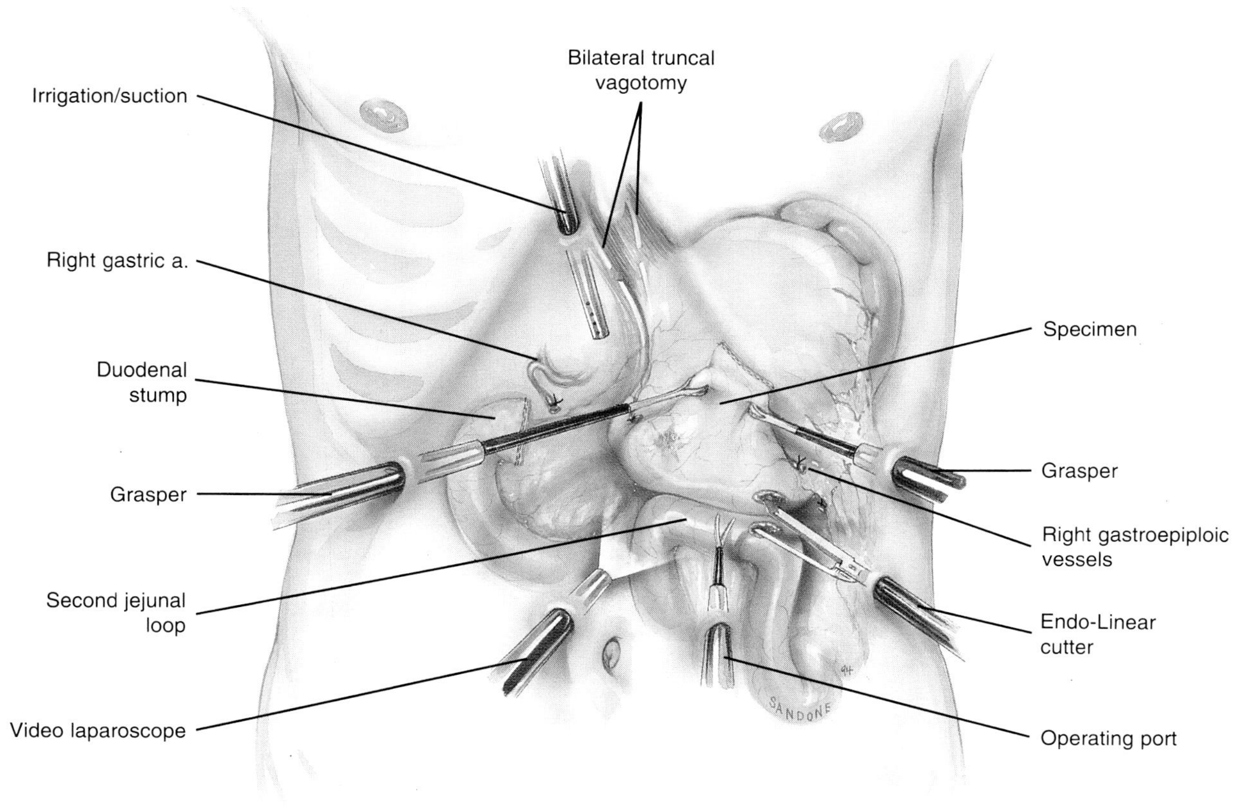

B

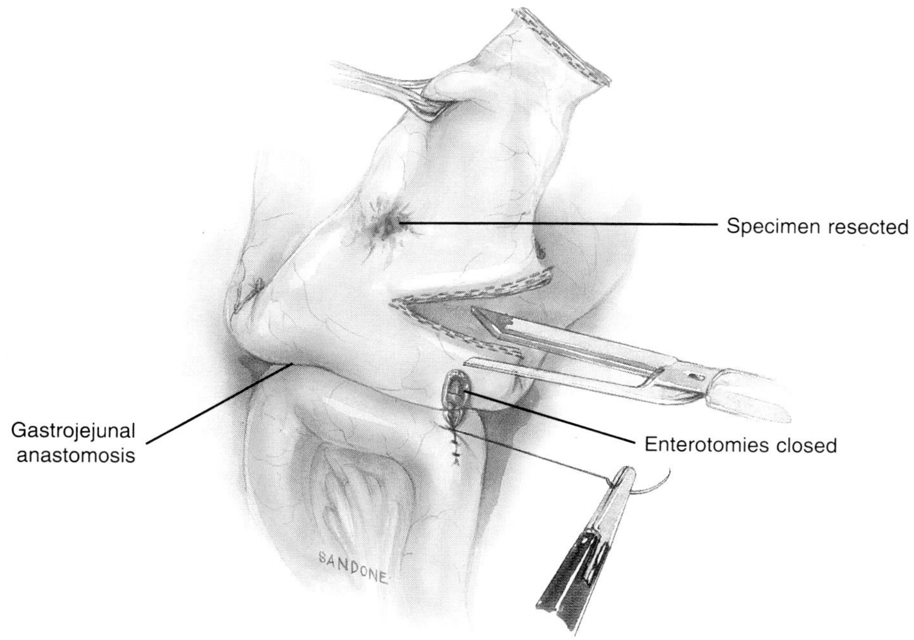

Fig. 15-8. A, Laparoscopic bilateral truncal vagotomy and antrectomy. **B,** Resection of gastric specimen after completion distal gastrectomy.

performing a stapled gastrojejunostomy. The enterotomies are then closed using continuous 3-0 Prolene sutures and curved needles. We do not recommend closing the enterotomies with staples since this may narrow the anastomosis.

The gastrectomy is completed by resection of the specimen. This can be difficult if the gastric wall is thick, as is usually the case in complicated gastric ulcers. The area is then irrigated generously and the trocars removed.

The postoperative course is the same as for any gastrectomy except the patient is able to ambulate freely on postoperative day 2 and is discharged from the hospital on the fourth or fifth day.

THORACOSCOPIC BILATERAL TRUNCAL VAGOTOMY FOR TREATMENT OF RECURRENT PEPTIC ULCERS (Figs. 5-9 and 5-10)

Thoracoscopic bilateral truncal vagotomy may be indicated for recurrent ulceration following a B2 gastrectomy. Adhesions from the first operation may preclude reoperation via an abdominal approach. If the recurrent peptic ulcer is benign, a thoracoscopic bilateral vagotomy may be the solution to this surgical problem.

A left-sided approach with the surgeon standing behind the patient is preferred. As with left lateral thoracotomy, the patient is given a general anesthetic, is positioned on his side, and the left lung is collapsed with a Carlens lumen tube. Four trocars are inserted in a triangular fashion with the thoracoscope between the two main operating trocars. The fourth trocar is used for the irrigation and suction device and may also serve as a palpation probe (Fig. 15-9).

Adhesions are divided and the pleura incised in front of the aorta. This allows dissection of the esophagus. The nasogastric tube can be used to localize the esophagus in the event of severe adhesions as well as an illuminated bougie (Bioenterics, Inc., Carpenteria, Calif.) or an endoscope. An atraumatic isolated hook can then be used. All the vagal nerves are dissected and divided. The white fibers are nerves and must not be confused with normal esophageal muscular fibers. When the operation is completed, the esophagus is peeled and freed from the nerve fibers. Hemostasis can be achieved by inserting a 4 by 4 inch gauze pad through one of the ports. Use of the electrocautery in the esophagus should be limited as much as possible to avoid the considerable danger of postoperative necrosis. The operation is completed by inserting a thoracic drain through one of the trocar ports and closure of the other ports.

CLINICAL RESULTS

As of September 31, 1993, we have performed 87 laparoscopic Taylor procedures for the treatment of chronic ulcer disease. The patients' mean age was 33 years (range 19 to 61 years). Forty-six patients were symptomatic for at least 4 years and averaged 2.8 relapses a year despite medical treatment with antacids, H_2 blockers, and/or omeprazole. Six patients had a history of bleeding ulcers that were controlled by medical treatment. None of these patients had complications such as hemorrhage or stenosis at the time of operation. Six patients were operated on because geographic or socioeconomic factors made long-term medical treatment impossible. No deaths occurred. Three patients had mild wound discharge, which was controlled medically. Three patients complained of postoperative fullness and were found to have bezoar formation, which resolved with papain administration, and one patient had post-

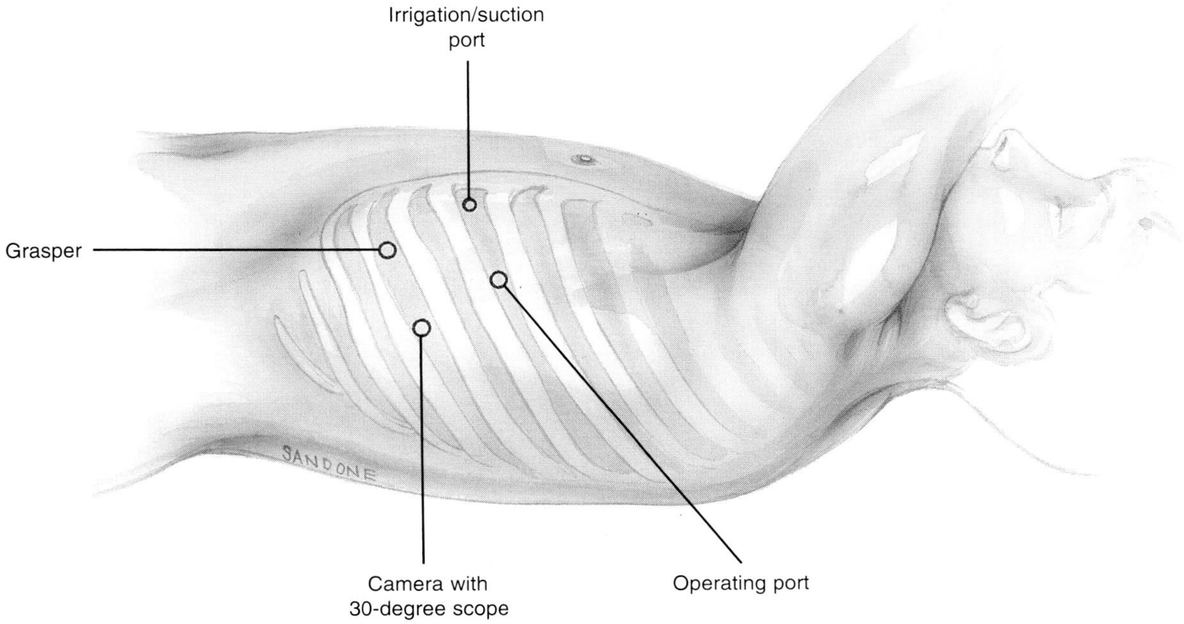

Fig. 15-9. Trocar placement for thoracoscopic vagotomy.

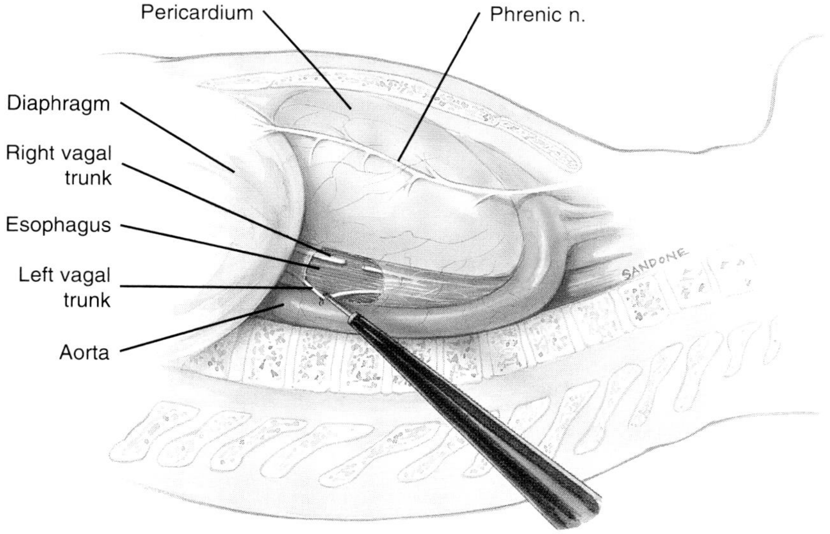

Fig. 15-10. Nerve dissection during thoracoscopic vagotomy.

operative reflux that required reoperation 2 months later. This patient had reflux before the operation. No postoperative functional disorders were found in any of the remaining 24 patients.

Endoscopic investigations performed 2 months postoperatively showed complete ulcer healing in all but three patients who had residual asymptomatic scars. Secretory studies at 2 months documented a decrease in basal and peak acid output of 79.3% ± 1.3% and 83.4% ± 1.2%, respectively. A late recurrence rate of 3.8% was noted at 51-month follow-up.

Taylor et al.[6] have reported a multicenter study of 605 patients operated on by 11 surgical teams using the same method. Postoperative mortality and morbidity was extremely low, with only one death (0.16%) from myocardial infarction. No patients had necrosis of the lesser curvature or gastric fistula. Ninety-four percent of the patients had Visick grades I or II. No patients had dumping syndrome, and only two complained of persistent diarrhea. Ulcers recurred in only 1.5% of the 481 patients operated on during this 5-year period.

Taylor's procedure is a simple and efficacious procedure that reduces acid secretion and is associated with a low 5-year recurrence rate of 3% to 6%, results that compared favorably with truncal vagotomy. The absence of secondary effects, particularly dumping, diarrhea, and gastric emptying disorders, was notable. Taylor's procedure was as effective as highly selective vagotomy in restoring gastric motility and reducing acidity. Others who have used this technique have reported that it is a reliable, consistent operation that produces good results. It should be noted that anatomic variations in Latarjet's nerve do not influence outcome.[19,21]

Conclusion

Laparoscopic vagotomy is as effective and safe as open vagotomy for the treatment of duodenal ulcer disease refractory to medical therapy and yields uniformly good results. This noninvasive technique represents a new horizon in the treatment of this common disease. Despite improvements in medical therapy, the recurrence rate for ulcer disease is approximately 90% a year without long-term medical treatment. Moreover, anti-ulcer drugs have not decreased the mortality rate or complications associated with ulcer disease, especially in the elderly. We believe that elective surgical treatment is a viable option to long-term maintenance therapy and therefore posterior truncal vagotomy with anterior seromyotomy is the procedure of choice if patients are selected as carefully as they are for open surgery. The results can be reproduced systematically and are not dependent on the individual surgeon's technique as is the case with highly selective vagotomy.[7] A prospective multicenter study is warranted to evaluate clinical outcome and cost effectiveness.

References

1. Graham DY. *Helicobacter pylori:* Its epidemiology and its role in duodenal ulcer disease. J Gastroenterol Hepatol 6:105-113, 1991.
2. George LL, Borody TJ, Andrews PO, et al. Cure of duodenal ulcer after eradication of *Helicobacter pylori.* Med J Aust 153:145-149, 1990.
3. Graham DY, Lew GM, Klein PD, et al. Effect of treatment of *Helicobacter pylori* infection on the long-term recurrence of gastric or duodenal ulcer: A randomized, controlled study. Ann Intern Med 116:705-708, 1992.

4. Hentschel E, Brandstater G, Dragosics B, et al. Effect of ranitidine and amoxicillin plus metronidazole on the eradication of *Helicobacter pylori* and the recurrence of duodenal ulcer. N Engl J Med 328:308-312, 1993.
5. Rauws EAJ, Tytgat GNG. Cure of the duodenal ulcer associated with eradication of *Helicobacter pylori*. Lancet 335:1233-1235, 1990.
6. Taylor TV, Gunn AA, MacLeod DAD, et al. Morbidity and mortality after anterior lesser curve seromyotomy and posterior truncal vagotomy for duodenal ulcer. Br J Surg 72:950-951, 1985.
7. Blackett R, Johnson D. Recurrent ulceration after highly selective vagotomy for duodenal ulcer. Br J Surg 68:705-710, 1981.
8. Hoffman J, Jensen HE, Christiansen J, et al. Prospective controlled vagotomy trial for duodenal ulcer. Results after 11 to 15 years. Ann Surg 209:40-45, 1989.
9. Taylor TV, MacLeod DAD, Gunn AA, et al. Anterior lesser curve seromyotomy and posterior truncal vagotomy in the treatment of chronic duodenal ulcer. Lancet 2:846-848, 1982.
10. Katkhouda M, Mouiel J. A new surgical technique of treatment of chronic duodenal ulcer without laparotomy by videocoelioscopy. Am J Surg 161:361-364, 1991.
11. Katkhouda N, Mouiel J. Laparoscopic treatment of peptic ulcer disease. In Hunter J, Sackier J, eds. Minimal Invasive Surgery. New York: McGraw-Hill, pp 123-130.
12. Katkhouda N, Mouiel J. Laparoscopic treatment of peritonitis. In Zucker KA, ed. Surgical Laparoscopy Update. St. Louis: Quality Medical Publishing, 1992, pp 287-300.
13. Mouiel J, Katkhouda N. Laparoscopic truncal and selective vagotomy. In Zucker KA, ed. Surgical Laparoscopy. St. Louis: Quality Medical Publishing, 1991, pp 263-279.
14. Taylor TV. Lesser curve superficial seromyotomy. An operation for chronic duodenal ulcer. Br J Surg 66:733-737, 1979.
15. Hill GL, Barker MCJ. Anterior highly selective vagotomy with posterior truncal vagotomy: A simple technique for denervating the parietal cell mass. Br J Surg 65:702-705, 1978.
16. Burge HW, Hutchinson JSF, Longland CJ, et al. Selective nerve section in the prevention of post-vagotomy diarrhea. Lancet 1:577, 1964.
17. Taylor TV. Experience with the Lunderquist Ownman dilator in the upper gastrointestinal tract. Br J Surg 70:445, 1983.
18. Daniel EE, Sarna SK. Distribution of excitatory vagal fibres in canine gastric wall to central motility. Gastroenterology 71:608-612, 1976.
19. Kahwaji F, Grange D. Ulcère duodénal chronique. Traitement par séromyotomie fundique antérieure avec vagotomie tronculaire postérieure. Presse Med 161:28-30, 1987.
20. OostVogel HJM, Van Vroonhoven TJMV. Anterior seromyotomy and posterior truncal vagotomy: Technic and early results of a randomized trial. Neth J Surg 37:69-74, 1985.
21. Triboulet JP. Progrès dans le traitement de l'ulcère duodenal: La séromyotomie avec vagotomie. In Mouiel J, ed. Actualités digestives medico-chirurgicales, 10th ed. Paris: Masson, pp 15-22.

Chapter

16

Laparoscopic Highly Selective Vagotomy

Leon G. Josephs, M.D.

Although the exact incidence of peptic ulcer disease in the United States is difficult to determine, it is estimated to occur in 19.3/1000 population.[1] Since the advent of H_2 antagonists and proton pump inhibitors, the volume of elective ulcer surgery has decreased significantly; unfortunately, we do not have an accurate estimate of the number of operative procedures performed electively for the treatment of peptic ulcer disease. However, there were 195,000 hospital admissions for peptic ulcer disease in 1986.[2]

Medical treatment of peptic ulcer disease does not provide optimal benefits. In addition to the known recurrence rate of 50% within 1 year after medication is discontinued, there are major problems related to side effects, poor compliance, and cost, which averages $1000 annually.[3]

Surgical therapy for peptic ulcer disease has fallen into disfavor largely because of the morbidity attending such a major operation and the postoperative complications related to either gastric resection or truncal vagotomy. Minimal access procedures avoid the morbidity associated with laparotomy, truncal vagotomy, and gastric resection. It has been shown that highly selective vagotomy is the least morbid of the successful peptic ulcer operations.[4] Since this procedure does not involve resection of, or entry into, the gastrointestinal tract, it is easily adapted to the laparoscopic approach. Our laboratory and clinical experience with a laparoscopic technique for performing highly selective vagotomy will be reviewed.

TECHNIQUE

The technique of laparoscopic highly selective vagotomy was initially developed using standard laparoscopic instrumentation and involves the insertion of five trocars (Fig. 16-1). The trocars are placed in the supraumbilical area, the right lower abdomen, the left lateral abdomen, and the right and left upper quadrants at the midclavicular line. A right epigastric port may be placed for retraction, instrumentation, and dissection if necessary. The liver is retracted cephalad, the greater curvature is retracted to the left lower quadrant, and the gastroesophageal junction is identified. It is usually not necessary to mobilize the left lateral segment of the liver. Identification of the

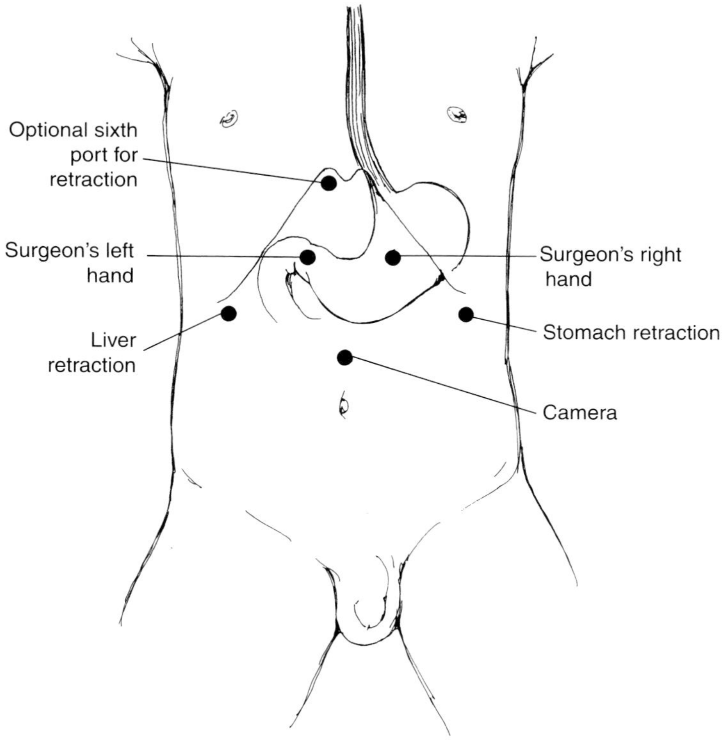

Fig. 16-1. Patient positioning and trocar placement for laparoscopic vagotomy. The patient is placed with the head elevated 45 degrees in a modified lithotomy position. The surgeon stands between the patient's legs. Five 10 mm ports are used; a sixth port can be placed in the subxiphoid region to aid in gastric or liver retraction if necessary.

gastroesophageal junction requires dissection of the right crus of the diaphragm and the peritoneum overlying the gastroesophageal junction using the electrocautery and scissors. Insertion of an esophageal dilator as well as a nasogastric tube is mandatory. If necessary, a flexible fiberoptic endoscope can be used to assist in identifying the gastroesophageal junction. The anterior vagal trunk is now visible and is dissected off the esophagus for future identification. Next the pyloroduodenal junction is identified and the anterior leaf of the peritoneum is incised along the gastrohepatic ligament up to the gastroesophageal junction (Fig. 16-2). The terminal branches of the anterior nerve of Latarjet are divided using hemostatic clips and/or bipolar cautery scissors. At this juncture the posterior vagal trunk is visible, and its terminal branches are divided using the same technique (Fig. 16-3). To facilitate the division of the posterior branches the left lower abdominal grasper is repositioned onto the lesser curvature of the stomach. The dissection of the anterior leaf is continued up the esophagus, dividing the terminal esophageal branches of the anterior vagus nerve (Fig. 16-4). The lesser curvature is inspected to ensure complete and accurate nerve division and hemostasis.

In animal experiments both anatomic and physiologic results using this methodology proved to be accurate, safe, and effective in decreasing acid secretion.[5]

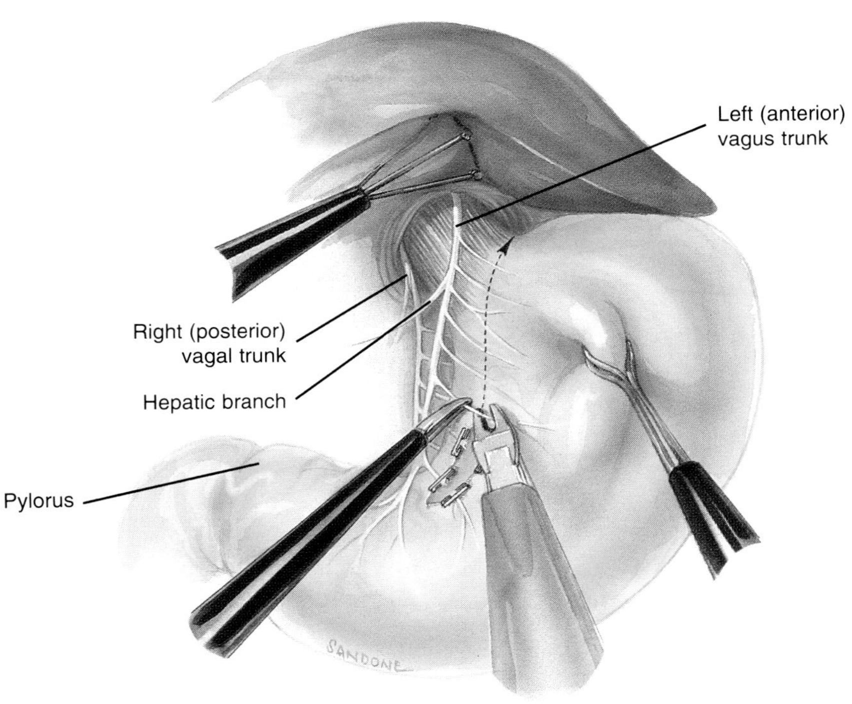

Fig. 16-2. Initially the anterior leaf of the gastrohepatic omentum is dissected 5 to 6 cm from the pylorus. Neurovascular bundles are carefully dissected circumferentially, clipped, and divided.

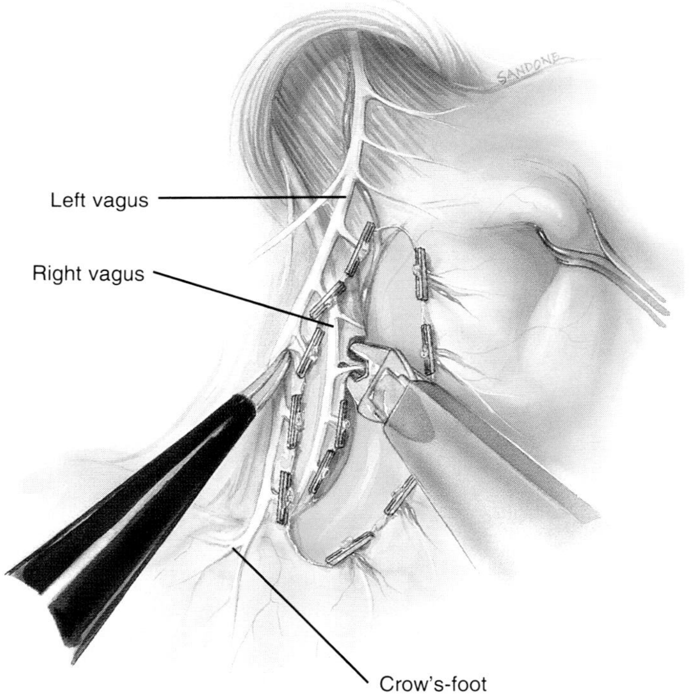

Fig. 16-3. Dissection of the gastrohepatic omentum. The lesser curve dissection is carried sequentially more posterior until the free lesser sac is entered.

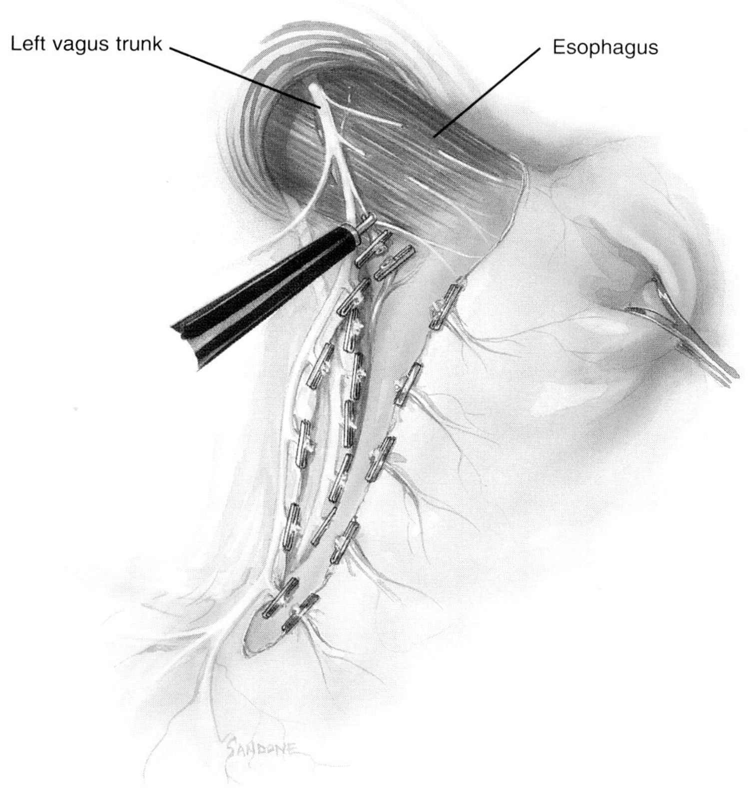

Fig. 16-4. The vagotomy is completed by carrying the vagal dissection 4 to 5 cm onto the lower esophagus. This dissection must be carried posterior for complete parietal cell vagotomy.

CLINICAL RESULTS

Despite the proven safety and efficacy of laparoscopic highly selective vagotomy, it has been difficult to gather sufficient clinical data. The identification of *Helicobacter pylori* as a possible causative agent in ulcer disease has further slowed referral for elective surgery. Our series includes 15 patients in whom laparoscopic highly selective vagotomy was completed after attempts were made in 21 patients. All patients had peptic ulcers documented by preoperative flexible endoscopy and had failed medical therapy. The technical aspects of the procedure were similar to those used in our earlier animal studies. The 30-degree telescope was used frequently but not routinely. Advances in instrumentation, particularly the liver retractor and grasping forceps, have increased the ease and safety of the procedure. The average operative time was 2 hours. In 12 of the 15 patients a true highly selective vagotomy was performed by dividing the anterior and posterior leafs. In three patients an anterior highly selective vagotomy coupled with a posterior truncal vagotomy was performed because of difficulties encountered. Six of the 21 procedures were converted to open surgery because of bleeding, obesity with poor anatomic landmarks, and cirrhosis with evidence of portal hypertension. Three of the six patients underwent open highly selective vagotomy. An alternative procedure was performed in the other three. The mean length of stay for patients undergoing laparoscopic highly selective vagotomy was 4 days and the mean time before these patients returned to work was 8 days.

One patient with severe diabetes mellitus developed postoperative gastroparesis that eventually required a drainage procedure. Ten patients had asymptomatic pneumomediastinum for 12 to 24 hours. The laparoscopic highly selective vagotomy patients have been followed up for a mean of 11 months. Twelve patients have undergone postoperative endoscopy that demonstrated complete ulcer healing. The remaining patients have not yet been evaluated endoscopically but are free of ulcer symptoms.

Highly selective vagotomy is a definitive and effective therapy for peptic ulcer disease and can be performed safely and accurately using laparoscopic techniques. Improvements in instrumentation, particularly for esophageal dissection and liver retraction, and surgical technique are making this procedure less formidable. It is essential to keep the dissection close to the lesser curvature of the stomach to avoid injuries of the descending branches of the left gastric artery and vein. If bleeding is encountered, it can be successfully controlled with laparoscopic techniques.

The primary criticism of highly selective vagotomy has been the associated recurrent ulcer rate secondary to an anatomically inaccurate dissection leading to incomplete denervation of the parietal cell mass. The wide range of incomplete vagotomies and the recurrent ulcer rates reported following both truncal and highly selective vagotomy are correlated to the individual surgeon's skills and experience.[6,7] The magnification provided by the laparoscopic procedure should increase the accuracy and therefore decrease the incidence of recurrent ulcers after laparoscopic highly selective vagotomy. In addition, the use of the intraoperative endoscopic Congo red test has been shown to increase the number of complete vagotomies, although its use is controversial.[8]

CONCLUSION

Highly selective vagotomy can be performed laparoscopically. Surgical therapy of peptic ulcer disease is effective, associated with a low recurrence rate, and obviates the need for maintenance drug therapy.[9] The major drawback to surgical therapy for peptic ulcer disease is the morbidity associated with laparotomy and with the sequelae of gastric resection. Long-term follow-up of highly selective vagotomy performed using conventional techniques has shown it to be the best option for the elective treatment of peptic ulcer disease. The large majority (85%) of patients have Visick grades of I or II at long-term follow-up (12 years) after undergoing highly selective vagotomy for the treatment of recalcitrant peptic ulcer disease.[10]

The cost of maintenance therapy with histamine antagonists as well as the morbidity of chronic medical therapy for the management of peptic ulcer disease is less than optimal and difficult to justify in this era of medical cost containment. If laparoscopic highly selective vagotomy can be successfully performed with minimal morbidity, a short length of stay, and rapid recovery, it may become the primary therapy for documented peptic ulcer disease.

REFERENCES

1. Collins JG. Prevalence of selected chronic conditions, United States, 1983-1985, advance data. Vital Health Stat 155:9, 1988.
2. Detailed diagnosis and procedures for patients discharged from short stay hospitals. Vital Health Stat 13(95):142, 1986.
3. Gear MWL. Proximal gastric vagotomy versus long-term maintenance treatment with cimetidine for chronic duodenal ulcer: A prospective randomized trial. Br Med J 286:98-99, 1983.
4. Johnston D, Blackett RL. A new look at selective vagotomies. Am J Surg 156:416-427, 1988.
5. Josephs LG, Arnold J, Sawyers J. Laparoscopic highly selective vagotomy: A porcine model. J Laparosc Endosurg 2:151-153, 1992.
6. Johnston D, Goligher JC. The influence of the individual surgeon and of the type of vagotomy upon the insulin test after vagotomy. Gut 12:963-967, 1971.
7. Adami HO, Enander LK, Enskog L, et al. Recurrences 1 to 10 years after highly selective vagotomy in prepyloric and duodenal ulcer disease. Ann Surg 199:393–394, 1984.
8. Donahue PE, Yoshida J, Richter HM, et al. Can the use of an endoscopic Congo red test decrease the incidence of incomplete proximal gastric vagotomy? Gastrointest Endosc 33:427-431, 1987.
9. Schirmer BD. Current status of proximal gastric vagotomy. Ann Surg 209:131-148, 1989.
10. Emas SM, Eriksson B. Twelve-year follow-up of a prospective, randomized trial of selective vagotomy with pyloroplasty and selective proximal vagotomy with and without pyloroplasty for the treatment of duodenal, pyloric and prepyloric ulcers. Am J Surg 164:4-12, 1992.

Part

V

Foregut Neoplasms

Chapter

17

Thoracoscopic Enucleation of Esophageal Leiomyoma

Alberto Peracchia, M.D. • Luigi Bonavina, M.D.
Romeo Bardini, M.D. • Marco Montorsi, M.D. • Andrea Segalin, M.D.

Although leiomyoma is the most common benign tumor of the esophagus, the incidence is 50 times lower than that of esophageal carcinoma.[1] It is seen most frequently in men in their fifties. This neoplasm is typically located in the lower or middle third of the esophagus (upper third in less than 10% of cases) and is solitary (multiple in less than 10% of cases). The tumor is generally an encapsulated, round to oval mass between 2 and 5 cm in diameter; occasionally a horseshoe-shaped or circumferential tumor is seen. Leiomyomatosis of the gastroesophageal junction in young females is rare.[2]

Tumor growth is slow. Occasionally a giant leiomyoma can cause ulceration of the overlying mucosa and possible bleeding. Reports describing sarcomatous degeneration of a leiomyoma are anecdotal.[3]

Dysphagia is the primary presenting symptom. Chest pain or substernal discomfort is a frequent complaint, possibly related to an associated motor disorder. However, almost half of the patients are asymptomatic, and the diagnosis of leiomyoma is made incidentally during investigation of other foregut symptoms. If a benign smooth muscle cell tumor is suspected on barium roentgenograms, endoscopy should be performed to rule out malignancy. If the mucosa overlying the mass is normal, a biopsy should not be performed since this complicates surgical removal. CT and endoscopic ultrasonography are useful for evaluating the density of the mass and identifying its relationship to the surrounding structures. Although no reliable criteria are available to differentiate benign and malignant submucosal tumors, small (<3 cm) echo homogeneous masses are likely to be benign.[4]

Indications for surgery are based on the presence of symptoms, the size of the mass, the inability to exclude a malignant process, and the presence of concomitant disease (epiphrenic diverticula, achalasia, or hiatal hernia) requiring treatment. The conventional surgical approach is enucleation of the tumor after splitting of the overlying muscle layer. This operation can be performed through a right thoracotomy for middle and upper third tumors and through a left thoracotomy for tumors of the lower thoracic esophagus. Huge esophageal leiomyomas and those located at the gastroesophageal junction may require esophageal resection and reconstruction.[5]

The trauma associated with thoracotomy seems inappropriate for the treatment of small, uncomplicated leiomyomas and makes it difficult for asymptomatic patients to accept this procedure. The minimally invasive surgical approach is gaining wide popularity in the treatment of esophageal disorders, and thoracoscopic enucleation of an esophageal leiomyoma is currently our technique of choice in these patients.

TECHNIQUE

The operation is carried out under general anesthesia with selective bronchial intubation. This allows complete lung collapse and offers a clear view of the posterior mediastinum. If a right thoracoscopic approach has been selected, as in most cases, the patient is placed on the operating table in the left lateral position with the arm held in abduction to ensure maximal superior displacement of the scapula. The operator stands on the right side of the patient, the first assistant on the left side, and the second assistant on the right side. Two video monitors are usually necessary to provide optimal visualization of the operative field by the surgeons. These are placed at both sides of the operating table close to the patient's head.

The position of the trocars is crucial. The first 10 mm trocar is placed in the intercostal space on the midaxillary line after open surgical dissection for introduction of a straight-viewing 0-degree wide-angle optic (Fig. 17-1). A pneumothorax can be created prior to inserting the trocar into the pleural space, reducing the risk of lung injuries. The intercostal space selected depends on the location of the leiomyoma. If the tumor is located in the upper thoracic esophagus, the optic is inserted in the seventh or eighth intercostal space caudad to the lesion. If the leiomyoma is situated in the lower thoracic esophagus, the trocar is placed in the fourth or fifth intercostal space. Two other 5 mm trocars are placed in the same intercostal space, usually the fifth, one on the anterior axillary line and the other posterior to this. These trocars accommodate dissecting instruments such as grasping forceps, scissors, or the hook diathermy. Occasionally the 5 mm trocar can be exchanged for a 12 mm trocar to allow insertion of a stapling instrument. An additional 10 mm port is usually needed on the midaxillary line at the sixth intercostal space for insertion of a lung retractor.

The mediastinal pleura over the tumor is opened. The dissection of the esophagus is limited to its lateral aspect. Dissection of the esophagus around its circumference is necessary only if the tumor is posterior or left sided. A plastic tape can be passed to facilitate traction and provide optimal exposure. When the leiomyoma is located in the upper third of the esophagus, it is necessary to isolate and divide the azygos vein to permit adequate exposure. This step can be accomplished using an endoscopic stapling device with a vascular cartridge introduced through the 12 mm trocar.

After precise identification of the tumor, the muscle layers of the esophagus are split longitudinally using cautery and scissors (Fig. 17-2). When the tumor appears, it is grasped with a forceps or better yet with a traction suture. The tumor is then pulled upward and the dissection is continued using sharp and blunt maneuvers (Fig. 17-3). Care must be taken to ensure the integrity of the vagi and to preserve the muscle fibers, which should be reapproximated at the end of the procedure.

As in open surgery, it is crucial that the esophageal mucosa, which sometimes is fragile, not be injured. Intraoperative esophagoscopy is especially useful for this purpose since it allows inflation and deflation of the esophagus, making it easy to iden-

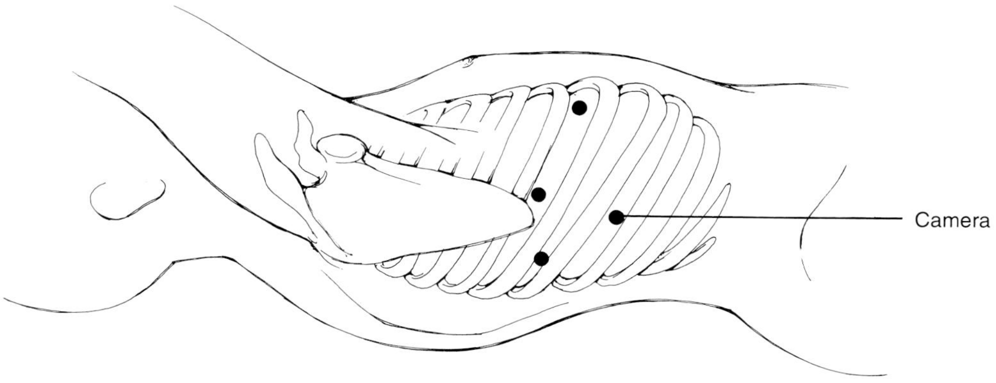

Fig. 17-1. Port positioning for dissection of esophageal leiomyoma.

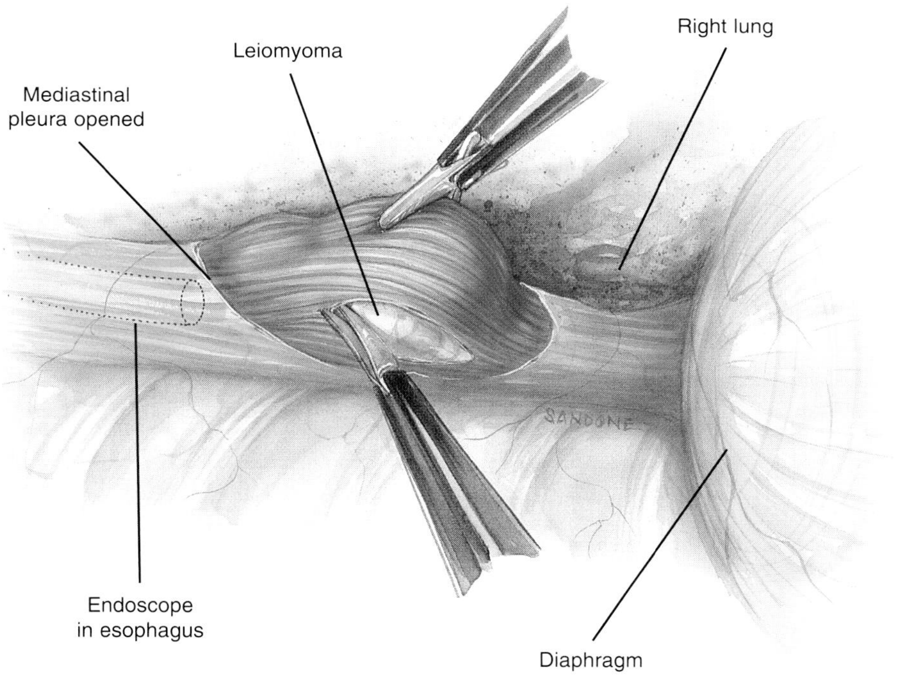

Fig. 17-2. Dissection of an esophageal leiomyoma through a right thoracoscopic approach.

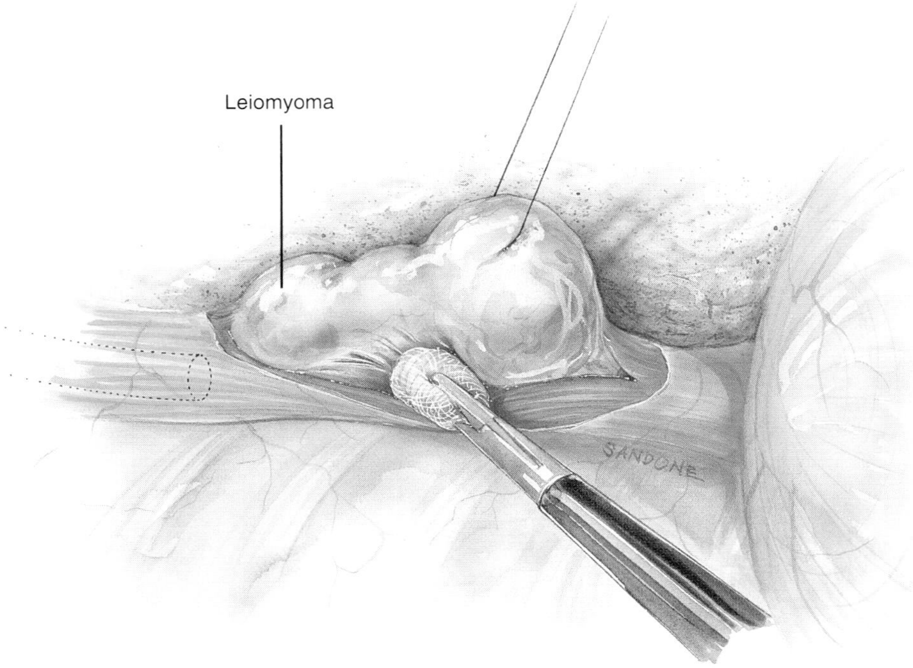

Fig. 17-3. Enucleation of a leiomyoma. A transfixing stitch is placed on the tumor to control the mass during the procedure.

tify the border between the mucosa and the leiomyoma. A minor perforation of the mucosa can be recognized immediately and repaired. With the nasogastric tube in place, the pleural cavity is now irrigated with warm saline solution and the integrity of the mucosa is checked with air insufflation.

Once the tumor has been completely enucleated, it is removed through the 12 mm cannula. If necessary, one of the trocar sites can be enlarged to allow the passage of large tumors. The muscular edges of the esophageal wall are then approximated with separate or running sutures (Fig. 17-4).

The operation is completed by positioning a chest tube through the posterior trocar site. A water-soluble contrast swallow is performed on the second postoperative day. The nasogastric tube is then removed and the patient can have a liquid diet. The patient is discharged on the sixth postoperative day.

Clinical Experience

Sixty-one operations for esophageal leiomyoma have been performed at our institution since 1976. Since November 1991 a right thoracoscopic approach has been undertaken in five men and one woman (mean age 48 years). All patients were symptomatic. Four patients had retrosternal pain or discomfort and two patients had dysphagia. The tumor was located in the lower middle thoracic esophagus in four patients and in the upper esophagus in the remaining two. A preoperative workup included a barium swallow study, CT scan, and endoscopic ultrasonogram.

The operation was successful in four patients. In two patients the procedure was

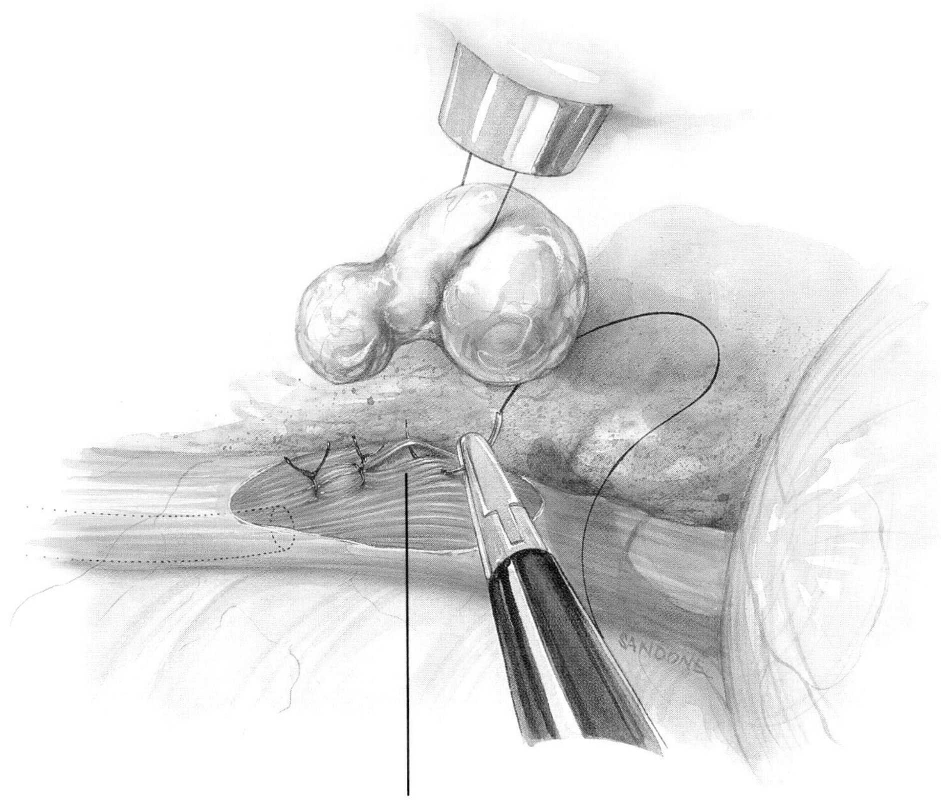

Fig. 17-4. After the leiomyoma is excised, the muscular wall is closed with interrupted sutures.

converted to a formal thoracotomy: in one of these the lung could not be excluded because of a large mediastinal goiter, and the other patient had a mucosal tear. The procedures lasted an average of 2½ hours. The size of the leiomyomas ranged from 2 to 6 cm. Two were horseshoe-shaped tumors.

No deaths occurred postoperatively. One patient in whom the muscle layer was not approximated developed a mucosal bulging at the level of the enucleation site. Manometry showed an area of segmental aperistalsis. Reoperation through a right thoracotomy was necessary because of persistent dysphagia and consisted of reapproximation of the muscle edges. Dysphagia resolved and the manometric abnormalities disappeared. Follow-up ranged from 3 to 20 months. Clinical results were satisfactory in all patients.

CONCLUSION

Surgical enucleation is the treatment of choice for esophageal leiomyoma. The conventional approach through a formal thoracotomy has the potential of causing excessive postoperative pain and patient discomfort. Moreover, the hospital stay and the recovery period are prolonged. A patient with a benign disease that requires simple enucleation should not be subjected to such a traumatic procedure. The same surgical results can be obtained using the video thoracoscopic approach with the added advantage of magnified vision of the operative field and less postoperative discomfort. The currently available thoracoscopic instruments allow safe and reliable dissection of the leiomyoma from the muscle and the mucosa. Preoperative attempts at endoscopic biopsy of the submucosal mass are responsible for most mucosal injuries. However, should a minimal mucosal tear occur during enucleation, it can be promptly repaired using fine sutures. We emphasize the need for reconstruction of the muscle layer of the esophagus after enucleation of the leiomyoma. As we have seen, a pseudodiverticulum may occur in an area of disorganized muscular anatomy, causing defective propulsive activity of the esophagus and dysphagia.

Reports of thoracoscopic treatment of esophageal leiomyoma are still anecdotal.[6,7] However, these reports confirm that esophageal leiomyoma represents an excellent indication for a minimally invasive approach, which may soon replace the conventional thoracotomy approach.

REFERENCES

1. Seremetis M, Lyons W, Deguzman V, Peabody J. Leiomyomata of the esophagus. An analysis of 838 cases. Cancer 38:2166-2177, 1976.
2. Lortat-Jacob J. Myomatoses localisees et myomatoses diffuses de l'oesophage. Arch Mal Appar Dig 39:519-524, 1950.
3. Johanet H, Marmuse J, Timores A, et al. Leiomyosarcome de l'oesophage, huit ans apres un diagnostic de leiomyome. Gastroenterol Clin Biol 15:780, 1991.
4. Rosch T, Lorenz R, Dancygier H, Von Wichert A, Classen M. Endosonographic diagnosis of submucosal upper gastrointestinal tract tumors. Scand J Gastroenterol 27:1-8, 1992.
5. Altorki N, Sunagawa M, Migliore M, Skinner D. Benign esophageal tumors. Dis Esoph 1:15-19, 1991.
6. Bardini R, Segalin A, Ruol A, Pavanello M, Peracchia A. Videothoracoscopic enucleation of esophageal leiomyoma. Ann Thorac Surg 54:576-577, 1992.
7. Gossot D, Fourquier P, El Meteinei M, Celerier M. Technical aspects of endoscopic removal of benign tumors of the esophagus. Surg Endosc 7:102-103, 1993.

Chapter

18

Endoscopic Resection of Intramucosal Esophageal Cancer

Mitsuo Endo, M.D. • Kimiya Takeshita, M.D.
Tatsuyuki Kawano, M.D. • Haruhiro Inoue, M.D.

The incidence of superficial cancer (T1) of the esophagus has been increasing steadily. Pathologic studies at our hospital have shown that mucosal cancer of the esophagus has a 4% incidence of lymph node metastasis and 10% incidence of vascular invasion, both acceptably low. In view of these findings we decided endoscopic resection in such cases was a viable option.

INDICATIONS

Pathologic studies of 235 T1 cancer resections at Tokyo Medical and Dental University between 1965 and 1992 have shown that 79 patients (34%) had mucosal cancer and 156 (66%) had submucosal cancer. The incidence of lymph node metastasis in patients with mucosal cancer was 4% as compared with 40% in patients with submucosal cancer. The incidence of vascular invasion was 10% in patients with mucosal cancer and 70% in patients with submucosal cancer (Table 18-1). Lymph node metastasis and vas-

Table 18-1. Depth of invasion of lymph node metastasis and vascular invasion in 235 patients with superficial esophageal cancer (1965-1992)

Depth of Invasion	No. of Patients	No. With Positive Nodes	No. With Vascular Invasion
Mucosal cancer			
Epithelium	22	0	0
Muscularis mucosae	57	3 (5.3%)	8 (14.0%)
	79	3 (3.8%)	8 (10.1%)
Submucosal cancer	156	62 (39.7%)	109 (69.9%)

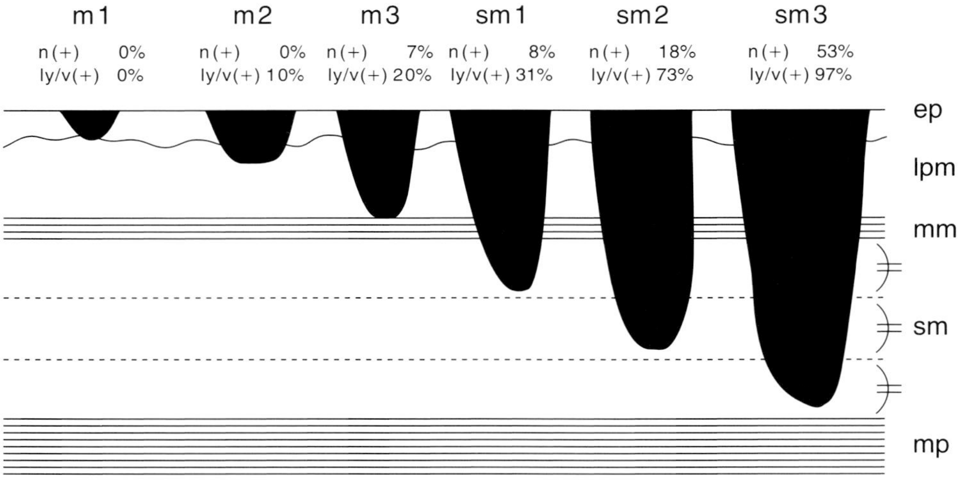

Fig. 18-1. Incidence of lymph node metastasis and vascular invasion by subdivided pathologic classification of T1 esophageal cancer. ep = epithelium; lpm = lamina propria mucosae; mm = muscularis mucosae; sm = submucosae; mp = muscularis propria.

cular invasion were observed in patients regardless of whether the muscularis mucosae or surrounding area was grossly invaded (Fig. 18-1).

The indications for curative endoscopic resection of esophageal cancer are as follows: mucosal cancer without gross invasion to the muscularis mucosae, less than 2 × 2 cm in size or less than one third the circumference of the esophagus, and absence of nodal involvement.

TECHNIQUE

At present we use two procedures for esophageal mucosal stripping: one involves capturing the mucosal lesion with grasping forceps[1] and the other is endoscopic resection using negative pressure at the tip of the endoscope.[2,3]

Grasping Forceps Procedure

A transparent tube 18 mm in diameter is used to cover the endoscope during the procedure. The distal part of the tube has an open slit. The snare forceps are inserted through the working channel of the covering tube and emerges from the center of the open slit. Grasping forceps are inserted through the working channel of the endoscope.

Before starting the procedure, the extent of the lesion is distinctly demarcated with Lugol's staining solution. Five to 15 ml of physiologic saline solution is injected submucosally with a syringe, which loosens the mucosa from the underlying muscle layer. The forward-viewing endoscope and covering tube are positioned close to the mucosal lesion of the esophagus. Grasping forceps are inserted through the working channel of the endoscope through an opened loop of a snare forceps and then inserted through the working channel of the covering tube.

The mucosal lesion is grasped with the forceps under direct vision and pulled into the opened loop of the snare forceps (Fig. 18-2) and through the slit of the

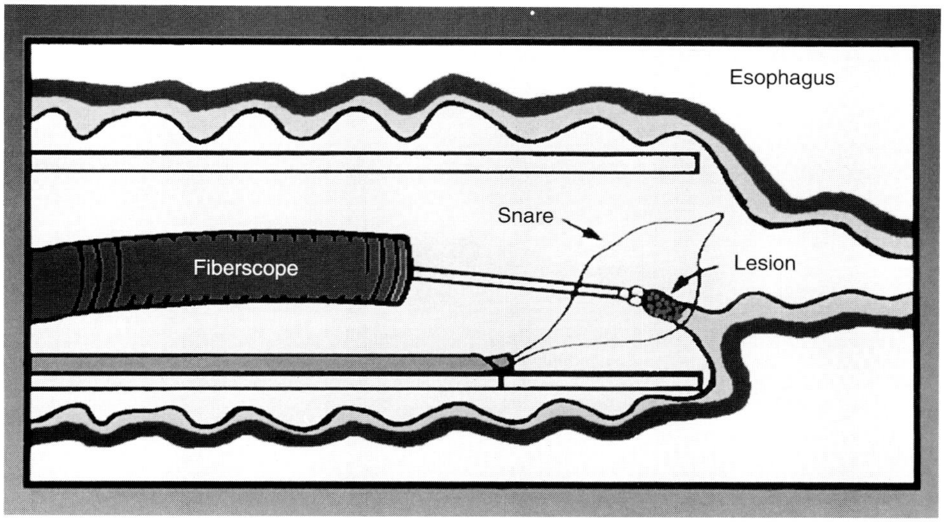

Fig. 18-2. The mucosal lesion is grasped with the forceps under direct vision through the opened loop of the snare forceps inserted through the working channel of the covering tube.

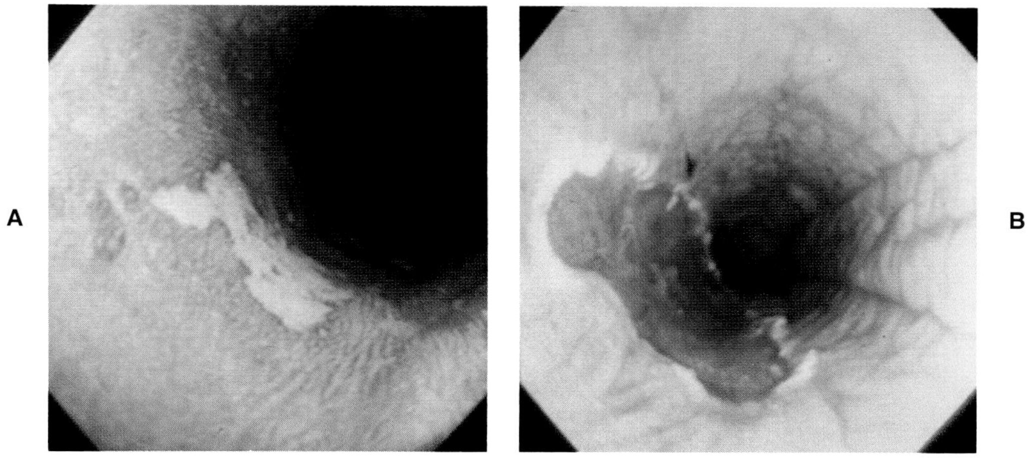

Fig. 18-3. A, Erosive lesion stained with Lugol's solution. **B,** Note the mechanically induced ulcer in the esophageal muscle layer.

covering tube. Thus the mucosa is completely separated from the underlying muscle layer of the esophagus prior to excision. The mucosa is then snared tightly and resected by means of blended cauterization current. The resected specimen is collected with the endoscope. The endoscope is reinserted through the covering tube and the procedure is repeated to resect more of the mucosa as needed.

After the procedure is completed, the esophageal muscular layer is readily seen (Fig. 18-3). Staining with Lugol's solution confirms that no lesion remains. The resultant ulcer heals within 1 month without any complications.

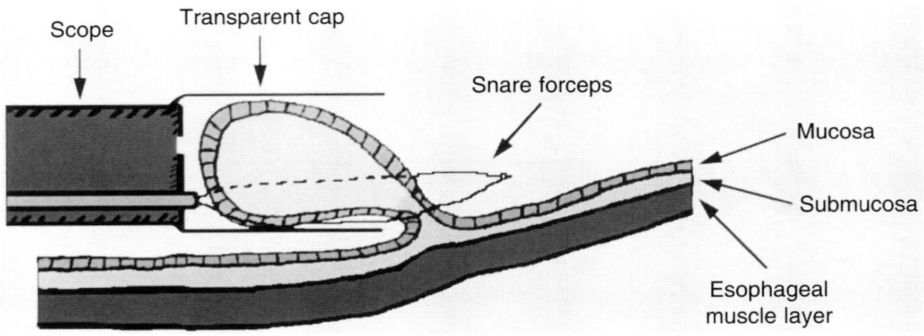

Fig. 18-4. Under negative pressure the esophageal mucosa protrudes like a polyp into the cap of the endoscope through the opened loop of the snare forceps.

Endoscopic Mucosal Resection Using Negative Pressure

A small cap is attached to the distal part of the conventional forward-viewing endoscope. Preparation for the procedure is the same as described above.

The snare forceps is inserted through the working channel of the endoscope and opened fully within the inner surface of the cap. Negative pressure is established at the tip of the endoscope by the suction mechanism. As a result, the esophageal mucosa protrudes like a polyp into the cap of the endoscope. The protruding mucosa is caught with the snare forceps, moved to and fro to ensure that only the mucosa is snared (Fig. 18-4), and resected with blended cauterization current. The resected specimen is collected within the cap. The procedure is repeated until a sufficient area of the mucosa has been resected. After the procedure is completed, the undersurface of the esophageal muscle layer is visible.

RESULTS

We have performed endoscopic resection of mucosal cancers in 17 patients. Histologic study confirmed that all patients had mucosal cancer. Of these, 12 patients had epithelial cancer and five patients had cancer of the lamina propria mucosae. The resected mucosa consisted of one fifth to four fifths of the circumference of the esophagus. Lesions in 12 patients were classified as erosive type (0-IIc) in seven patients, as flat type (0-IIb) in four, and as slightly elevating type (0-IIa) in one All patients had a complete local response and no postoperative complications were seen. The longest follow-up has been 3 years 8 months, with no recurrence seen to date.

DISCUSSION

Minimally invasive surgery for esophageal cancer is indicated only in patients with mucosal cancer in whom extensive examination fails to reveal lymph node metastasis. We usually perform either a transhiatal or endoscopic resection in such cases. If the tumor is found to extend to the submucosa, transthoracic esophagectomy and lymph node dissection are necessary since lymph node metastases are frequently encountered in submucosal lesions.[4]

When a lesion suspected to be mucosal cancer is less than 2 cm in size and lymph node metastases are excluded preoperatively, endoscopic resection can be considered. Lymph node metastases were observed in only 4% of our patients with mucosal cancer, including those with unsuspected invasion into the muscularis mucosae histologically. Mucosal cancer with gross invasion into or near the muscularis mucosae contraindicates endoscopic resection even if the lesion is small.

Transhiatal esophagectomy for esophageal cancer should be performed when a lesion suspected to be mucosal cancer has a circumference that covers three fourths of the esophagus or if there are multiple lesions but no lymph node metastasis is documented preoperatively.

Endoscopic mucosal resection was first performed using the same strip-off biopsy method for early cancer of the stomach.[5] Other modalities of endoscopic resection of mucosal cancer of the esophagus have also been reported.[6,7]

We believe our snare procedure has the advantage of providing larger mucosal specimens. Endoscopic resection offers good visibility of the esophageal muscular layer, provides larger mucosal specimens, and prevents the muscular layer from being damaged.

Current statistics show that the 5-year survival rate for resected mucosal cancer is 100%, excluding death from other disease. For submucosal cancer, the rate is 62%. In our series of 17 patients undergoing endoscopic resection there have been no recurrences and no complications at the longest follow-up of 3 years 8 months. The only recurrence was observed in a patient with submucosal cancer.[4]

Minimally invasive surgery appears to be a safe and effective procedure in selected patients. Long-term follow-up data will available in the future.

REFERENCES

1. Inoue H, Endo M. Endoscopic esophageal mucosal resection using a transparent tube. Surg Endosc 4:198-201, 1990.
2. Inoue H, Takeshita K, Hori H, Muraoka Y, Yoneshima H, Endo M. Endoscopic mucosal resection with a cap-fitted panendoscope for esophagus, stomach and colon mucosal lesions. Gastrointest Endosc 39:58-62, 1993.
3. Kawano T, Miyake S, Yasuno M, Takamatsu S, Katoh S, Nakamura H, Sugihara K, Hatano M, Yoshino K, Takeshita K, Inoue H, Yamagiwa A, Endo M. A new technique for endoscopic esophageal mucosectomy using a transparent overtube with intraluminal negative pressure (np-EEM). Dig Endosc 3:159-167, 1991.
4. Endo M, Ide H, Yoshino K, Yoshida M. Diagnosis and treatment of early esophageal cancer. In Siewert JR, Holscher AH, eds. Diseases of the Esophagus. Berlin: Springer-Verlag, 1986, pp 375-380.
5. Tada M, Karita M, Yanai H, Kawano H, Takemoto T. Evaluation of endoscopic strip biopsy therapeutically used for early gastric cancer. Stomach Intestine 23:373-385, 1988 (in Japanese).
6. Makuuchi H, Machimura T, Sugihara T, Sasaki T, Mitomi T. Endoscopic diagnosis and treatment of mucosal carcinomas of the esophagus. Endosc Dig 2:447-452, 1990 (in Japanese).
7. Momma K, Sakaki N, Yoshida M. Endoscopic mucosectomy for precise evaluation and treatment of esophageal intraepithelial cancer. Endosc Dig 2:501-506, 1990 (in Japanese).

Chapter

19

Transmediastinal Endodissection

Rudolf Bumm, M.D. • Arnulf H. Hölscher, M.D.
J. Rüdiger Siewert, M.D., F.A.C.S.

The incidence of adenocarcinoma of the esophagus has been increasing in the United States as well as in Europe.[1,2] Alcohol and nicotine abuse are known predisposing factors for squamous cell carcinoma. Diet has also been implicated in the geographic distribution of this disease.[3] The risk factors for adenocarcinoma, however, are different; an increased incidence is seen in Caucasians, males, and those with columnar epithelium (Barrett's esophagus). Although Barrett's epithelium has been linked to reflux esophagitis, it is not clear if treatment decreases the risk of malignancy.

Early detection and diagnosis of esophageal malignancy are essential to successful treatment. Multimodality treatments have proved increasingly efficacious, but tumor resection at an early stage still offers the best hope for a permanent cure.

OPTIONS FOR ESOPHAGEAL RESECTION

Esophageal resection can be accomplished using a variety of techniques ranging from radical en bloc procedures to minimally invasive methods. Each has certain advantages and disadvantages.

En Bloc Resection

Transthoracic en bloc removal of the thoracic esophagus and the adjacent lymphatic structures of the posterior mediastinum with a resection line lateral to the azygos vein is the recommended method for removal of esophageal squamous cell carcinoma (Fig. 19-1). Studies have demonstrated a high incidence of mediastinal lymph node metastases from tumors at all esophageal levels.[4] Superior long-term results have been demonstrated when lymphadenectomy is performed.[4-6]

Since this operation involves three body cavities, it should be reserved for patients without major risk factors. Reconstruction requires patient repositioning, thus prolonging the operating time. Improvements in intensive care technology have reduced the morbidity and mortality of this operation in the past decade,[7] but pulmonary complications, age, and comorbid conditions represent significant risks.[8]

Transhiatal Esophagectomy

Transhiatal esophagectomy is an alternative that avoids thoracotomy and accomplishes the esophagectomy in a shorter time (Fig. 19-2). Since periesophageal tissues can be

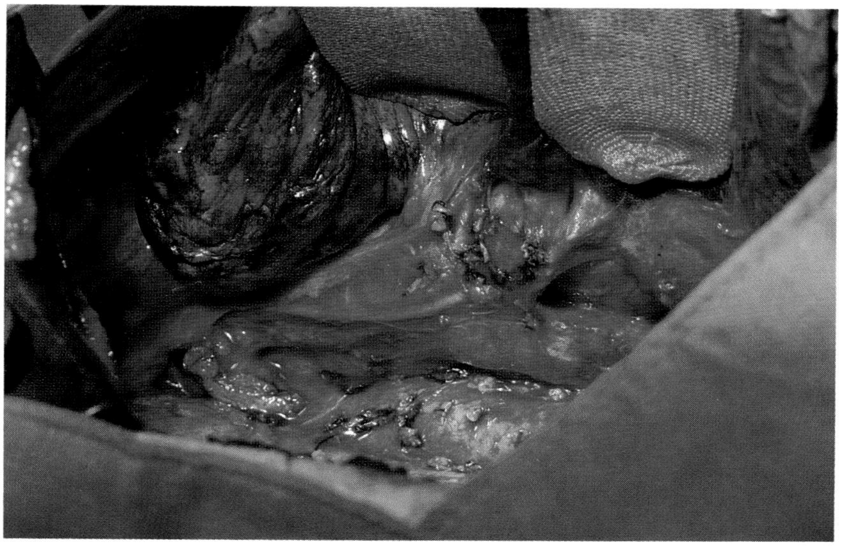

Fig. 19-1. En bloc resection of the thoracic esophagus via a right posterolateral thoracotomy. The specimen has been resected with adjacent lymph nodes as well as the azygos vein. This operation is the standard surgical technique for squamous cell carcinoma of the esophagus. The aorta, the tracheal bifurcation, and the right upper lobe are visible.

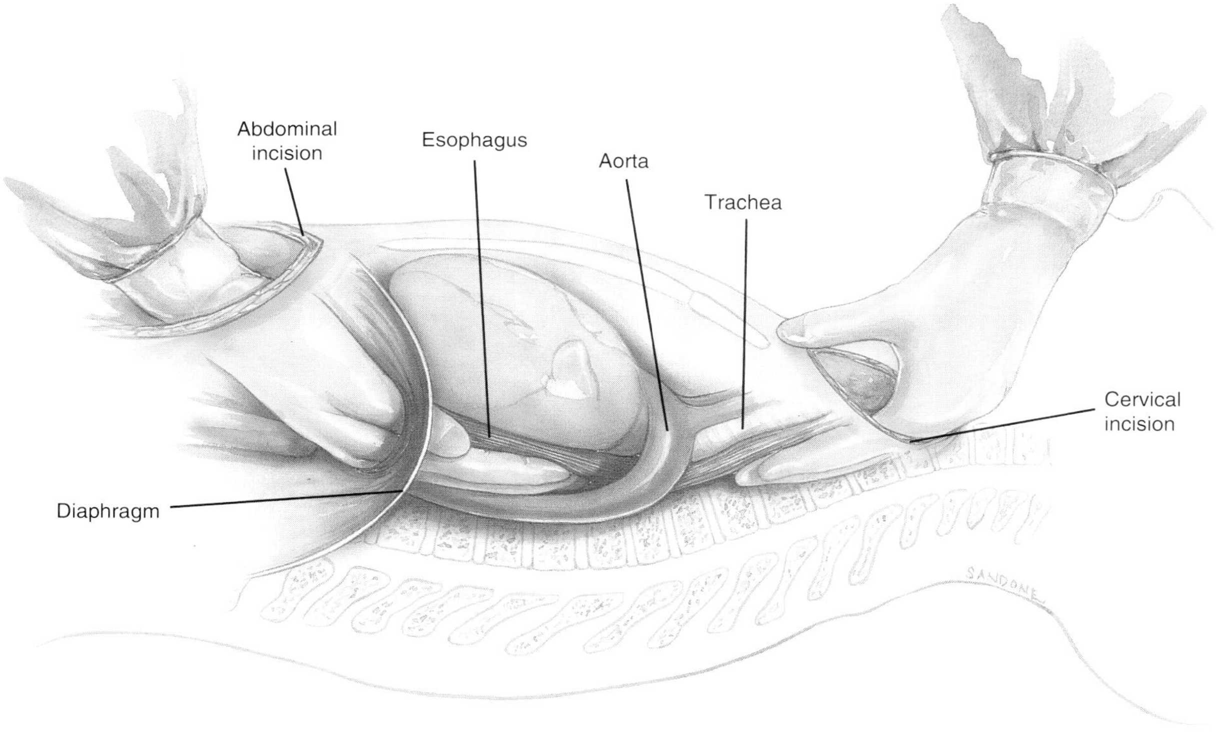

Fig. 19-2. Conventional technique of blunt dissection of the thoracic esophagus during transhiatal esophagectomy. The area of the tracheal bifurcation cannot be controlled visually.

divided by blunt dissection, advocates claim that the risk of arterial bleeding is minimized. Morbidity and mortality rates are quite low at centers experienced in performing transhiatal esophagectomy,[9] but the overall incidence of life-threatening complications including mediastinal bleeding, tracheal tears, and recurrent nerve palsy reported in the literature is high.[4-16] We believe this to be attributable to the limited visual control above the level of the tracheal bifurcation. It is in this area that the risk of injury to surrounding structures increases dramatically.

Although transhiatal esophagectomy is not considered curative,[15] it has been widely used for all types of esophageal carcinoma, primarily because the extent of resection was considered to have little effect on long-term outcome. We do not share this view. We use transhiatal esophagectomy to treat most patients with adenocarcinoma of the esophagus because removal of the lymph nodes in the lower mediastinum can be performed safely via the open hiatus.

Improvement in the transhiatal approach is needed and is contingent on improved visualization of the operative field, refinement of microsurgical instruments, controlled hemostasis, and better access to mediastinal structures and lymph nodes.

Endodissection

Transhiatal esophagectomy usually requires two incisions: an abdominal (inverse T) laparotomy and a left-sided neck incision for the esophagogastric anastomosis. In 1990 Buess et al.[17] described a mediastinoscope that could be inserted and manipulated through the cervical incision. This device inspired us to develop an instrument for endoscopic surgical dissection called an endodissector. It features a specially shaped tissue dilator at the tip of the instrument, a multifunctional, 360-degree rotating handle, and a working channel for introduction of instruments. Vision and illumination are provided by two built-in fiberoptic light bundles.

OPERATIVE PROCEDURE

Instrumentation

A mediastinoscope (Fig. 19-3), a video endoscopy unit, and suitable instruments are required (H. Plank, Munich, and Karl Storz, Tuttlingen, Germany). Mounting the mediastinoscope takes approximately 10 to 15 minutes. The mediastinoscope has a tissue dilator at the tip for creating a hollow space in the mediastinum. This dilator has several openings for the fiberoptic bundle, the working channel, and flushing and suction devices. It is shaped to allow it to ride on the esophagus during the initial dissection. The instrument is manipulated by a handle that can be rotated 360 degrees, which allows circumferential dissection of the esophagus in the mediastinum. The fiberoptic bundle is connected to an endocamera, a xenon light source (Karl Storz), and monitors. Instruments such as monopolar electrocautery, biopsy forceps, and microscissors can be introduced through the working channel.

Position of Patient and Surgeons

The rigid mediastinoscope requires that the patient be positioned to allow an optimal "angle of attack" (Fig. 19-4). The patient is placed supine with the right arm stabilized at a 90-degree angle to permit access by the anesthetist. The head is turned to the right and the neck is retroflected approximately 30 to 40 degrees. The patient's shoulder is positioned on the left edge of the operating table to increase the maneu-

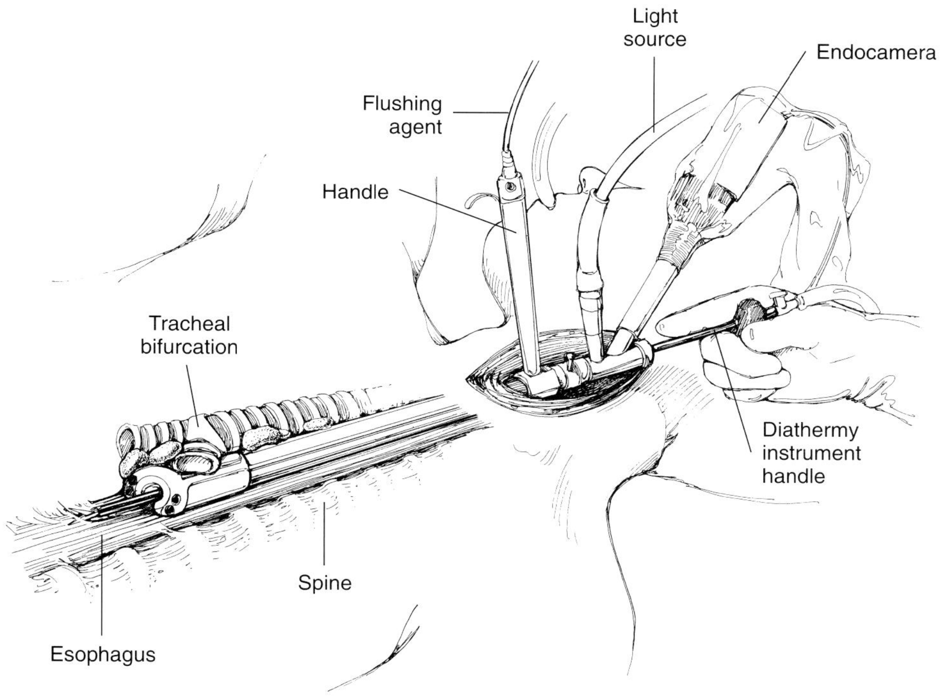

Fig. 19-3. Mediastinoscope used for endodissection. The tip of the instrument carries a dilatation olive that creates a hollow space in the mediastinum. The olive can be rotated 360 degrees to allow dissection of the sides of the esophagus.

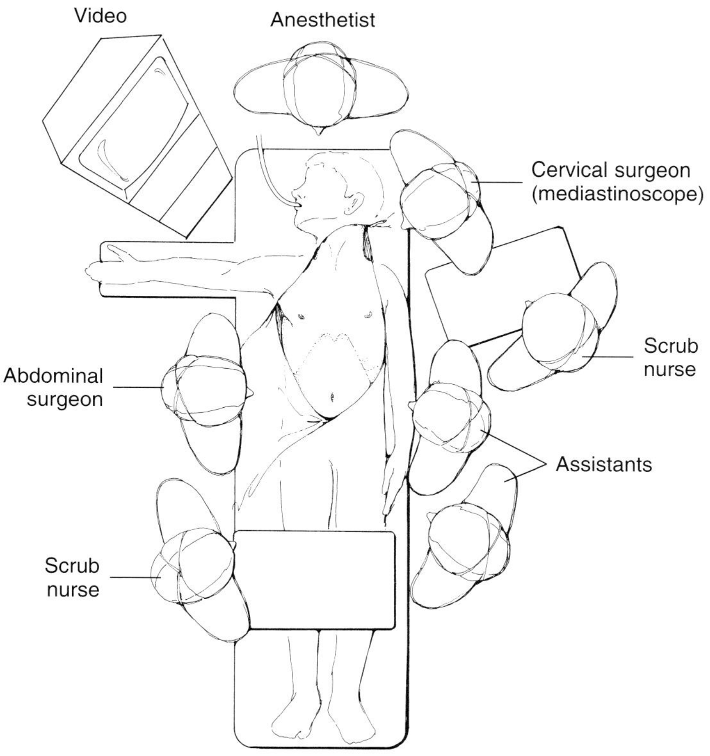

Fig. 19-4. Position of patient, nurses, and surgeons and arrangement of operating room tables.

verability of the mediastinoscope. A Stuhler retractor is mounted on a specially modified suspension. The abdominal surgeon stands on the right side of the patient and the two assistants on the opposite side, leaving enough space for the cervical surgeon, who usually works alone.

Technique

Disinfection of the skin and intravenous antibiotic coverage are used in the event that a sternotomy becomes necessary. The endodissection is carried out via a left cervical approach, as described previously.[18] A 10 to 15 cm incision is made at the anterior edge of the sternocleidomastoid muscle. The carotid artery and the jugular vein are exposed after division of the omohyoid muscle, and the recurrent laryngeal nerve is identified after division of the inferior thyroid artery. The esophagus, which is intubated with a thick rubber tube, is carefully exposed circumferentially and elevated with silicone tubing. The anterior surface of the cervical esophagus and the space between the esophagus and trachea are divided by blunt finger dissection. After the mediastinoscope is assembled, the tip of the instrument is carefully inserted into the upper mediastinum. This maneuver is critical because at this stage of the dissection the paraesophageal tissues are poorly visualized and anatomic orientation can be difficult. Placing moderate tension on the esophageal bougie can facilitate this portion of the procedure.

The anterior surface of the esophagus is dissected using the suction device, the electrocautery, and the microscissors. Dissection with the electrocautery and microscissors should be performed in multiple, staged steps since the structures behind the tissue being dissected are difficult to identify. During the remainder of the dissection the esophageal surface should be kept in view, and the periesophageal tissues should be placed under moderate tension by anterior movement of the mediastinoscope. Tissue bridges can then be divided easily with the electrocautery or microscissors. The back wall of the trachea is usually characterized by the sharp edges of its inferior surface and should be manipulated with great care to avoid injury. The area of the tracheal bifurcation (Fig. 19-5) is an important landmark for both surgical teams and should be inspected frequently during the procedure. If mediastinal tissue layers make recognition difficult, they can be removed. Laterally the paratracheal and parabronchial lymph nodes are readily identifiable by their characteristic anthracotic pigmentation. Biopsy specimens can be obtained as necessary. The left recurrent laryngeal nerve is only visible if the overlying paratracheal tissues are removed.

During anterograde dissection only a small area is under visual control and the endoscopic view is often impaired by fluid collection. Continuous rinsing of the operative field as well as intermittent flushing of the optical front end is mandatory so that the instrument does not have to be redrawn from the mediastinum. Instruments should be manipulated with great care in view of the limited degree of freedom and because manuevers must be performed within the axis of vision. The mediastinoscope is turned 180 degrees and the instrument is inserted behind the esophagus for dissection of the back wall (Fig. 19-6). This step is usually simple since there is no danger of damaging vital organs and the instrument can be advanced rapidly. The mediastinoscope is then adjusted to begin dissection of the left lateral and right lateral sides. The left-sided dissection is usually more difficult because of adherence to the left main bronchus. In addition, the esophagus has to be dissected from the descending aorta. If bleeding occurs, it will most likely be in this region. The right-sided dissection is not difficult,

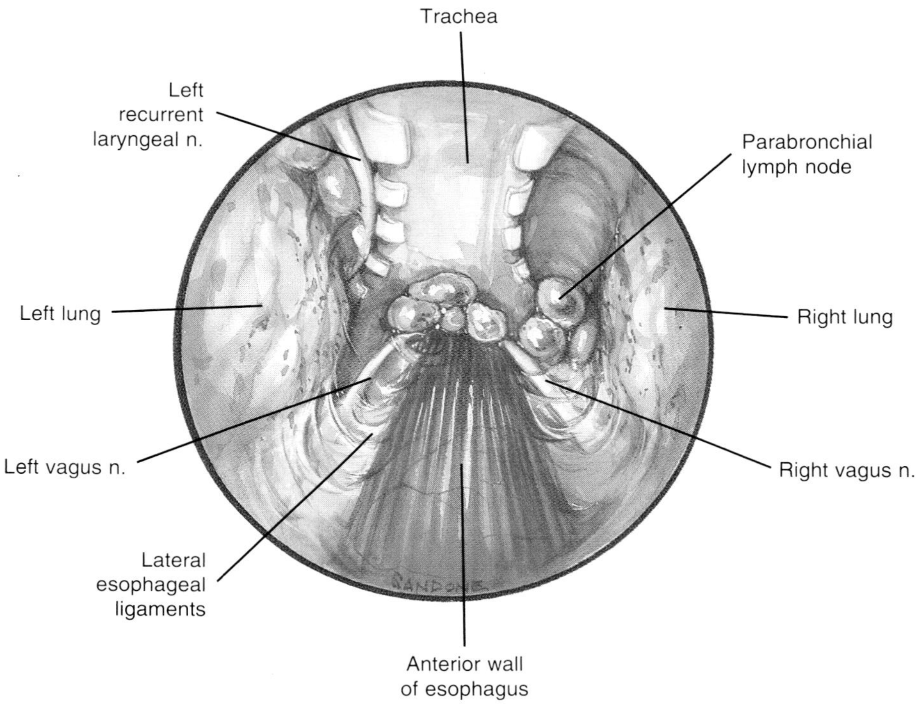

Fig. 19-5. Intraoperative appearance of the anterior esophageal surface and the relevant anatomic structures.

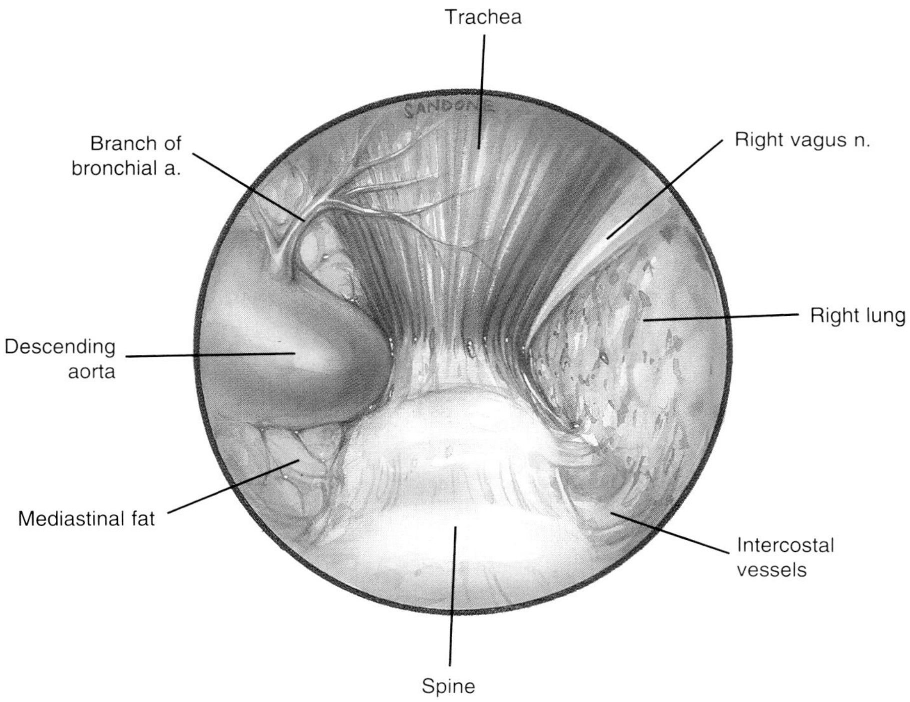

Fig. 19-6. Intraoperative appearance of the posterior esophageal surface and the relevant anatomic structures.

but care must be taken not to damage the azygos vein during the final steps. The pleural layer is frequently opened in this region, but drainage is seldom required.

The mediastinoscope is again inserted into the anterior compartment and advanced as far as possible. The abdominal surgeon is asked to open the hiatus and to control the position of the instrument. Remaining tissue bundles are incised bilaterally. Opening the hiatus earlier usually results in flooding of the mediastinum with peritoneal fluids, which impairs endoscopic vision.

The systemic blood pressure and cardiac rhythm are not altered if the mediastinoscope does not compress the pericardium. If this occurs, only minor changes are seen as compared with those associated with the use of retractors in the lower mediastinum. Endodissection seems to reduce the length of time retractors must be used.

The cervical team should not be overly aggressive in dissecting the lower esophagus or the tumor. A better angle of vision is afforded transhiatally, and the inferior esophagus can be excised along with periesophageal tissues and adherent lymph nodes. The cervical team can assist the abdominal team by focusing the light from the fiberoptic bundle so that the abdominal field can be visualized, which is especially helpful during transhiatal dissection. After the specimen is extracted, the time span necessary for preparation of the gastric interposition should be used for systematic removal of mediastinal lymph nodes and final hemostasis. In the event of technical failure the abdominal team can continue the operation (conventional blunt dissection) without the need for repositioning the patient or greater surgical exposure.

Management of Potential Complications

Initial concerns about complications have not materialized. The cervical team should be prepared for the possibility of a major injury occurring during dissection. If orientation is lost, the instrument should be retracted until the esophageal surface can be identified by its longitudinal muscle fibers. In the presence of arterial bleeding the optical end of the instrument should be flushed and the bleeding source localized and coagulated with the electrocautery. If bleeding is profuse, the instrument should be retracted after localization of the bleeding site and the cervical access used for mediastinal tamponade. The patient is then monitored for 10 to 20 minutes and the pack removed so that an endoscopic approach can be continued. Care should be taken to drain the right pleural cavity to prevent a hemothorax from developing. If the second attempt fails, the hiatus is opened by the abdominal team and the source is located transhiatally. If this fails, the bleeding has to be controlled through a right posterolateral thoracotomy.

In the event of bronchial injury the abdominal team should continue to prepare the stomach. After the abdomen is closed, the patient is brought to a left lateral position and the bronchial leak is sutured through a right posterolateral thoracotomy. The gastric interposition is then fixed over the injured area for additional coverage.

Clinical Experience

Endodissection was evaluated in a defined cohort of patients. No patients with advanced tumors or mediastinal tumor masses were included. All of the study patients would have been scheduled for transhiatal esophagectomy. We do not believe transhiatal esophagectomy and endodissection are indicated as a general treatment for patients with squamous cell carcinoma unless en bloc removal of the thoracic esophagus and adjacent lymph nodes cannot be performed. Thus only patients with squamous cell carcinoma in whom en bloc resection was contraindicated were included in this series.

Transmediastinal endodissection was tested in animal experiments between November 1990 and April 1991. From April 1991 until July 1993 we used endodissection rather than conventional transhiatal esophagectomy for all patients except those with carcinoma at or above the tracheal bifurcation and patients with advanced carcinoma. All patients underwent preoperative staging, including endoscopy, endosonography, and computed tomography, as well as operative risk assessment that included pulmonary function, ECG stress, and creatinine clearance tests.

We have performed endodissection on 50 patients to date (40 men and 10 women whose median age was 62 years, range 35 to 80 years). Of these, 33 patients (66%) had adenocarcinoma of the distal esophagus and 13 patients (20%) had squamous cell carcinoma. The median time required for endodissection was 45 minutes (range 40 to 60 minutes); the operative time decreased sharply during the study period.

Four patients died in the hospital within 30 days (8%). No fatality was directly related to endodissection. One patient with advanced liver cirrhosis had an esophageal rupture that was treated by esophagectomy. Despite multiple risk factors, we believe surgery was the best treatment option for this patient because of impending right-sided empyema. Endodissection was complicated by preexisting scars in the periesophageal tissues secondary to radical sclerosing treatments. The esophagus was finally removed without damage to the tracheobronchial system or mediastinal vessels. However, the patient died of hepatic failure during the early postoperative period. One patient died of septic organ failure caused by gastric necrosis, the third patient developed acute cardiorespiratory failure 14 days after the operation, and the fourth patient died of acute pulmonary embolism after discharge from the intensive care unit.

Relatively few serious intraoperative complications occurred (Table 19-1). The

Table 19-1. Complications directly related to endodissection observed in 50 consecutive patients (April 1991 to July 1993)

Complication	Management	No. of Patients	%
Insufficient view, technical failure	Conventional transhiatal esophagectomy	1	2
Significant mediastinal bleeding	Transhiatal ligation of intercostal vein	1	2
Early postoperative bleeding	Wound revision	1	2
Injury of right main bronchus	Transthoracic approach, suture	1	2
Esophageal tear during endodissection (muscular layer only)	Endodissection continued	5	10
Esophageal tear during endodissection (mucosal layer)	Transhiatal blunt dissection	2	4

most significant was an injury of the right main bronchus during lymph node dissection that was successfully managed by thoracotomy, esophagectomy, and bronchial suture. In one patient, bleeding from a right intercostal vein could not be stopped endoscopically. Transhiatal ligation successfully controlled the bleeding without the need for thoracotomy.

Trial I: Comparison of Endodissection and Transhiatal Esophagectomy

To compare the rate of postoperative complications a retrospective study was conducted in which the first 30 patients who had undergone endodissection were compared with 30 patients undergoing conventional transhiatal esophagectomy between 1986 and 1990.[18] The study was designed as a matched-pair analysis controlling for tumor stage, operative risk analysis, and age of patients.

The overall mortality was not significantly different for the two groups (6.6% vs. 13.3%). There were fewer postoperative pulmonary complications in the endodissection group (13.3% vs. 30%, $p < 0.05$) (Fig. 19-7). The rate of other complications was similar (Fig. 19-8). Two patients (6.6%) developed postoperative hoarseness secondary to left vocal cord palsy, which was confirmed by laryngoscopy. In one of these patients the recurrent nerve was injured during the cervical anastomosis; in the other patient the cause of recurrent nerve palsy remained undefined and occurred despite endodissection.

Trial II: Comparison of Endodissection to Conventional Transhiatal Esophagectomy and Transthoracic En Bloc Resection

Endodissection appears to be less stressful to the patient than conventional transhiatal esophagectomy or transthoracic esophagectomy. To document this observation we compared 15 patients who underwent endodissection and complete peri- and postoperative cardiopulmonary monitoring with 15 patients undergoing either transhiatal or transthoracic esophagectomy. The groups were matched according to tumor stage, operative risk analysis, and age of patients. Surprisingly, patients undergoing transthoracic esophagectomy had the best peri- and postoperative values for intrapulmonary shunt pressure, left ventricular function, and pulmonary artery pressure. However, this physiologic difference did not affect the postoperative course. Patients undergoing endodissection and transhiatal esophagectomy spent fewer days in the intensive care unit and had shorter intervals of intubation and mechanical ventilation than patients undergoing transthoracic esophagectomy without endodissection.

It was also apparent from this study that the total duration of anesthesia and the length of operation were considerably longer (almost 100%) in patients undergoing transthoracic esophagectomy than in those who had transhiatal esophagectomy. Although we thought that endodissection would shorten the transhiatal esophagectomy procedure, analysis of the operating time did not show any significant difference.

Cardiopulmonary monitoring gives no indication that endodissection is less stressful than conventional transhiatal esophagectomy. Furthermore, the data suggest that the decreased rate of postoperative pulmonary complications detected in trial I cannot be explained by a reduction of pulmonary or cardiac operative trauma in comparison with transhiatal esophagectomy.

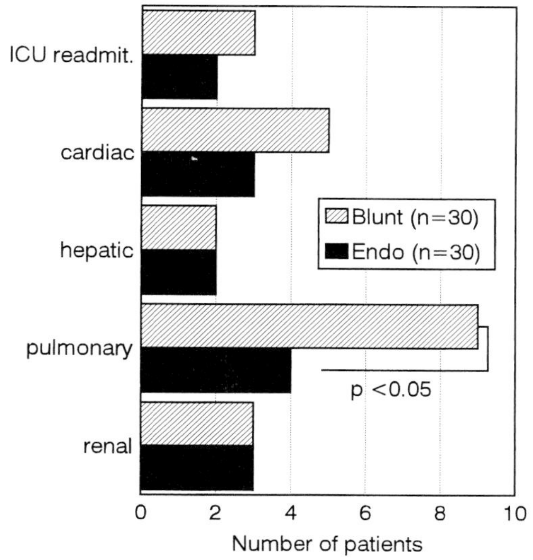

Fig. 19-7. Complications encountered in the intensive care unit in a prospective study comparing 30 patients undergoing endodissection and 30 patients undergoing conventional transhiatal esophagectomy. The rate of pulmonary complications was higher in patients who had conventional transhiatal esophagectomy. All other complications were comparable.

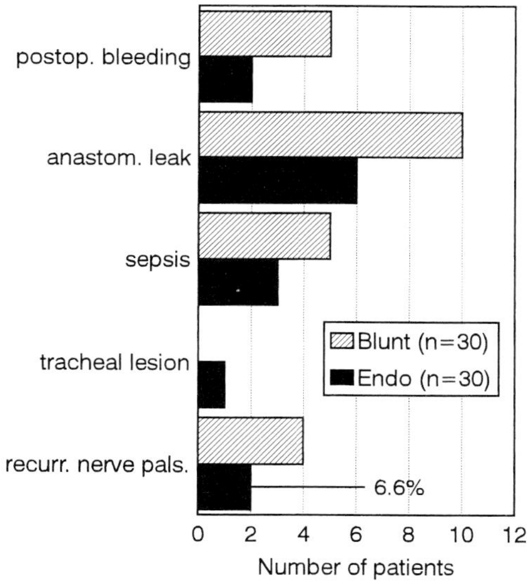

Fig. 19-8. Postoperative complications encountered in a prospective study comparing 30 patients undergoing endodissection and 30 patients undergoing conventional transhiatal esophagectomy. The rate of recurrent nerve palsy was only 6.6% in patients undergoing endodissection.

DISCUSSION

The primary goal of minimally invasive surgery is to reduce the surgical access necessary for therapeutic manipulation and to increase the postoperative well-being of the patient by reducing tissue trauma. Minimally invasive surgery is thus synonymous with minor access surgery. In our view this approach is justified in patients with malignant disease only if the benefits can be achieved without compromising the principles of oncologic surgery. Consequently, minor access surgical techniques in cancer of the foregut have few indications to date (see Chapters 18 and 20).

Endodissection per se does not reduce surgical trauma, and rather than being classified as a minor access procedure it should be considered a video-assisted esophagectomy because the surgical access is the same. Endodissection has been performed in many patients with minor perioperative morbidity and no mortality, demonstrating that the method is feasible and safe. The most significant complication encountered was a lesion of the right main bronchus, which was successfully treated and possibly could be avoided today because of safer anatomic orientation. Indications for the procedure must be strictly observed. Mediastinoscopic dissection should only be attempted in patients with a healthy esophagus. Tumor dissection is dangerous and may impair the patient's prognosis.

A systematic lymphadenectomy cannot be performed with the instruments currently available because dissection of the esophagus requires direct visualization. The risk of mediastinal bleeding at resection lines, including periesophageal tissue and lymph nodes, would be too great. The use of clip applicators is not advised because they can be easily dislocated by the tip of the mediastinoscope. On the other hand, we have observed that removal of isolated mediastinal lymph nodes is relatively easy although time consuming.

Trial I revealed that postoperative pulmonary complications are fewer in the endodissection group, possibly because of the low rate of recurrent nerve palsy observed after endodissection.[18] This is in contrast to recurrent nerve palsy rates of 10% to 25% after conventional transhiatal esophagectomy.[10-16] The reason is not yet clear; however, meticulous dissection during cervical access could be a factor as well as the minimal tissue traction created by the tissue dilator at the tip of the mediastinoscope compared with the hand and finger dissection used in conventional transhiatal esophagectomy. We believe the low rate of recurrent nerve palsy is important in preventing pulmonary complications secondary to silent aspiration.

Peri- and postoperative pulmonary monitoring of patients undergoing endodissection in trial II failed to demonstrate a benefit in terms of pulmonary shunt volume, pulmonary artery pressures, or cardiac output compared with conventional transhiatal esophagectomy. In this series, patients undergoing transthoracic esophagectomy had the best peri- and early postoperative monitoring values despite prolonged ventilation and intensive care unit stays. The latter are the first indicators that endodissection may be the preferred surgical technique in older patients with squamous cell carcinoma who are at increased pulmonary risk.

In summary, we believe endodissection is a valuable technical modification of transhiatal esophagectomy that should be considered primarily in patients with adenocarcinoma of the lower esophagus. The primary advantage of this technique is that it adds visual control to an operation heretofore performed blindly in a critical anatomic compartment. Further studies are needed to evaluate the potential of endodissection in treating advanced esophageal tumors as well as for the removal of lymphatic tissue.

REFERENCES

1. Beattie EJ, Bloom ND, Harvey JC. Esophagus. In Beattie EJ, Bloom ND, Harvey JC, eds. Thoracic Surgical Oncology. New York: Churchill Livingstone, 1993, pp 185-199.
2. Siewert JR. Esophageal cancer from the German point of view. Jpn J Surg 191:11-20, 1989.
3. Day NE, Munoz N. Esophagus. In Schottenfield D, Fraumenti JF, eds. Cancer Epidemiology and Prevention. Philadelphia: WB Saunders, 1982, p 195.
4. Akiyama H, Tsurumaru M, Kawamura T, Ono Y. Principles of surgical treatment for carcinoma of the esophagus: Analysis of lymph node involvement. Ann Surg 1944:438-446, 1981.
5. Siewert JR, Hölscher AH, Roder J, Bartels H. En Bloc Resektion der Speiseroehre beim Oesophaguskarzinom. Langenbecks Arch Chir 373:367-376, 1988.
6. Skinner DB, Belsey RHR. En bloc resection for neoplasms of the esophagus and the cardia. J Thorac Cardiovasc Surg 85:59-71, 1983.
7. Muller JM, Erasmi H, Stelzner M, Zieren U, Pichlmaier H. Surgical therapy of esophageal carcinoma. Br J Surg 77:845-857, 1990.
8. Fan ST, Lau WY, Yip WC, Poon GP, Yeung C, Lam WK, Wong KK. Prediction of postoperative pulmonary complications in esophagogastric surgery. Br J Surg 74:408-410, 1987.
9. Orringer MB. Transhiatal esophagectomy without thoracotomy for carcinoma of the thoracic esophagus. Ann Surg 200:282-288, 1984.
10. Barbier PA, Becker CD, Wagner HE. Esophageal carcinoma: Patient selection for transhiatal esophagectomy. A prospective analysis of 50 consecutive cases. World J Surg 12:263-269, 1988.
11. Finley RJ, Grace M, Duff JH. Esophagogastrectomy without thoracotomy for carcinoma of the cardia and the lower part of the esophagus. Surg Gynecol Obstet 160:49-56, 1985.
12. Finley RJ, Inculet RI. The results of esophagogastrectomy without thoracotomy for adenocarcinoma of the esophagogastric junction. Ann Surg 2104:535-543, 1989.
13. Hankins JR, Attar S, Coughlin TR, Miller JE, Hebel JR, Suter CM, McLaughlin CM. Carcinoma of the esophagus: A comparison of the results of transhiatal versus transthoracic resection. Ann Thorac Surg 47:700-705, 1989.
14. Orringer MB. Transhiatal esophagectomy for esophageal carcinoma. In Siewert JR, Hölscher AH, eds. Diseases of the Esophagus. New York: Springer Verlag, 1987, pp 390-393.
15. Siewert JR, Hölscher AH, Horvarth OP. Transmediastinale Oesophagektomie. Langenbecks Arch Chir 367:203-213, 1986.
16. Steiger Z, Wilson RF. Comparison of the results of esophagectomy with and without thoracotomy. Surg Gynecol Obstet 153:653-656, 1981.
17. Buess G, Becker HD, Mentges R, Teichmann R, Lenz G. Die endoskopisch mikrochirurgische Dissektion der Speiseroehre. Chirurg 61:308-311, 1990.
18. Bumm R, Hölscher AH, Feussner H, Tachibana M, Bartels H, Siewert JR. Endodissection of the thoracic esophagus: Technique and clinical results in transhiatal esophagectomy. Ann Surg 2161:97-104, 1993.

Chapter

20

Minimal Access Surgery for Cancer of the Foregut and Pancreas

Dilip Parekh, M.D.

The introduction of the computer chip camera in 1986 allowed the coupling of the laparoscope to a video system and led to a revolution in the application of this technology for surgery of intra-abdominal organs. Initially laparoscopic procedures for abdominal malignancy were largely confined to diagnosis of metastatic disease in patients with ascites of unknown origin. Recent developments in minimally invasive surgery have expanded the role of laparoscopy in the diagnosis and treatment of abdominal malignancies. Improvements in laparoscopic equipment and the availability of laparoscopic ultrasonography have led to a reevaluation of its role in staging patients with foregut and pancreatic malignancies.

Minimal access surgery techniques can provide palliative treatment for patients with advanced malignancies with the significant benefits of rapid convalescence and discharge from the hospital for those whose life expectancies may be limited. The use of therapeutic laparoscopy may also result in earlier entry of patients into adjuvant or therapeutic chemoradiation protocols. Minimally invasive surgery's reduced immunosuppressive effect may favorably alter tumor growth. On the other hand, disadvantages of minimal access surgery include longer operative times and a significant learning curve for mastering the techniques of tumor removal. The adequacy of resection as compared with open techniques is a continuing concern. We will review the emerging role of minimal access surgery in the diagnosis and treatment of foregut malignancies, although it must be emphasized that an objective comparison with standard open techniques is impossible in view of the limited data available from control studies to date. It is unclear at present whether minimal access techniques can permit the extent of resection possible with open techniques to effect a cure in patients with foregut cancer. Nor has the incidence of port site recurrences been adequately addressed. Virtually no data are available on survival rates after minimal access surgery in comparison to open surgery. We believe that widespread, indiscriminant use of minimal access techniques for *curative* resection of lesions of the foregut cannot be condoned at present and should be limited to controlled clinical trials.

Advantages and Disadvantages of Minimal Access Surgery for Foregut Malignancies

Advantages

Reduced tissue trauma
Reduced wound infections, postoperative analgesia, deep vein thrombosis, and respiratory complications
Reduced hospital stay
?Reduced immunosuppressive effect

Disadvantages

Controlled data unavailable for comparison to open procedures
Significant learning curve for mastering techniques
Need for technologic improvements to ensure adequate resection of foregut cancers
Lack of data on incidence of port site recurrences

New methodologies must adhere to certain time-honored principles in the surgical management of gastrointestinal cancers.

1. Adequate proximal and distal margins must be obtained to prevent local recurrence. Gastric and esophageal cancers commonly spread via submucosal lymphatics. A curative procedure requires at least a 10 cm proximal and distal margin for esophageal cancer and a 5 cm margin for gastric cancer.
2. All margins must be negative (i.e., a circumference of normal tissue must be removed with the cancer).
3. The regional lymph nodes and any adjacent organs involved should be resected en bloc with the tumor.

Indiscriminate use of laparoscopic procedures for foregut malignancies may violate these principles and adversely affect the outcome. In the following discussion we will emphasize the application of these principles to each foregut organ and reiterate that a laparoscopic procedure for cancer is only justified if these principles are not compromised during resection of the tumor.

ESOPHAGEAL CANCER

Minimal access surgery may have applications in the treatment of esophageal neoplasms. Thoracoscopic[1] and endoscopic[2] dissection of the esophagus has been performed successfully and may be a therapeutic option in patients requiring esophagectomy.[1] Endosurgical esophagectomy offers some potential advantages over a transhiatal esophagectomy.[2] The vascular supply to the esophagus can be transected under direct vision, which should significantly decrease postoperative bleeding from the mediastinum; injury of the recurrent laryngeal nerve should be minimized with the endoscopic procedure; and both middle and lower esophageal lesions can be resected.[3] It is not yet clear if these theoretical advantages can be translated into greater clinical benefits.

Selection of Surgical Approach

Emphasis should be placed on appropriate selection of patients for curative en bloc esophagectomy.[3] Transhiatal or endoscopic resection could be offered to those in whom palliation is the only therapeutic option. Lymph node metastases are not adequately treated by endosurgical or transhiatal esophagectomy since a formal thoracic lymphadenectomy cannot be accomplished with these procedures. Surgery is limited to removing the primary tumor in the anticipation that adjuvant therapy will eradicate locoregional and systemic disease.[3] Endosurgical methods of esophagectomy are therefore limited to the palliative treatment of esophageal malignancy.

Survival following surgical removal of a carcinoma arising in the distal esophagus or cardia depends on the method of resection. Patients with early lesions (i.e., tumors limited to the esophageal wall with four or less involved nodes) have significantly better survival rates after extended en bloc resection.[3] Evidence increasingly suggests that survival rates following transhiatal resection are inferior to those following curative en bloc esophagogastrectomy and lymphadenectomy in properly selected patients.[3] There are several possible explanations for the failure of a transhiatal resection to achieve the results obtained with en bloc resection in favorably staged patients:

1. Dissemination of tumor cells during blunt dissection of the thoracic esophagus
2. Failure to leave an adequate distal tumor margin in an effort to preserve the full length of the stomach to ensure gastrointestinal continuity with the cervical esophagogastrostomy, resulting in recurrent disease along the gastric suture line[4]
3. Transfer of unrecognized perigastric metastatic nodes to the thorax during the gastric pull-up
4. Leaving residual nodal metastases in the mediastinum, splenic hilum, and celiac axis

An en bloc esophagogastrectomy effectively eliminates all of these possible causes of recurrence. Procedures focusing only on removal of the primary tumor (such as transhiatal thoracic or endoscopic esophagectomy) can only be considered palliative procedures.

Selection of Patients for Surgical Approach

En Bloc Esophagectomy

Age <75 years
Early tumors of distal esophagus
No significant cardiovascular or pulmonary disease

Endoscopic or Transhiatal Esophagectomy

Tumor penetrating through esophageal wall
Metastases to regional lymph nodes
Age >75 years
Significant cardiovascular or pulmonary disease
Intraoperative staging showing cavitary spread of tumor, extension of tumor through mediastinal pleura, multiple gross lymph node metastases, or microscopic evidence of lymph node involvement at margins of en bloc resection (i.e., low paratracheal, porta hepatis, subpancreatic, or periaortic lymph nodes)

Open transhiatal esophagectomy is a safe procedure. Bleeding, recurrent laryngeal nerve paralysis, and tracheal injuries, complications associated with transhiatal esophagectomy, may be avoided by endoscopic esophagectomy. At present open transhiatal esophagectomy for distal esophageal cancer is still preferable to a laparoscopic transhiatal approach. With time, an endosurgical procedure may be a reasonable alternative.

GASTRIC CANCER

It is estimated that in 1992 there were 24,000 new cases of gastric cancer and 13,000 deaths from this disease. An interesting epidemiologic change in the United States and Europe has been the decrease in distal gastric tumors and a shift of the disease proximally, as evidenced by the increase in cancers of the cardioesophageal junction. The principles of treatment of patients with proximal gastric cancers are the same as for those with esophageal cancer.

Extent of Resection

Although the appropriate surgical procedure for patients with gastric cancer is a subject of controversy,[4-7] it is not likely that laparoscopic gastric resection will emerge as a therapeutic option in the curative setting. In Japan an aggressive operative approach to patients with gastric cancer, including an extended lymphadenectomy, is advocated.[4,5] The standard procedure for gastric cancer in Western countries has not routinely included extended lymphadenectomy. The Japanese experience suggests that a gastrectomy with an extended lymphadenectomy (R_2 or R_3 gastrectomy) removes occult nodal disease and achieves better locoregional control.[4,5] The Japanese have consistently reported better survival stage for stage for gastric cancer in comparison to reports from Western countries. In 1981 Kodama et al.[4] reported a 45% 5-year survival rate for patients with advanced gastric cancer following gastrectomy and regional lymph node dissection. This was significantly better than that reported in patients undergoing simple gastrectomy, who had an 18% 5-year survival rate. Inokuchi[5] states that the primary factor responsible for the dramatic improvement in the survival of patients with gastric cancer in Japan has been the standardization of the operative method to include extensive lymph node dissection. Investigations in other countries have shown similar results. In a prospective study from Chile, Csendes et al.[6] reported a series of 253 patients with stage III gastric cancer who underwent R_1 gastrectomy and limited lymphadenectomy vs. those undergoing radical gastrectomy with extended lymph node dissection (R_2 or R_3). The 5-year survival was 23% in patients who had extended lymph node dissection vs. 7.6% for those who had simple gastrectomy only. Limited data from the West also corroborate that extended lymph node dissection may improve survival in patients with gastric cancer. Lawrence and Shiu[7] reported a 76.4% disease-free 5-year survival rate in 60 patients with early gastric cancer following extended gastrectomy. Three of eight patients with nodal metastases survived 5 years or longer, including one with N2 nodal disease. Siewert et al.[8] from Germany recently reported that R_2 gastrectomy resulted in significantly improved outcome compared with patients who underwent simple gastrectomy.

There is evidence that extended lymphadenectomy with radical gastric resection results in less locoregional failures in patients with advanced gastric cancers. Simple resection for gastric cancer results in locoregional recurrence rates of 10% to 25%.

The gastric remnant and the adjacent gastric bed were the only sites of recurrent disease in 53% of patients who had relapses.[9] Meyer and Pichlmayr[10] reported that 20% to 30% of local recurrences originated from the perigastric lymphatic tissue. Papachristou and Fortner[11] observed 257 gastric cancer patients from the time of resection to death. They found a 25% incidence of local recurrence in the field of the gastrectomy. On the contrary, radical gastrectomy is associated with a low incidence of locoregional and nodal failure. In a study of 7060 cases of gastric cancer treated by radical gastrectomy, Nakajima et al.[12] found a 6.8% incidence of recurrence in the gastric stump or in the adjacent gastric bed and a 3.8% incidence of nodal recurrence. Even for early gastric cancer (T1 lesions) the pattern of recurrence shifted away from nodal recurrence in those patients undergoing R_2 resection.

These studies strongly support radical gastrectomy and extended lymphadenectomy as the preferred procedure for gastric cancer. Two large prospective randomized studies comparing R_1 to R_2 gastrectomies are currently under way in the United Kingdom and in the Netherlands. It is anticipated that the results from these studies will clarify whether R_2 gastrectomy with extended lymph node dissection is the procedure of choice.

We recommend an R_2 radical gastrectomy with extended lymph node dissection as the standard procedure for gastric cancer in patients with stage I to III disease. Patients with stage IV disease with liver or peritoneal metastases probably do not benefit from this procedure and a simple palliative gastrectomy may be the best choice. In this setting laparoscopic gastrectomy may have future potential.

Indications for Laparoscopy

The primary role of laparoscopy in the management of gastric cancer involves the staging and diagnosis of peritoneal or liver metastases. The technique of exploratory laparoscopy described subsequently in this chapter for pancreatic cancer is used. As mentioned, although the technique for laparoscopic gastrectomy has been described, we do not advocate laparoscopic resection for curable gastric cancer.

In patients with advanced or unresectable gastric cancer a palliative procedure such as a gastrojejunostomy for gastric outlet obstruction or feeding gastrostomy or jejunostomy may be indicated and performed using advanced laparoscopic techniques.

Selection of Patients With Gastric Cancer for Laparoscopy

Diagnostic Laparoscopy

Ascites
Metastases
Altered liver function tests
Abnormal pelvic examination

Therapeutic Laparoscopy

Palliative gastrectomy
Feeding gastrostomy or jejunostomy
Palliative gastrojejunostomy

PANCREATIC CANCER

Pancreatic cancer is now the fourth leading cause of death from cancer in the United States after lung, colorectal, and breast cancer. Current trends indicate that approximately 28,000 new cases will be diagnosed and 25,000 patients will die annually from this disease in the United States. The overall 5-year survival rate is less than 5% and the outcome of pancreatic cancer has not improved over the past five decades.

Extent of Disease

Patients with pancreatic cancer fall into three distinct subgroups: patients with resectable disease, patients with locally advanced unresectable disease (involvement of major vascular structures, including the portal vein and superior mesenteric artery), and patients with metastatic disease. These subgroups are associated with different outcomes and require different management strategies.

Resectable Pancreatic Cancer. At present, cancer of the body and tail of the pancreas is generally considered incurable. Tumors of the head of the pancreas remain localized in some 5% to 25% of cases. Significant progress has been made in the past two decades in the treatment of patients with resectable cancer of the head of the pancreas. Mortality rates following resection have decreased from 25% in the 1960s to less than 5% at present. In addition, the 5-year survival has improved from less than 10% three decades ago to about 20% today.[13,14] Resection offers the only chance for cure, and it is our firm belief that this option should be aggressively pursued in every patient who presents with a diagnosis of pancreatic cancer. In recent studies selected subgroups of patients receiving postoperative chemoradiation therapy have been shown to have improved survival rates. Five-year survival rates of 30% to 40% have been reported.[13]

Locally Advanced Unresectable Pancreatic Cancer. This subgroup of patients have extrapancreatic extension of the tumor with involvement of the portal vein and/or superior mesenteric artery. These patients are generally not offered surgical resection since resection of the major vascular structures is thought to be associated with a prohibitive morbidity rate. On the other hand, the outcome for these patients has been shown to be different from that for patients with metastatic pancreatic cancer. Studies have demonstrated that 45% of patients with advanced regional disease are alive at 1 year, with an occasional 5-year survivor recorded.[15] Furthermore, aggressive neoadjuvant chemoradiation therapy may prolong survival and permit resection of the cancer in some patients.[16]

Metastatic Pancreatic Cancer. Metastatic pancreatic cancer has a poor prognosis that has not changed despite decades of intense investigation. The median survival in these patients is 3 to 6 months. No combination of chemotherapy and radiation treatment has proved to be effective in this group of patients.[17]

Staging

It is quite clear that the therapeutic approach to pancreatic cancer depends on the stage of the disease. Accurate preoperative staging of pancreatic cancer is important for appropriate management.

Abdominal Computed Tomography (CT). CT remains the gold standard for the initial diagnosis and staging of patients with pancreatic cancer. Pancreatic masses as small as 2 cm in diameter can be detected and may indicate extrapancreatic spread and liver metastases. Percutaneous biopsies may be performed under CT guidance to obtain a pathologic diagnosis. Liver metastases larger than 2 cm in diameter are easily identified by CT; however, approximately one third of patients have metastatic deposits smaller than 1 cm in size that cannot be detected by CT.[14] Furthermore, peritoneal and omental metastases are common and usually measure only 1 to 2 mm in diameter. These can be diagnosed only by direct visualization.[16] The high frequency with which small metastatic deposits less than 1 cm in diameter are found in patients with pancreatic cancer is characteristic of gastrointestinal tumors.[16] In addition, when an endobiliary prosthesis is in place prior to CT staging, it can produce significant artifacts that limit the ability of CT to accurately assess local disease progression.

Not only is the value of CT limited in staging unrecognized metastatic disease, it is also relatively insensitive for predicting resectability. Warshaw et al.[16] reported the preoperative staging of 88 patients referred for treatment of potentially curable pancreatic adenocarcinomas to the Massachusetts General Hospital from July 1985 to March 1989. A dynamic CT scan was 92% accurate in predicting unresectability, whereas it was only 45% correct in predicting resectability. This study suggests that surgical exploration of a lesion thought to be resectable on CT would lead to unnecessary laparotomy in some 40% to 50% of cases. Further, CT prediction of unresectability may lead to a significant number of patients with resectable lesions going undetected.

In summary, CT cannot identify small metastatic tumor nodules, which are particularly prevalent in patients with pancreatic cancer, and often understages or overstages the extent of local invasion, largely because of its lack of accuracy in predicting vascular invasion. The primary usefulness of CT is thus limited to the initial diagnosis of pancreatic cancer and detection of obvious liver metastases. MRI has not been shown to be superior to CT.

Angiography. Angiography has become a routine investigation in some centers to stage patients with pancreatic cancer. The use of CT and angiography has improved resectability rates from 20% in earlier studies to 50% to 70% of patients at present. Dooley et al.[18] reviewed the use of angiography in 90 patients with pancreatic cancer. In 62 patients the vessels were patent on angiography; only three of these had vascular involvement at surgery. Of 11 patients in whom either the portal vein or superior mesenteric artery was completely occluded, the tumor was not resectable in any patient. Angiography showed vessel encasement in a third group of 17 patients. Six of these patients were found to have resectable disease. Because angiography is an invasive procedure, noninvasive alternatives such as color-flow Doppler or duplex scanning have aroused interest in recent years.[19-20] We have found that duplex scanning is reliable for detecting vascular occlusion and it has replaced angiography at our institution. Angiography is used in selected patients only.

Endoscopic and Laparoscopic Ultrasonography. Endoscopic and laparoscopic ultrasonography are new technologies that allow direct local imaging of the tumor[21,22] and may signal more effective staging of pancreatic cancer in the future. The accuracy of direct imaging of the pancreas by ultrasound is demonstrated by the experience with intraoperative ultrasound at laparotomy. Intraoperative ultrasonography has a

Table 20-1. Diagnostic accuracy of laparoscopy and laparoscopic ultrasonography in determining resectability of pancreatic or ampullary cancers

	Laparoscopy (n = 28)	Laparoscopy and Laparoscopic Ultrasonography (n = 26)
Sensitivity	100% (10/10)	90% (9/10)
Specificity	44% (8/18)	88% (14/16)
Accuracy	64% (18/28)	88% (23/26)

From John TG, Garden OJ. Assessment of pancreatic cancer. In Cuesta MA, Nagy AG, eds. Minimally Invasive Surgery in Gastrointestinal Cancer. Edinburgh: Churchill Livingstone, 1993, pp 95-111.

sensitivity of 94.1%, a specificity of 86.4%, and an overall accuracy of 89.7% in assessing resectability of pancreatic cancer.[23] This is significantly better than a combination of all preoperative studies, which have an overall accuracy of only 64.1% for diagnosing portal vein invasion.[23]

Preliminary reports on endoscopic and laparoscopic ultrasonography are promising. Endoscopic ultrasonography is superior to transabdominal ultrasound and CT for assessment of resectability of pancreatic cancer.[21] The involvement of the portal venous system as judged by surgical exploration was correctly assessed by endoscopic ultrasonography in 95% of cases as opposed to 85% for angiography, 75% for CT, and 55% for abdominal ultrasonography. Endoscopic ultrasonography correctly predicted portal venous infiltration found at surgery in 10 out of 11 patients; CT and angiography were significantly less accurate. This study concluded that endoscopic ultrasonography is the single most sensitive procedure for staging pancreatic cancer.[21]

The value of endoscopic ultrasonography for staging pancreatic cancer is limited by the technical difficulties of adequately imaging the pancreas through the stomach and the duodenum. Laparoscopic ultrasonography is a simpler technical procedure, although experience with this modality is limited. John and Garden[24] found that laparoscopic ultrasonography, however, was sensitive, specific, and accurate for staging pancreatic cancer (Table 20-1). If wider experience with laparoscopic ultrasonongraphy supports the limited findings to date, CT followed by laparoscopy and laparoscopic ultrasonography may prove to be the best method of staging pancreatic cancer.

Laparoscopy. Laparoscopy has been advocated as a routine preoperative investigation to assess resectability in patients with pancreatic cancer. Its major contribution to date has been in identifying patients with small metastatic deposits on the surface of the peritoneum or liver. Warshaw et al.[16] demonstrated that a combination of preoperative CT, angiography, and diagnostic laparoscopy predicted resectability in 75% of cases, the best sensitivity reported to date. There are, however, three major criticisms of staging laparoscopy: (1) Its value has been questioned as a routine investigation in all patients with pancreatic cancer. The Johns Hopkins group, in particular, has found that CT and angiography predict resectability in about 70% of patients,[13] a number similar to that reported by Warshaw et al.[16] (2) Although metastatic deposits on the surface of the liver may be visualized, lesions deeper in the parenchyma cannot be adequately imaged by diagnostic laparoscopy. (3) Laparoscopy does not address the difficulties of assessing the extent of disease outside the pancreas, particularly involvement of major vessels such as the portal vein, superior mesenteric vein, and superior mesenteric artery. Some of the criticisms may be overcome if ongoing work with laparoscopic ultrasonography establishes its role in assessing vascular and liver involvement.

Selection of Surgical Approach

Current surgical practice dictates resection in all patients with localized cancer of the head of the pancreas. Patients not considered for pancreaticoduodenectomy include those in whom liver metastases is documented on preoperative CT, laparoscopy shows peritoneal dissemination or liver metastases, imaging studies clearly document occlusion of the portal vein or superior mesenteric artery, or advanced cardiorespiratory disease is present.

In the absence of these four criteria we believe that surgical exploration is warranted in all patients since curative resection provides the only chance for long-term survival. In patients with metastatic disease biliary stents should be placed by endoscopic techniques. Patients with metastases generally are not candidates for chemoradiation therapy since no survival benefit has been demonstrated. Surgical gastroenterostomy is not indicated in the presence of metastatic disease unless the patient has symptomatic gastric outlet obstruction.

Palliative Surgical Procedures for Unresectable Pancreatic Cancer. Palliative procedures for unresectable pancreatic cancer include biliary decompression, relief of gastric outflow obstruction, and pain control. The standard surgical approach in patients who are found to have unresectable tumors at exploration is a biliary bypass. Most surgeons would also advocate performing a gastrojejunostomy, although its routine use is controversial.[17,25,26]

In patients without metastatic disease who are not candidates for resection because of portal vein or superior mesenteric artery involvement, palliative biliary bypass using either an open or laparoscopic technique is indicated. Because of the risk of cystic duct obstruction, laparoscopic cholecystojejunostomy should be considered only if the entry of the cystic duct is at least 1.5 cm above the site of involvement of the common duct.

The choice of choledochojejunostomy or a cholecystojejunostomy has been long debated in the literature.[17] Choledochojejunostomy is often preferred because of the risk of recurrent jaundice from tumor progression and infiltration and obstruction of the cystic duct following cholecystojejunostomy. Minimally invasive surgery makes this choice particularly relevant. Laparoscopic cholecystojejunostomy is technically less demanding and more expeditious. The potential for recurrent jaundice has been poorly addressed in the literature. It would seem that at worst fewer than 5% to 10% of patients with a cholecystojejunostomy will develop recurrent jaundice.[17] A comparison of cholecystojejunostomies and choledochojejunostomies performed at Memorial Sloan Kettering showed no difference in the length of time it took for bilirubin levels to decrease to normal or overall mortality.[17] Singh et al.[25] found that cholecystojejunostomy was as effective as choledochojejunostomy. An adequate tumor-free distance between the entry of the cystic duct into the bile duct and the upper limit of the tumor is essential if a laparoscopic cholecystojejunostomy is performed to bypass biliary obstruction.

Of particular concern has been the late occurrence of gastric outlet obstruction as a terminal event in many patients.[17,25,26] A prophylactic gastrojejunostomy may improve survival, suggesting that the nutritional consequences of late duodenal obstruction may contribute to early mortality.[17] In reviewing the experience at the University of California, Los Angeles, Singh et al.[25] found that in 22% of patients with advanced pancreatic cancer, gastric outlet obstruction was the terminal event if a prophylactic gastrojejunostomy had not performed. Data on the role of prophylactic gastrojejunostomy are difficult to interpret since patients with locally advanced and metastatic disease are not identified in most studies. Because the median survival of patients with metastatic pancreatic cancer is only 3 months, gastroenterostomy is not indicated unless there are symptoms of gastric outflow obstruction. When treated aggressively with chemoradiation therapy, patients with locally advanced unresectable pancreatic cancer have a median survival of 10 months and 45% are alive at the end of 1 year. A substantial number of these patients will develop duodenal obstruction if a gastric bypass procedure is not performed at the time of the initial surgery.[16,25,26] It is our practice to perform a prophylactic gastrojejunostomy routinely in patients with locally advanced unresectable pancreas cancer in the absence of metastatic disease.

Surgical Techniques

Diagnostic Laparoscopy. A 2 cm incision is made in the periumbilical region and extended into the peritoneal cavity using an open technique. A Hasson cannula is introduced through this incision and the abdomen is insufflated with CO_2. The laparoscope is introduced and an initial survey of the abdomen is performed. If metastatic deposits are seen in the peritoneal cavity or in the liver, a second 5 mm trocar is inserted at the appropriate position to perform a biopsy. Frozen sections of the tumor deposits should be obtained to confirm metastatic deposits.

If no metastatic deposits are seen on the initial survey, we explore the abdomen further. Additional trocars are inserted as needed. A detailed laparoscopic examination of the abdominal cavity includes careful examination of the posterior aspect of the anterior abdominal wall, the right pericolic gutters, the pelvis, and the left pericolic gutters. The bowel is retracted and the superior and inferior surfaces of the liver are examined carefully. To examine the inferior surface of the liver a fan-shaped liver retractor is used to pull the liver upward. One of the criticisms of the laparoscopic examination in comparison to open surgery is the inability to palpate the liver parenchyma to detect metastases. Laparoscopic ultrasonography may be used as a substitute for the surgeon's hand. The 6 MHz articulated laparoscopic probe allows for adequate imaging over the dome of the liver. The probe is introduced through a 10 mm port to image the anterior and superior surfaces of the liver. The base of the transverse mesocolon and the area around the ligament of Treitz are common sites of metastasis. The greater omentum is grasped with two Babcock clamps and curled back onto itself until the transverse colon with its mesocolon is exposed. The omentum is then pushed back over the stomach into the upper quadrant of the abdomen. At this stage the patient is placed in a reverse Trendelenburg position, and the loops of small bowel lying along the base of the transverse mesocolon are gently swept down

Table 20-2. Incidence of unsuspected peritoneal and/or liver metastases discovered during laparoscopy in patients presenting with pancreatic and ampullary cancer reported in the literature

Reference	Tumor Location	No. of Patients
Warshaw et al.[16]	Head of pancreas	15/55 (27%)
	All pancreatic and ampullary	27/88 (31%)
Cuschieri et al.[27]	Head of pancreas and ampullary	3/15 (20%)
Warshaw et al.[28]	All pancreatic and ampullary	17/40 (43%)
Watanabe et al.[29]	All pancreatic	8/16 (50%)

in the pelvis using the fan retractor. If Babcock clamps are used to elevate the transverse colon, the entire length of the transverse mesocolon can be easily visualized. As one moves laterally the ligament of Treitz comes into view.

The ventral surface of the pancreas is examined through the lesser sac. Two Babcock clamps are introduced through ports in the right and left side of the abdomen and the stomach is tented up to expose the thinned area on the lateral aspect of the greater omentum. This provides easy access into the lesser sac. Large omental vessels are ligated with endoclips. The lesser sac is exposed widely. Adhesions between the posterior aspect of the stomach and the pancreas are taken down and the full length of the pancreas exposed. Any pancreatic lesions are examined carefully. Involvement of the hepaticogastric omentum is readily assessed by this technique.

A laparoscopic ultrasound probe may be passed over the ventral surface of the pancreas, the size of the lesion mapped, and the portal vein, superior mesenteric vein, and the superior mesenteric artery imaged through the ventral surface of the pancreas. The pancreas is scanned in both longitudinal and transverse planes. We use an articulated probe to examine for regional lymph node enlargement, including portal nodes. The probe is passed over the gastrohepatic ligament along the superior aspect of the stomach and through the lesser sac along the superior surface of the pancreas to image splenic, hepatic, and celiac nodes. The probe is then passed over the periaortic region to check for aortic node involvement.

Criteria for resectability include the absence of metastatic disease or obvious vascular invasion (Table 20-2). In those patients whose disease is judged to be resectable, a standard Whipple procedure is performed by open laparotomy.

Laparoscopic Bypass Procedures for Advanced Pancreatic Cancer. Laparoscopic techniques have been described for cholecystojejunostomy and gastrojejunostomy in patients with advanced unresectable or metastatic pancreatic cancer.[30-32] At present it is unclear whether laparoscopic cholecystojejunostomy offers any significant advantages over endoscopic stenting. Although techniques have been described for laparoscopic choledochojejunostomy, it is unlikely that this procedure will gain widespread acceptance because of its technical complexity. As mentioned, laparoscopic cholecystojejunostomy should only be performed if the cystic duct enters the common hepatic duct at least 1.5 cm above the tumor. Such invasion is a common cause of

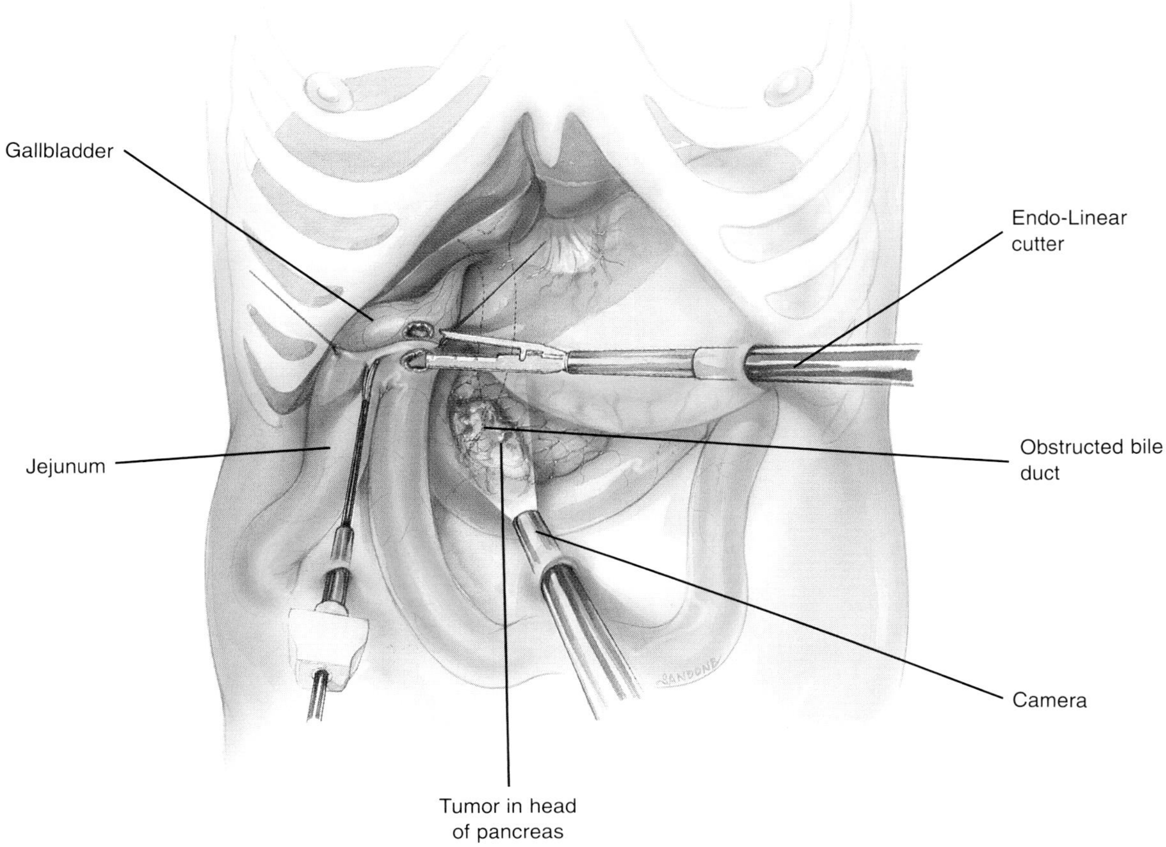

Fig. 20-1. Laparoscopic cholecystojejunostomy using a linear stapler. A side-to-side cholecystojejunostomy is created in a fashion analogous to that used for gastrojejunostomy.

recurrent jaundice and failure of palliation following surgical cholecystenterostomy. Endoscopic stenting with metal expandable stents should be used if the cystic duct common junction is close to the tumor. Two techniques have been reported for laparoscopic cholecystojejunostomy. Shimi et al.[30] described a handsewn anastomosis performed completely laparoscopically, and Fletcher [31] performed laparoscopic cholecystojejunostomy using a stapling device.

Cholecystojejunostomy. Because endoscopic stent placement is an alternative means of palliation, laparoscopic cholecystojejunostomy is only justified if the morbidity rate is less than 4% and the mortality rate is less than 2% (Fig. 20-1).

An appropriate site is selected on the jejunum, which is then brought up to the fundus of the gallbladder. Extracorporeally placed sutures are used to approximate the fundus of the gallbladder to the jejunum. A 1 cm incision is made in the jejunum and gallbladder, and a vascular gastrointestinal stapling device is introduced and fired. The opening left when the stapling device is removed is closed by firing the stapler again.

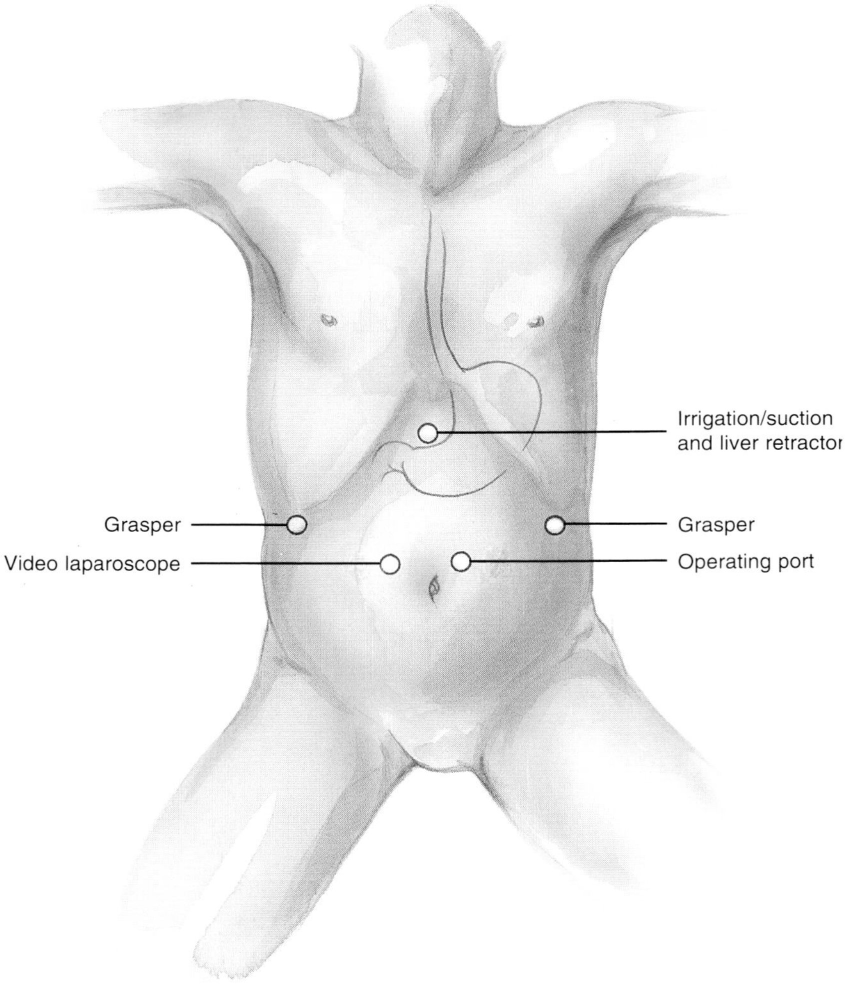

Fig. 20-2. Trocar placement for bilioenteric or gastroenteric bypass.

Gastrojejunostomy. Experience with laparoscopic gastroenterostomies is more limited. Mouiel et al.[29] reported the first two cases in the literature. A description of this procedure follows.

The port sites shown in Fig. 20-2 are used. A convenient site is selected on the jejunum approximately 10 to 15 cm distal to the ligament of Treitz. The jejunum is grasped with Babcock clamps and brought up to an antecolic position and apposed to the stomach. A gastrojejunostomy to the anterior surface of the stomach rather than the posterior wall of the stomach is technically easier to accomplish using laparoscopic techniques. Two extracorporeal sutures are then placed to anchor the jejunum to the anterior wall of the stomach (Fig. 20-3). A 1 cm incision is made on the medial aspect of the jejunum and stomach using the hook diathermy. A 60 mm endoluminal linear stapler introduced into the incisions made in the stomach and jejunum is closed and fired. A side-viewing 30-degree laparoscope is used to assess the anastomotic site and to exclude bleeding. The possibility of narrowing the jejunal lumen during closure of

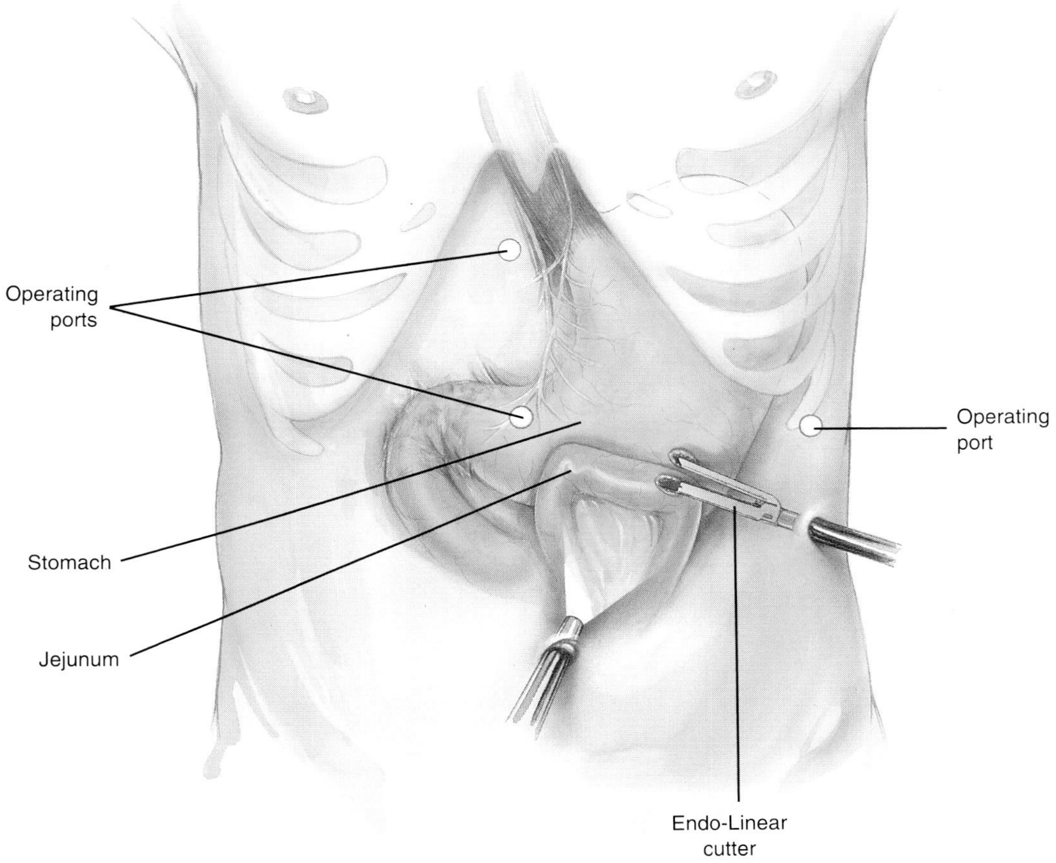

Fig. 20-3. Laparoscopic gastrojejunostomy. The anastomosis can be placed either on the anterior (as shown) or the posterior wall of the stomach. Stay sutures are placed at either end of the anastomosis to approximate the proximal jejunum and stomach. The anastomosis is then created with an endoscopic linear stapler.

the defect after removing the stapling device is of concern. An Endo GIA stapling device is used to fire two lines of staples perpendicular to each other to close the defect in a triangular fashion. If this is technically difficult, the remaining defect may be sutured closed laparoscopically or closed via a small minilaparotomy incision.

REFERENCES

1. Dallemagne B, Weerts JM, Jehaes C. Thoracoscopic esophageal resection. In Cuesta MA, Nagy AG, eds. Minimal Invasive Surgery in Gastrointestinal Cancer. New York: Churchill Livingstone, 1993, pp 59-68.
2. Becker HD, Buess GF, Mentges BR, et al. Esophagectomy. Adv Surg 26:397, 1993.
3. Hagen JA, Peters JH, DeMeester TR. Superiority of extended en bloc esophagogastrectomy for carcinoma of the lower esophagus and cardia. J Thorac Cardiovas Surg 106:850, 1993.
4. Kodama Y, Sugimachi K, Soejima K, et al. Evaluation of extensive lymph node dissection for carcinoma of the stomach. World J Surg 5:241, 1981.
5. Inokuchi K. Prolonged survival of stomach cancer patients after extensive surgery and adjuvant treatment: An overview of the Japanese experience. Semin Surg Oncol 7:333, 1991.

6. Csendes A, Amat J, Alam E, et al. Five-year survival rate of patients with advanced gastric carcinoma submitted to subtotal or total gastrectomy with or without extensive lymph node dissection. Rev Med Chil 111:889, 1993.
7. Lawrence M, Shiu MH. Early gastric cancer: Twenty-eight year experience. Ann Surg 213:327, 1991.
8. Siewert JW. Personal communication.
9. Diggory RT, Cuschieri A. R2/3 gastrectomy for gastric carcinoma: An audited experience of a consecutive series. Br J Surg 72:146, 1985.
10. Meyer HJ, Pichlmayr R. Patterns of recurrence in relation to therapeutic strategy in gastric cancer. Scand J Gastroenterol 22(Suppl 133):45, 1987.
11. Papachristou DN, Fortner JG. Local recurrence of gastric adenocarcinomas after gastrectomy. J Surg Oncol 18:47, 1981.
12. Nakajima T, Hishi M, Kajitani T. Improvement in treatment results of gastric cancer with surgery and chemotherapy: Experience of 9700 cases in the Cancer Institute Hospital, Tokyo. Semin Surg Oncol 7:365, 1991.
13. Cameron JL, Pitt HA, Yeo CJ, et al. One hundred and forty-five consecutive pancreaticoduodenectomies without mortality. Ann Surg 217:430, 1993.
14. Crist DW, Cameron JL. The current status of the Whipple operation for periampullary carcinoma. Adv Surg 24:21, 1992.
15. Gastrointestinal Tumor Study Group: Treatment of locally unresectable carcinoma of the pancreas: Comparison of combined modality therapy (chemotherapy plus radiotherapy) to chemotherapy alone. JNCI 80:751, 1988.
16. Warshaw AL, Gu Z-Y, Wittenberg J, et al. Preoperative staging and assessment of resectability of pancreatic cancer. Arch Surg 125:230, 1990.
17. Brennan MJ, Kinsella TJ, Casper ES. Cancer of the pancreas. In DeVita VT, Hellman S, Rosenberg SA, eds. Cancer: Principles and Practice of Oncology, vol 1, 4th ed. Philadelphia: JB Lippincott, 1993, pp 849-882.
18. Dooley WC, Cameron JL, Pitt HA, et al. Is preoperative angiography useful in patients with periampullary tumors? Ann Surg 211:649, 1990.
19. Foley WD, Erickson SJ. Color Doppler flow imaging. AJR 156:3, 1991.
20. Looser C, Stain SC, Baer HU, et al. Staging of hilar cholangiocarcinoma by ultrasound and duplex sonography: A comparison with angiography and operative findings. Br J Radiol 65:871, 1992.
21. Rosch T, Braig C, Gain T, et al. Staging of pancreatic and ampullary carcinoma by endoscopic ultrasonography. Gastroenterology 102:188, 1992.
22. Murugiah M, Paterson-Brown S, Windsor JA, et al. Early experience of laparoscopic ultrasonography in the management of pancreatic carcinoma. Surg Endosc 7:177, 1993.
23. Machi J, Sigel B, Zaren HA, et al. Operative ultrasonography during hepatobiliary and pancreatic surgery. World J Surg 17:640, 1993.
24. John TG, Garden OJ. Assessment of pancreatic cancer. In Cuesta MA, Nagy AG, eds. Minimally Invasive Surgery in Gastrointestinal Cancer. New York: Churchill Livingstone, 1993, pp 95-111.
25. Singh SM, Longmire WP, Reber HA. Surgical palliation for pancreatic cancer: The UCLA experience. Ann Surg 212:132, 1990.
26. Sarr MG, Cameron JL. Surgical management of unresectable carcinoma of the pancreas. Surgery 91:123, 1982.
27. Cuschieri A, Hall AW, Clark J. Value of laparoscopy in the diagnosis and management of pancreatic cancer. Gut 19:672, 1978.
28. Warshaw AL, Pepper JB, Shipley AW. Laparoscopy in the staging and planning of therapy for pancreatic cancer. Am J Surg 151:76, 1986.
29. Watanabe M, Takatori Y, Veki K, et al. Pancreatic biopsy under visual control in conjunction with laparoscopy for diagnosis of pancreatic cancer. Endoscopy 21:105, 1989.
30. Shimi S, Banting S, Cuschieri A. Laparoscopy in the management of pancreatic cancer: Endoscopic cholecystojejunostomy for advanced disease. Br J Surg 79:317, 1992.
31. Fletcher DR. Palliative surgery in pancreatic cancer. In Cuesta MA, Nagy AG, eds. Minimal Invasive Surgery in Gastrointestinal Cancer. New York: Churchill Livingstone, 1993, pp 112-121.
32. Mouiel J, Katkhouda N, White S, et al. Endolaparoscopic palliation of pancreatic cancer. Surg Laparosc Endosc 2:241, 1992.

Part

VI

Acute Foregut Problems and New Therapeutic Approaches

Chapter

21

Minimally Invasive Approaches to Upper Gastrointestinal Perforations

Adrian E. Ortega, M.D. • Eduardo T. Froes, M.D.

In the past four decades the management of peptic ulcer disease has undergone a remarkable evolution worldwide. Changing patterns in demographic variables, incidence, prevalence, and causation are emerging, making minimally invasive approaches to the management of peptic ulcer disease more appealing.

Peptic ulcer disease is common in Western countries, with a reported prevalence of 6% to 15%.[1] In 1978 more than 300,000 patients in the United States were hospitalized for this disease; 5% of them had perforations.[2] This complication continues to account for 5% to 10% of admissions related to peptic ulcer disease.[3] Although the number of patients admitted to hospitals for peptic ulcer disease over the past 20 years has steadily declined, the prevalence of complications, namely perforation and bleeding, has remained constant overall.[1,4] In some countries, however, operations for perforations have declined by 50%.[5]

Demographic factors have changed. The young to middle-aged man with a history of peptic ulcer disease is no longer the typical patient. The more likely demographic profile is that of an older, chronically ill patient who is often taking ulcerogenic medication. The male:female ratio has also decreased.[1] The number of patients requiring elective surgery for peptic ulcer disease has declined,[1] in part because of more effective medical treatment.

The etiology of peptic ulcer perforation remains obscure. However, alcohol use, smoking, postoperative stress, and ulcerogenic medications, including nonsteroidal anti-inflammatory agents, have been implicated.[1,2,6] The role of acid hypersecretion in the pathogenesis of perforation is increasingly being challenged, calling into question the need for definitive acid reduction therapy in the treatment of peptic perforation.

The increasing prevalence of older, chronically ill patients whose ulcer diathesis is related to factors other than acid hypersecretion is the strongest argument for a less invasive approach to treatment.

DIAGNOSIS

The clinical presentation of peptic ulcer perforation is generally straightforward, consisting of abrupt onset of severe epigastric abdominal pain that becomes generalized. Eliciting a history of tobacco use, alcohol consumption, and medication is important. The presence of similar antecedent symptoms and use of antacids, H_2 blockers, etc. should also be noted. Physical examination generally reveals either localized or generalized peritonitis. The diagnostic hallmark is free air on upright chest x-ray or lateral decubitus abdominal films. Pneumoperitoneum is present in 70% of cases of peptic ulcer perforation.[1] Other causes of extraluminal free air include perforated diverticulitis and less often appendicitis. Although the diagnosis is usually not difficult, elderly patients may present a greater diagnostic challenge.[1,3,4]

The classic confirmatory test for peptic perforation is a Gastrografin contrast study to demonstrate the ulcer or ulcer-related stigmata and to determine whether the ulcer has sealed. Failure of this contrast study to detect an ulcer or other related radiographic signs of peptic ulcer disease such as duodenal deformity and scarring mandates further investigation to exclude other causes of a perforated viscus prior to operative intervention. Given its propensity for producing electrolyte imbalance secondary to hypertonicity,[7] Gastrografin contrast in elderly patients must be used with caution.

Laparoscopy is emerging as an alternative modality for the management of peptic perforation because of its diagnostic capabilities as well as its therapeutic benefits.[8]

PRINCIPLES OF TREATMENT

Treatment options depend on the site of origin of the perforation. Because ulcers arising in the juxtapyloric region are thought to share a common pathophysiology with duodenal ulcers, they are discussed under the treatment of duodenal ulcers. The successful management of both conditions mandates early aggressive resuscitation. Broad-spectrum antibiotics to cover gram-positive and gram-negative organisms and nasogastric suction are generally instituted.

Duodenal Ulcers

The treatment of perforated duodenal ulcers remains controversial. Both operative and nonoperative options are available. Donovan et al.[9] championed selective or nonoperative management of perforated duodenal ulcers. This approach is considered appropriate in patients in whom an ulcer and/or ulcer stigmata can clearly be identified on contrast examination and those in whom the ulcer is not leaking freely. Acute perforations, that is, those occurring in patients without a long-standing ulcer diathesis, are considered more likely to seal spontaneously and nonoperative treatment may be considered. Selective treatment is also recommended for patients with significant comorbid conditions that make the operative risk prohibitive.

The operative management of perforated duodenal ulcers seems most appropriate in patients with chronic ulcers and in those with an unsealed perforation. Traditional operative options include simple closure, truncal vagotomy and drainage, truncal vagotomy and antrectomy, and simple closure with highly selective vagotomy.

Simple closure is generally favored for acute perforation, particularly in patients using ulcerogenic medications, as well as in poorer risk patients, including those with severe systemic comorbidity and those with significant and/or long-standing peritoneal contamination. Highly selective vagotomy is a poor choice for prepyloric ulcers given the unacceptable recurrence rate reported by several investigators.[1,10] Otherwise the choice of procedure depends primarily on the surgeon's experience and familiarity with each technique.

Gastric Ulcers

Ulcers occurring in the stomach above the incisura angularis constitute a clinical entity distinctly different from those occurring in the prepyloric regions. The principles of treatment of the latter are the same as for duodenal ulcers. Unlike duodenal ulcers, gastric ulcers must be regarded as carcinomatous until proved otherwise. Perforated gastric ulcers are malignant in 7% to 15% of cases.[11,12] This fundamental principle distinquishes the treatment of gastric and duodenal ulcers. Moreover, gastric ulcers are associated with a significantly higher mortality than their duodenal counterparts. The mortality rate in patients with perforated gastric ulcers varies from 10% to 40%.[11]

The classic approaches to gastric perforation are excision with pathologic examination or gastric resection with or without vagotomy. The relative merits of each approach are controversial, even with respect to the safest option in any given patient. In general the condition of the patient, the size of the ulcer, and its location ultimately determine the appropriate course of action.

History of Laparoscopic Approaches

Mouret et al.[13] reported the laparoscopic treatment of five patients with perforated peptic ulcers in 1990. Fibrin sealant and an omental patch were used with generally satisfactory results in three of these patients. Costalat et al.[14] dissected the ligamentum teres and then pulled it into the stomach endoscopically in 10 patients with anterior ulcerated perforations. Deyo[15] performed a simple closure using a figure-of-eight stitch and omental patch (Graham) in four patients. A number of case reports in the literature note generally good results with this same approach. The largest series was reported by the Belgian Group of Endoscopic Surgery and described the preliminary results in 30 patients who underwent primary treatment consisting of closure and placement of an omental patch.[16] In two patients the procedure was converted to open laparotomy. There was one death secondary to multiple organ failure, two pulmonary infections, and one subphrenic abscess. Patients resumed their regular diets by the fourth postoperative day on average. No further interventions were necessary and no cases of ulcer recurrence were noted, although the longest follow-up was only 5 months. This study is ongoing and longer follow-up results are awaited.

Swanström and Deyo[17] treated 13 patients with perforated ulcers via oversewing and a Graham patch. Four of these patients who met the criteria for chronic or refractory ulcer disease also underwent laparoscopic highly selective vagotomy. No wound infections, intra-abdominal abscesses, or ulcer recurrences were noted at a follow-up of 4 to 28 months. One patient underwent antrectomy for gastric outlet obstruction and one had a mediastinal abscess drained percutaneously. These investigators concluded that laparoscopy is effective for diagnosing and treating patients who present with suspected perforated ulcers. The merits of this approach are the ability to visualize and irrigate the total abdomen, a decreased incidence of wound morbidity and ileus, and shorter hospital stays. Obviously further study of long-term results is necessary to evaluate the efficacy of laparoscopic highly selective vagotomy and other modifications such as posterior truncal vagotomy with either anterior seromyotomy, anterior highly selective vagotomy, or anterior linear gastrectomy.[18-21] Other more traditional approaches, including truncal vagotomy with pyloroplasty or some other drainage procedure, are theoretically possible, but we have no personal experience with these techniques and no case reports of such treatment of peptic ulcer perforations have appeared in the literature to date.

Procedure for Endosurgical Closure

Patient Selection

Individuals with documented unsealed acute perforations in whom a definitive anti-ulcer procedure is not necessary appear to be the most appropriate candidates for simple laparoscopic closure of perforations. Cardiopulmonary comorbidity should be taken into consideration, although careful hemodynamic monitoring complemented by arterial blood gas assessment intraoperatively should permit safe laparoscopic intervention in most cases. Patients suspected of having a perforated viscus without an obvious source are also candidates for diagnostic laparoscopy since it allows differentiation of a perforation from a peptic ulcer and from other causes.

Patient Positioning and Trocar Placement

Either the Lloyd-Davies modified lithotomy position with the surgeon standing between the patient's legs or the more conventional supine position is appropriate for diagnostic laparoscopy for a suspected perforated peptic ulcer. The camera monitors are placed lateral to the patient's shoulders on each side. Given the potential for imflammatory adhesions throughout the abdomen, we recommend an open peritoneoscopy technique using a Hasson trocar placed periumbilically. This trocar serves as the camera port. A 10 or 11 mm port is placed in the right pararectus position at the level of the Hasson trocar. A fan-type retractor may be introduced through this port to elevate the left lateral segment of the liver. An additional 10 or 11 mm port is placed in the left subcostal area for insertion of atraumatic graspers to remove any inflammatory adhesions from the operative field (Fig. 21-1).

Simple Closure

A duodenal or prepyloric perforation can be closed with simple sutures. With the camera positioned in the midline, needle graspers and suture are introduced through the left subcostal and right pararectus trocars. The perforation may be closed with simple nonabsorbable 6-inch sutures tied intracorporeally (Fig. 21-2). Alternatively, 36-inch (or longer) sutures can be used for extracorporeal knot(s). Only one to three sutures are usually required for the typical punctate perforation of the duodenum. In a similar fashion a piece of omentum is sutured over the repair using either intra- or extracorporeal knot(s) (Fig. 21-3). The abdominal and pelvic cavities are thoroughly irrigated with multiple liters of warm saline solution. The trocar wounds are closed in a conventional manner.

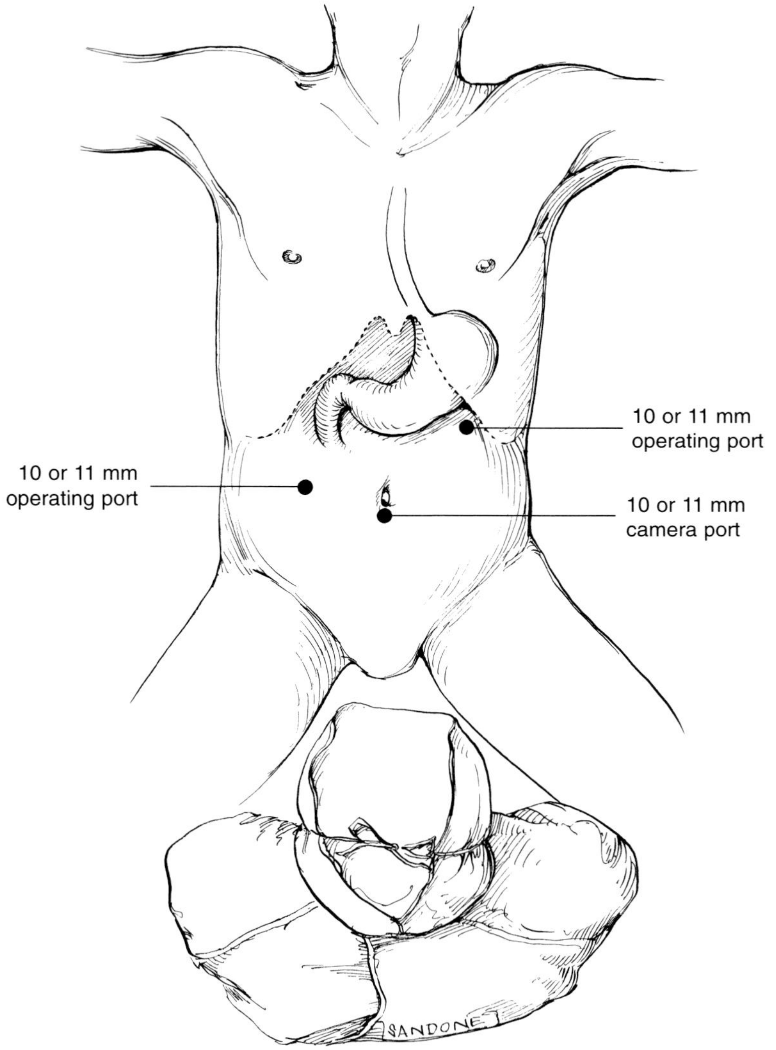

Fig. 21-1. Trocar placement. The initial examination of the abdominal cavity requires three trocars. The infraumbilical port is used for the video laparoscope. A fan retractor may be necessary to elevate the left lateral segment of the liver. A two-handed suturing technique is performed with instruments passed through the right pararectus and left subcostal ports.

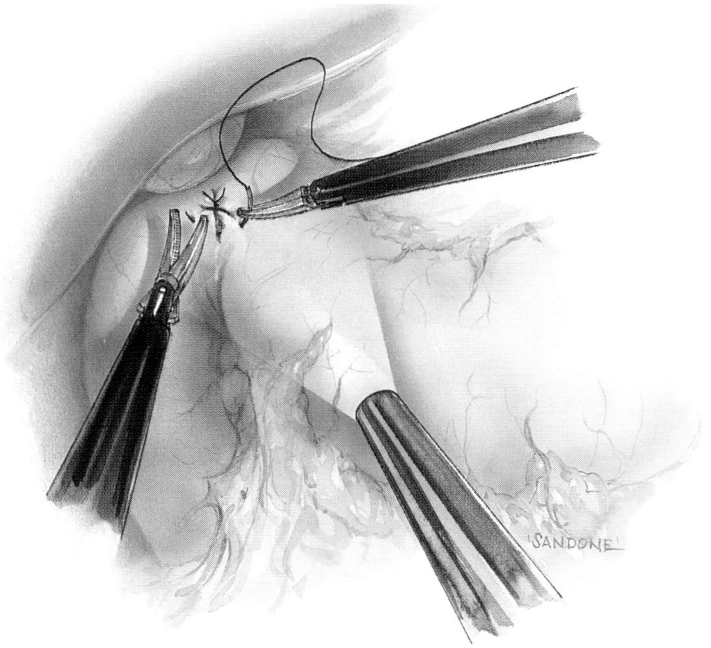

Fig. 21-2. Duodenal perforations may be closed using simple interrupted sutures tied either intra- or extracorporeally.

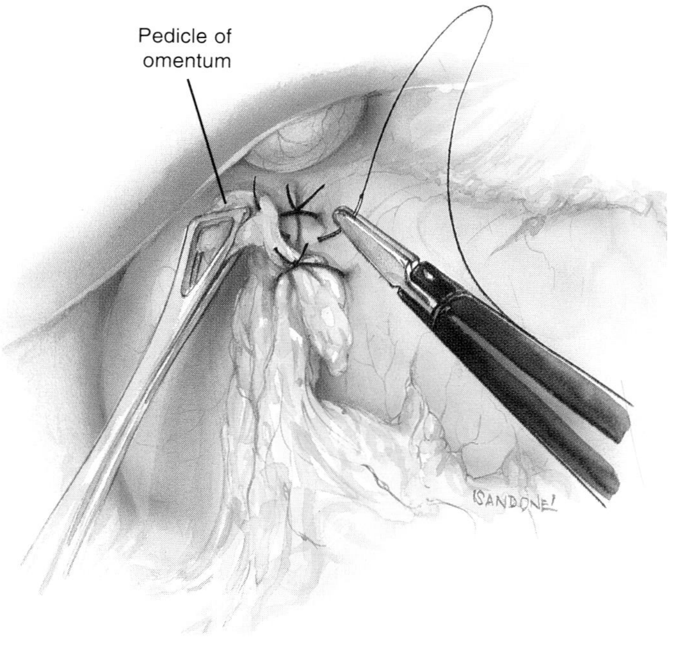

Fig. 21-3. Suturing of a pedicle of omentum completes the laparoscopic Graham patch.

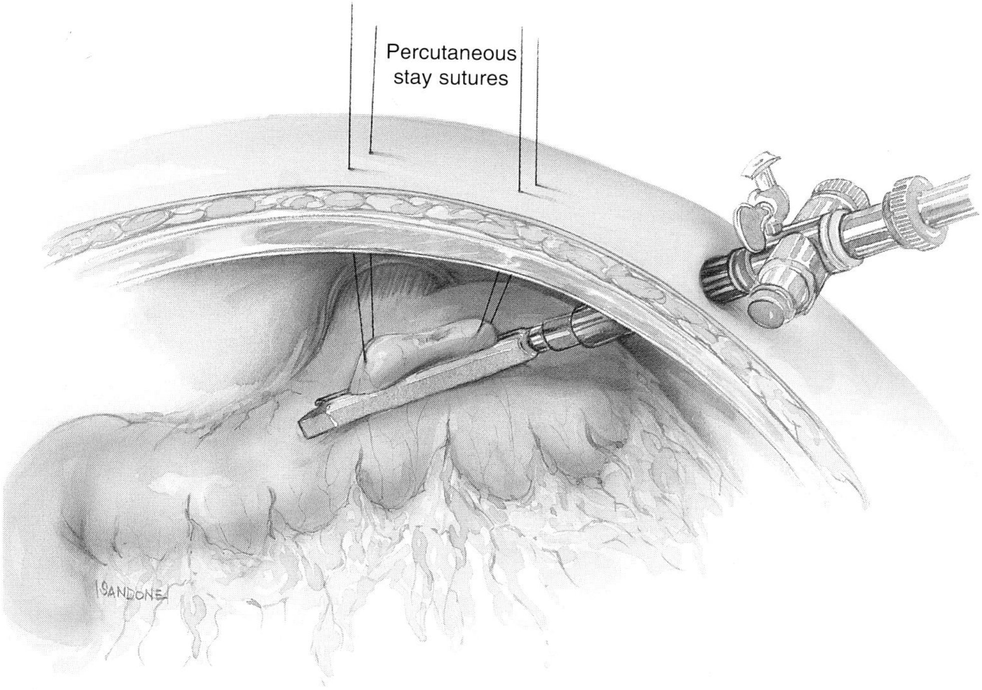

Fig. 21-4. Wedge excision of a gastric ulcer is facilitated by suspending the anterior wall of the stomach with percutaneously placed sutures on Keith needles. The percutaneously placed stay sutures also facilitate closure of the defect with a linear stapling device.

Excision of an Anterior Gastric Ulcer

Because of the inherent risk of carcinoma associated with gastric ulcers, we are reluctant to recommend simple closure of a perforation of the stomach. A reasonable laparoscopic approach consists of excision of an anterior ulcer using electrocautery. A trocar setup similar to that described previously is used to confirm the diagnosis. An additional 10 or 11 mm port is placed in a subxiphoid position to grasp the stomach over the ulcer. Visualization of the entire extent of the ulcer is aided by concomitant endoscopic visualization from within the stomach. The gastrotomy is closed after placement of two or three stay sutures on Keith needles passed percutaneously to align the gastrotomy and facilitate application of a linear stapler (Fig. 21-4). Depending on the size of the linear stapler to be used, the left subcostal trocar is exchanged for a larger 12 to 18 mm port for introduction of the stapler. Because of the risk of contaminating and/or seeding the abdominal wall with neoplastic cells, the excised tissue is placed in a plastic bag and retrieved through a port site. The ulcer is submitted for pathologic examination, and the abdominal cavity is thoroughly irrigated.

Postoperative Care

Anecdotal experience suggests that patients undergoing laparoscopic closure of peptic ulcer perforations have less ileus than those undergoing laparotomy and simple closure; however, decisions on whether to use nasogastric tubes and the length of time they are kept in place as well as intravenous antibiotics postoperatively should be made on a case-by-case basis.

CONCLUSION

Changes in the demographic and pathophysiologic patterns of peptic ulcer disease are making minimally invasive approaches to upper gastrointestinal perforations increasingly appealing. Nondefinitive treatments consisting of simple closure of duodenal perforations and wedge excision of gastric perforations appear to be most amenable to laparoscopic technology. Minimally invasive procedures for definitive ulcer treatment will require critical analysis when more extensive follow-up data become available.

REFERENCES

1. Jordan PH Jr, Morrow C. Perforated peptic ulcer. Surg Clin North Am 68:315-329, 1988.
2. Boyd EJS, Wormsley KG. Etiology and pathogenesis of peptic ulcer disease. In Haubrich WS, Kalser MH, Roth JLA, Schaffner F, eds. Bockus Gastroenterology. Philadelphia: WB Saunders, 1985, pp 1013-1059.
3. Rabinovic R, Manny J. Perforated duodenal ulcer in the elderly. Eur J Surg 157:1121-1125, 1991.
4. Gunchefski L, Flancbaun L, Brolin R, Frankel A. Changing patterns in perforated peptic ulcer disease. Am J Surg 56:270-274, 1990.
5. Gustavsson S, Nyren O. Time trends in peptic ulcer surgery, 1956 to 1986: A nationwide survey in Sweden. Ann Surg 210:704-709, 1989.
6. Kulber DA, Hartunian S, Schiller D, Morgestein L. The current spectrum of peptic ulcer in the older age group. Am J Surg 56:737-741, 1990.
7. Lee CHF, Yip AWC, Lam KHM. Pneumogastrogram in the diagnosis of perforated peptic ulcer. Aust N Z J Surg 63:459-461, 1993.
8. Cheschire N, Darzi A, Menzies-Gow N, Guillow P, Jandmonson JRT. Preliminary results of laparoscopic repair of perforated duodenal ulcer. Br J Surg 79(Suppl): 944, 1993.
9. Donovan AJ, Vinson TL, Mulsby GO, Gewin J. Selective treatment of perforated duodenal ulcer. Ann Surg 189:627-634, 1979.
10. Johnston D, Lyndon PJ, Smith RB, Humphrey CS. Highly selective vagotomy without a drainage procedure in the treatment of hemorrhage, perforation, and pyloric stenosis due to peptic ulcer. Br J Surg 60:790-797, 1973.
11. Hodnett RM, Gonzalez F, Lee C, Nance FC, Deboisblanc R. The need for definitive therapy in the management of perforated gastric ulcers. Ann Surg 29:36-39, 1989.
12. Hewitt RM, Krige J, Bornman PC. Perforated gastric ulcer: Resection compared with simple closure. Am J Surg 59:669-673, 1993.
13. Mouret P, Francois Y, Vignal J, Barth X, Lombart-Platet R. Laparoscopic treatment of perforated peptic ulcer. Br J Surg 77:1006, 1990.
14. Costalat G, Dravet F, Noel P, Alquier Y. Coelioscopic treatment of perforated gastroduodenal ulcer using the ligamentum teres hepatis. Surg Endosc 5:154-155, 1991.
15. Deyo GA. Laparoscopic management of perforated duodenal ulcer. Presented at the International Minimal Access Surgery Symposium, Kansas City, Mo., Nov. 17-19, 1991.
16. Vereecken L. Laparoscopic treatment of perforated gastroduodenal ulcer. Presented at the Society of American Gastrointestinal Endoscopic Surgeons, Phoenix, Ariz., March 31-April 3, 1993.
17. Swanström L, Deyo G. Laparoscopic repair of perforated ulcer: Treatment, algorithm, and follow-up. Presented at the Society of American Gastrointestinal Endoscopic Surgeons, Phoenix, Ariz., March 31-April 3, 1993.
18. Katkhouda N, Mouiel J. A new technique of surgical treatment of chronic duodenal ulcer without laparotomy by videocoelioscopy. Am J Surg 161:361-364, 1991.

19. Kum CK, Goh P. Laparoscopic truncal vagotomy and anterior highly selective vagotomy—a case report. Singapore Med J 33:302-303, 1992.
20. Zucker KA. Combined laparoscopic cholecystectomy and selective vagotomy. Laparosc Endosc 1:45-49, 1991.
21. Josephs LG, Arnold GH, Sawyers JL. Laparoscopic highly selective vagotomy. J Laparoendosc Surg 2:151-153, 1992.

Chapter

22

Development of Endo-Organ Surgery and Potential Clinical Applications

Charles J. Filipi, M.D. • Gerold J. Wetscher, M.D. • Tom R. DeMeester, M.D.
Jeffrey H. Peters, M.D. • Ronald A. Hinder, M.D., Ph.D.
Robert J. Fitzgibbons, Jr., M.D.

Gastroesophageal reflux disease, benign and malignant gastric neoplasms, and upper gastrointestinal bleeding secondary to peptic ulcer disease are common health problems in the United States. More than 400,000 patients are hospitalized annually for gastric or duodenal ulceration, and the American Gastroenterology Association estimates that treatment for peptic ulcer disease costs $6 billion annually. In addition, one fourth of the population report symptoms of heartburn at least monthly.

The success of laparoscopic cholecystectomy has led to other limited-access operations associated with reduced postoperative pain and an earlier return to normal activity. Laparoscopic Nissen fundoplication,[1] the endoluminal removal of superficial esophageal malignancies,[2] and laparoscopic truncal or proximal gastric vagotomy[3] are examples of this approach for upper gastrointestinal problems. Despite the reduced morbidity associated with laparoscopic surgery, open procedures for the treatment of gastroesophageal reflux disease, peptic ulcer disease, and gastric neoplasms are still common. The morbidity and mortality associated with open surgical correction of these disorders prompted us to develop a novel method of treatment by obtaining surgical access to the stomach. This endoscopic approach may also be appropriate for procedures such as small bowel endoscopy, excision of benign gastric ulcers, and antral mucosectomy.

Reports of minimally invasive procedures for the treatment of foregut disorders continue to proliferate. Rubber band ligation of esophageal varices,[4] closure of small gastric wall perforations,[5] removal of gastric polyps by scoop cauterization,[6] endoscopic sphincterotomy,[7-9] biliary stent placement,[10] hemostatic techniques for bleeding peptic ulcers,[11-13] and bleeding duodenal diverticula[14] are all effective endotherapeutic maneuvers. The ability to manipulate tissues is reduced with these procedures because of space confinement and instrument limitations. Access to the stomach for more extensive intraluminal procedures has been envisioned for several years but never extended to clinical practice.

In 1991 Frimberger and Classen[15] reported a prototype technique for creating large gastrostomies for the performance of intraluminal procedures. They used a metallic operative port 11.5 mm in diameter and 150 mm in length. The benefits of this port were immediately apparent and provided safe access to the gastric lumen. The disadvantage was that the metallic 2.5 cm diameter intraluminal retaining ring required a secondary procedure for removal. Way[16] has recently reported performing pancreatico-cystogastrostomies in five patients using a new expandable 5 mm intragastric operative port (Innerdyne Medical, Mountain View, Calif.). This port has a small balloon to secure it within the gastric lumen and requires laparoscopic suturing of the gastric openings after removal. Jennings et al.[17] reported an animal investigation using intragastric surgery for construction of a gastroesophageal valve. Their technique includes traction on the squamocolumnar junction and retrograde staple application to secure the valve.

DEVELOPMENT OF ENDO-ORGAN TECHNIQUES

Laboratory investigation into the feasibility of endoscopic operative construction of a nipple valve was initiated in 1990 at Creighton University. A Greenfield filter was first used for traction on the distal esophagus in the hope of pulling it into the gastric lumen sufficiently to fix the valve with staples. Various other invagination techniques and instruments have been used and fixation methods investigated. Development of the endoscopic antireflux procedure has produced many meaningful results, which will be reviewed in detail later in this chapter. The primary considerations for construction of an effective endoscopic nipple valve include durability and secure intra-abdominal positioning. With invagination (pushing of the distal esophagus into the stomach), tension occurs if a 3 to 4 cm nipple valve is constructed and thus durability is a major concern. A shorter valve has been demonstrated in the laboratory to retract into the esophageal lumen. A size 60 F bougie within the esophageal lumen is necessary to prevent an excessively tight wrap,[18] which increases the probability of retraction because of its large size. Therefore a longer valve is necessary, which in turn increases tension at the fixation points.

Although the coaxial forces on the nipple valve we developed have not been scientifically measured, ex vivo tests have quantitated the amount of tension that will cause pull-out failure of various size staples and sutures. We have concluded that coaxial traction forces are applied first at the most proximal fasteners where the primary load is distributed. Regardless of the configuration of the staples, we were unable to distribute the load sufficiently to prevent the first staple or suture from failing, which in turn creates an unzipping effect on the remaining sutures or staples. A shorter valve may be more effective because the tension on the most proximal fastener will not be as great. If a smaller diameter bougie is used under less tension, the valve may not invert back into the esophagus. The developmental steps will be reviewed later and further considerations concerning valve formation discussed. As refinements of instruments and techniques proved successful for the endoscopic antireflux procedure, developmental work on disposable operative ports began.

Three prototypes for a large-diameter percutaneous gastrostomy were used sequentially in the laboratory. The dilating assembly was also altered on the basis of laboratory findings. Numerous revisions have now made the operative port easy and safe to introduce. It became apparent with this new form of access that additional operative procedures were possible.

In addition to the endoscopic antireflux repair, laboratory protocols were established for upper gastrointestinal bleeding and excision of gastric mucosal and full-thickness gastric lesions. Port placement for lesions in different portions of the stomach was varied. Because of the room afforded in the gastric lumen, satisfactory positioning of the port was usually possible. Criteria were developed to determine the frequency with which optimal port positioning was obtainable. Mucosal resection and closure with interrupted sutures were easy to perform without limiting the extent of the mucosectomy. Intraluminal suture closure of mucosal defects in virtually every portion of the stomach was possible. It became apparent that intragastric bleeding could be controlled by this technique. The difficulty in suturing in the confined space of the duodenum, however, has prompted us to pursue further instruments and refinements in technique.

Posterior duodenal ulcers are the most common cause of upper gastrointestinal bleeding.[19] Bleeding often originates from the gastroduodenal artery or one of its branches and is usually severe and life threatening.[20] Techniques for visualization, exposure, suturing, and stapling in the duodenum are also under investigation. A clinical protocol for selected cases of upper gastrointestinal bleeding is under development, and as instruments and devices become available a pilot study will be implemented.

We will outline the background, techniques, and results of our laboratory work to date. Clinical application awaits FDA approval of devices and instruments.

ENDO-ORGAN ACCESS

Background

The first open gastrostomy was performed by Sedillot[21] in 1849. Gastrostomies were initially performed in children who had swallowed caustic material and to palliate malignant bowel obstructions and gastric outlet obstructions secondary to peptic ulcer disease. Because many of these patients were malnourished and had significant comorbid conditions, the mortality rate was high.

In 1981 Ponsky and Gandevev[22] published their report entitled "Percutaneous Endoscopic Gastrostomy: A Nonoperative Technique for Feeding Gastrostomy." Conditions such as compromised oral alimentation, neurologic impairment, and trauma are indications for percutaneous endoscopic gastrostomy. The most common contraindication to percutaneous endoscopic gastrostomy tube placement is a progressive comorbid condition leading to compromised life expectancy. Discretion is required and difficult decisions are necessary in many of these circumstances.

Other procedures such as percutaneous endoscopic jejunostomy and even percutaneous cecostomy for pseudo-obstruction of the colon[23] have more recently received acceptance. Additional applications for percutaneous endoscopic gastrostomy include placement of a transgastric jejunostomy or duodenostomy tube for administration of medications or refeeding of bile, access for retrograde dilatation of esophageal strictures, management of gastric volvulus, and pancreatic pseudocyst drainage.[24]

Complications of percutaneous gastrostomy include aspiration, peritonitis, hemorrhage, peristomal wound infection, gastrocolic fistula, and occasionally migration of the device out of the stomach. Although these complications are uncommon, the mortality rate is 5%, primarily because the associated commorbid conditions are severe in nature.

Operative Port Design Replacement and Introduction

The increased diameter and the need for 5 and 10 mm instruments to be passed numerous times through the gastrostomy presented several interesting challenges. To gain access for this procedure a larger diameter port (Fig. 22-1) was used that had an inner balloon foam rubber stent to prevent inadvertent removal. Size was the greatest concern since esophageal injury secondary to pulling the port through the mouth and esophagus was a potential complication if tube diameter was excessive. A size 60 F dilator (2 cm diameter) can be introduced through the normal adult esophagus without difficulty. The greatest outer diameter of the operative port with the balloon collapsed is 2 cm. The diameter varies between 2 cm at the collapsed balloon level to 1.65 cm on the shaft. No evidence of esophageal injury was observed in 17 pigs after 38 operative port placements.

Intraoperative dislodgment from the stomach can be a problem, in some circumstances necessitating conversion to an open procedure. To prevent this occurrence a bolster that attaches to the port was developed along with a foam rubber stent within the balloon to secure the port in the stomach even if the balloon de-

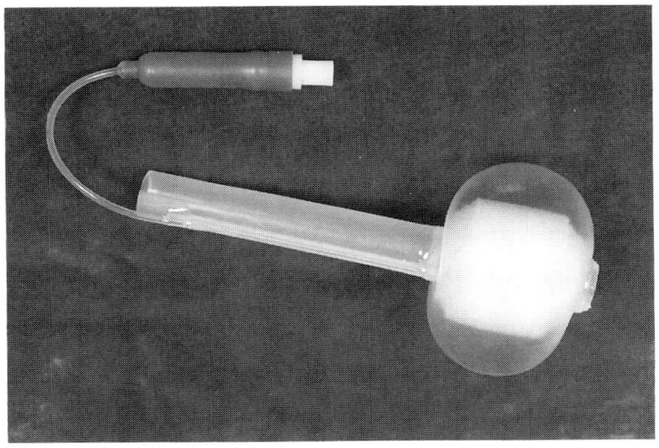

Fig. 22-1. Operative port developed for intraluminal gastric access.

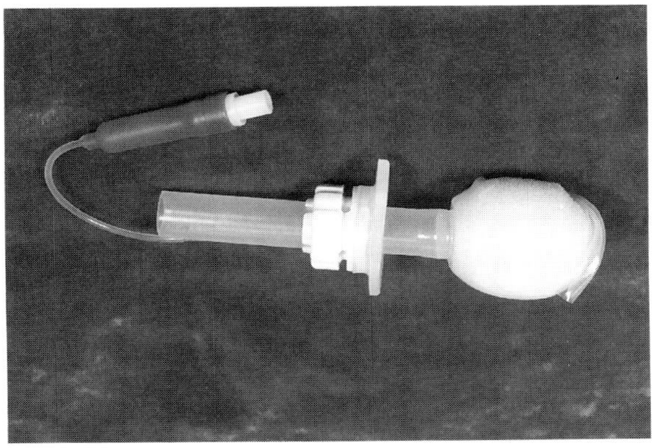

Fig. 22-2. The intraballoon stent remains distended despite the ruptured balloon shown here, thereby preventing port dislodgment from the gastric lumen.

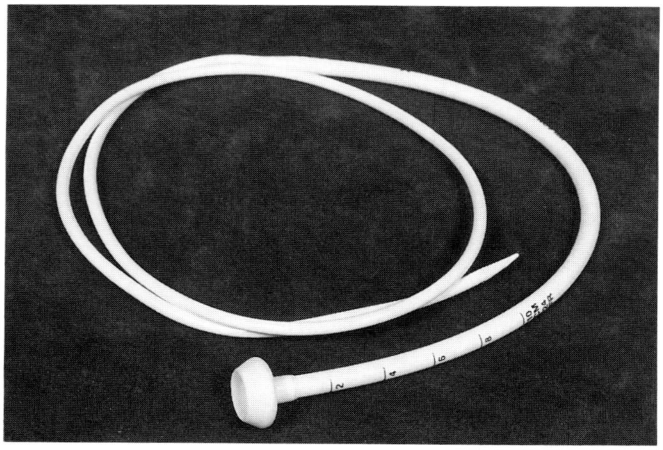

Fig. 22-3. Percutaneous gastrostomy tube used for replacement of the operative port.

flates (Fig. 22-2). Five of 38 operative ports used during experimental operations have been accidentally deflated during laboratory operative procedures. One was inadvertently extracted despite the foam rubber stent. The force to extract with and without the balloon inflated was measured after the operative procedure as 11.1 and 2.3 pounds, respectively.

An additional consideration with a large-diameter port is the possibility of a gastric fistula. A replacement tube (Fig. 22-3) may easily be introduced after use of the larger diameter tube. Leakage from the gastric lumen can also be prevented by introducing Brown/Mueller T-fasteners (Medi-Tech, Inc., Watertown, Mass.) adjacent to the smaller replacement tube. Direct suture closure can be accomplished by pulling the stomach wall above the skin level with a Sen retractor. The hooks on the retractor are placed through the operative port prior to its removal. In a heavy patient the ports can be removed after aspiration of all gastric contents and laparoscopic instruments introduced through the abdominal wall openings created by the operative ports for laparoscopic closure of the gastric openings. Finally, if the operative port needs to be left in place for follow-up, endoscopy, or gastric decompression, a gastric fistula may result if the port is left in too long. Clinical trials will determine optimal maintenance techniques and complication rates.

Two ports are required for most procedures. The technique is identical for each access port. After endoscopic insufflation of the stomach and transillumination a loop guidewire is introduced into the stomach and pulled out the mouth and through a bite block. Traction on the guidewire exiting the abdominal wall is applied after the operative port dilator assembly is attached. It is advisable at this interval to replace the endoscope for localization of the port. The skin incision is 2.5 cm in length and is made prior to pulling the dilator port assembly through the abdominal wall.

A No. 15 knife blade is used on a standard knife handle. With the long axis of the knife kept close to that of the dilator a sufficient amount of deep fascia is incised using a slot within the tapered portion of the dilator assembly. When the distal portion of the port is above the skin level, the port's balloon is inflated with 60 ml of saline solution after endoscopically confirming that the balloon portion is in the gastric lumen. Further traction is applied and the ring bolster is placed. To prevent gastric secretions from extruding from the port, a seal cap is fitted onto the port and instruments are then introduced for operative manipulation.

ENDOSCOPIC ANTIREFLUX PROCEDURE

Background

Gastroesophageal reflux disorders are diagnosed in over 600,000 people in the United States each year and approximately 30,000 undergo antireflux surgery. Since 1935 the gross and histologic changes of esophagitis have been attributed to reflux of gastric peptic juices. Hiatal hernia was often blamed for this disorder because of its frequent association with the classic symptom complex of heartburn and regurgitation. The causal relationship of hiatal hernia and gastroesophageal reflux disease was finally refuted in the 1960s when manometric studies suggested that a weak lower esophageal sphincter[25] was the etiologic basis and with the realization that over half of the patients with hiatal hernia did not show objective evidence of reflux.

Surgery for gastroesophageal reflux disease has evolved from simple hiatal hernia reduction and closure of the diaphragmatic crura using various forms of fundoplication (Nissen, Hill, and Belsey Mark IV). These operations effectively control gastric reflux[26]; however, each has an associated 1% mortality and a 10% to 30% postoperative morbidity. Failure to control reflux occurs in 10% to 15% of patients. Iatrogenic splenic injury and subsequent splenectomy or inadvertent perforation of the esophagus are the operative complications most often associated with postoperative mortality. Technical alterations such as a short fundoplication over a 60 F bougie have decreased postoperative dysphagia and significantly reduced the need for postoperative dilatation.[18]

Jennings et al.[17] published a report describing a transgastric endoscopic approach for construction of an antireflux valve. Six pigs underwent endoscopically guided, large-diameter gastrostomy placement and introduction of a traction hook into the gastroesophageal junction for intussusception of the distal esophagus into the gastric fundus. The intussuscepted tissue was fixed with a modified linear stapler and the valve tested was assessed with an acid reflux test. Although the pigs did not survive, investigation revealed that the operative procedure was possible and the valve did prevent reflux during anesthesia.

Other minimally invasive methods for recreating a competent lower esophageal sphincter have been reported. McGouran and Galloway[27] induced scar formation at the cardia with the Nd:YAG laser. Nine dogs were tested. One configuration of scar formation did increase valvular competence as measured by yield pressure (the intragastric pressure needed to force the valve open). The operation was designed to restore or preserve the abdominal length of the lower esophageal sphincter and augment the average resting pressure by an extrinsic pressure phenomenon. Their efforts did not lead, however, to a consistently effective valvular mechanism.

In summary, surgeons view the failure at the lower esophageal sphincter mechanistically and internists point to an intrinsic myogenic factor as the likely cause. Despite good data to support a defective cardia as the frequent and correctable pathology,[28] the rate of referral remains low in part because of this debate. Gastroenterologists cite postoperative morbidity and mortality rates and maintain the perpetual hope that the next generation of prokinetic agent or acid inhibitor will provide long-term, inexpensive, and effective medical therapy.

A noninvasive operation that would reduce morbidity and create an effective barrier against acid reflux would be appealing to clinicians. At the University of Southern California and Creighton University a transluminal operation conducted in the laboratory through two large-diameter percutaneous gastrostomies is under investigation. Instrument and technique refinements have made this operation possible and new fixation devices are now being tested. Laboratory techniques and results will be described.

Laboratory Technique

The goal of the phase I laboratory investigation was to develop an invagination and nipple-valve fixation technique at the gastroesophageal junction. Seventeen mongrel dogs were followed from 1 to 12 months. Manometry and endoscopy were performed preoperatively and postmortem examination was completed in all animals. Interval postoperative manometry was performed when endoscopy revealed a complete valve. Operative access was initially obtained by open laparotomy and introduction of standard laparoscopic trocars into the gastric lumen. A pursestring suture at the entry site prevented CO_2 gas leakage. Through the previously described operative ports a 10 mm laparoscope was introduced through port A (Fig. 22-4) and the fixation device (stapler or suture passer) through the remaining port (B). The invaginator shown in Fig. 22-5 was introduced transorally over a taut guidewire and positioned at the gastroesophageal junction. The needle constellation was deployed just distal to the squamocolumnar junction and a 4 to 5 cm invagination produced by pushing the proximal end while visualizing the distal instrument via an intragastric laparoscope. Invagination was attempted by transgastric placement of a Kimray-Greenfield filter (Medi-Tech, Inc.) in two preliminary animal experiments.

Five animals underwent valve fixation with a linear stapler (Endo GIA, United States Surgical Corp., Norwalk, Conn.). With the cutting blade removed, one jaw of the stapler was introduced into the esophageal lumen after invagination. In two animals valve formation was attempted with direct suturing of invaginated tissue. A prototype helical needle (Ethicon, Inc., Somerville, N.J.) was developed for this purpose. The outer diameter of the helix was 10 mm, being confined by the inner diameter of the operative port. A two-channel suture passer (Ethicon, Inc.) with a proximal drive wheel (Fig. 22-6) was used to place 2-0 Prolene full-thickness U-stitches. This device was able to penetrate the tissue and was easy to introduce into the stomach and over the invaginated gastroesophageal junction. Seven laboratory experiments were completed using this device. An additional animal that did not survive underwent nipple-valve reconstruction with a prototype stapler (Ethicon Endo-Surgery, Cincinnati, Ohio). This instrument placed box-shaped staples using a 0.01-inch diameter wire.

Results

The Greenfield filter was ineffective because the traction hook wires collapsed the esophagus while pulling it. Dislodgment of the hooks also occurred. The invaginator

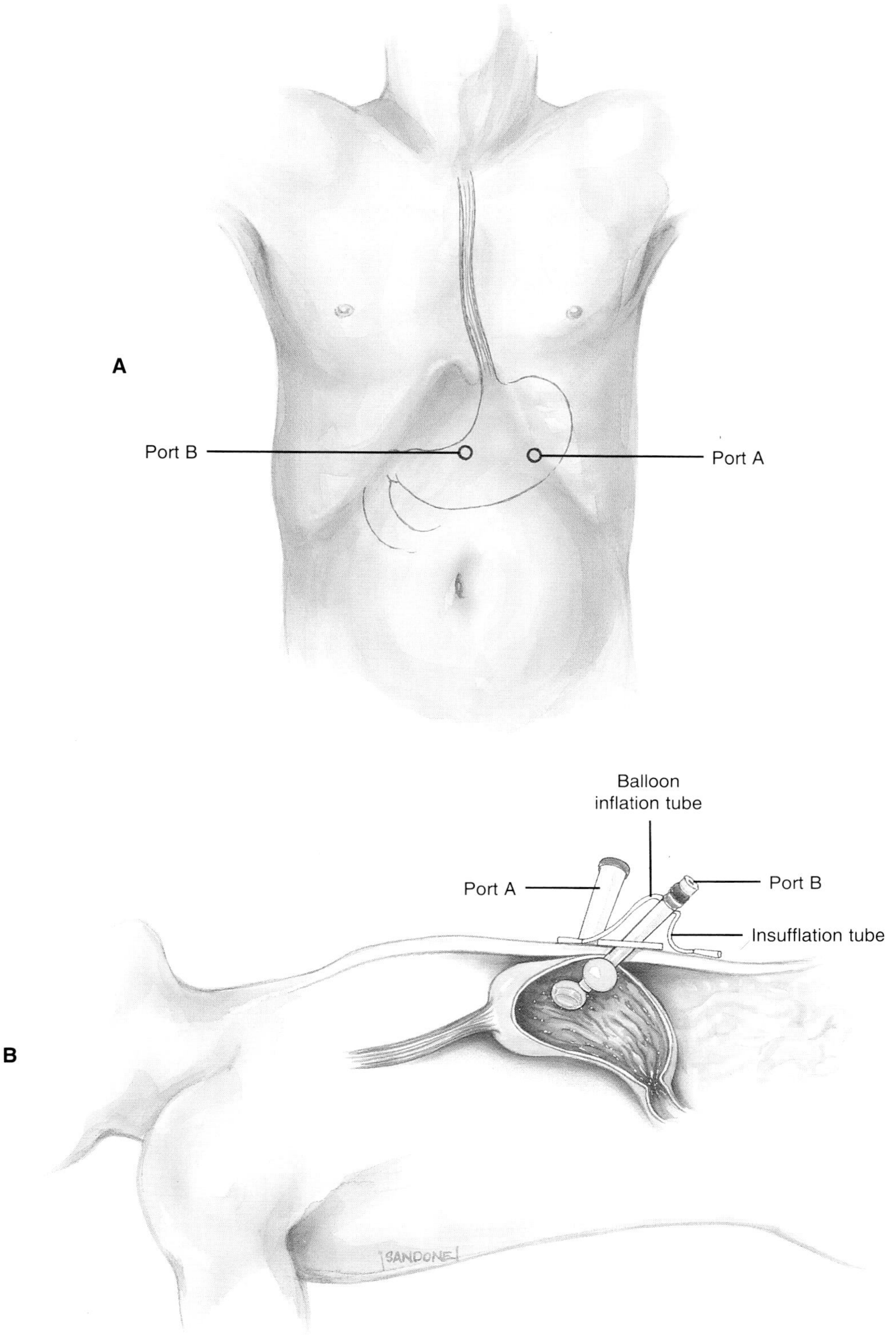

Fig. 22-4. Laboratory endoscopic antireflux procedure port sites. **A,** Cutaneous placement. **B,** Transgastric view.

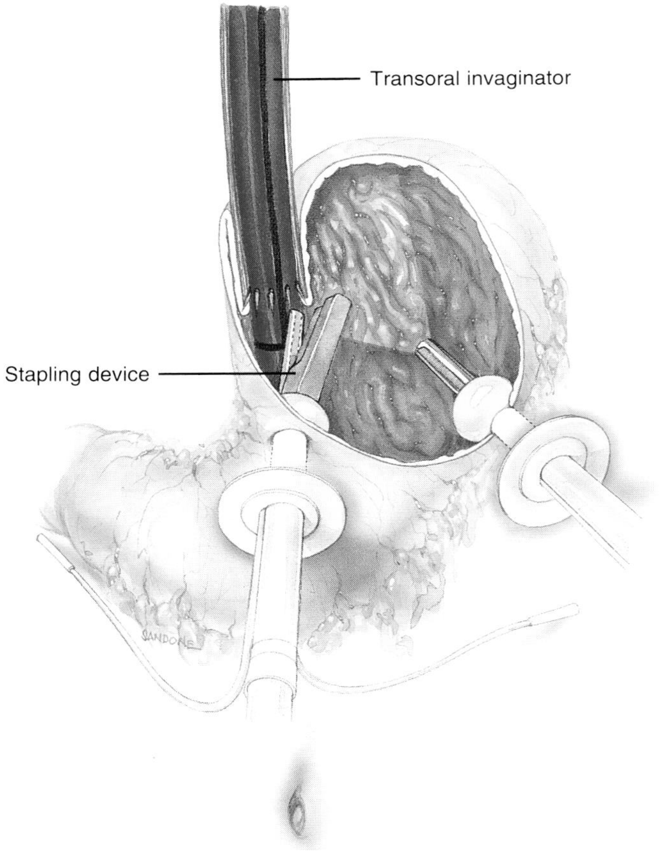

Fig. 22-5. Esophageal invaginator.

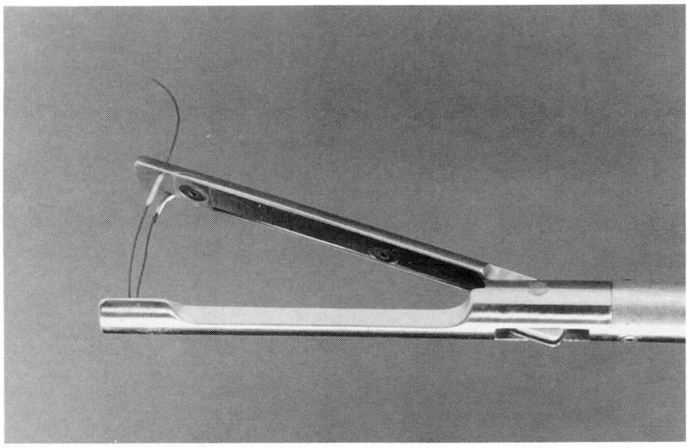

Fig. 22-6. Suture passer used to place a 2-0 monofilament U-stitch through the double-cuffed invagination.

Table 22-1. Results of valve fixation techniques

Fixation Method	No. of Dogs	Completed Valve	Length of Valve Competence	Manometric Values	Reason for Valve Failure
Linear stapler	5	3	1-2 wk	Increase in LES average resting pressure of 10 mm Hg	Inadequate invagination, 2 dogs Inadequate stapler tissue gap, 3 dogs
Helical needle (direct suturing)	2	0	NA	NA	Inadequate needle size
Suture passer	8	6	6-10 wk	Increase in LES average resting pressure of 10 mm Hg	Suture breakage, 1 dog Diaphragm suture placement, 1 dog Tissue pull-out, 4 dogs
Single-fire stapler	1	1	Animal killed immediately postop	Not measured	NA

LES = lower esophageal sphincter.

shown in Fig. 22-5 provided 360-degree 4 to 5 cm invagination in 14 of 15 dogs tested. One complication occurred. In this animal, perforation at the gastroesphageal junction required open suturing for closure of the defect. Mishandling of the suture passer was the probable causative factor, although rotational movement of the invaginator may have contributed. No postoperative evidence of esophageal leakage was observed in any experimental animals. The invaginator was easy to manipulate, could be guided into place without difficulty, and could be disengaged from the distal esophagus without complication.

Valve formation when using the linear stapler (Endo GIA) was observed postoperatively in three animals (Table 22-1), but excessive tissue prevented jaw closure in one animal and inadequate invagination in another made tissue approximation impossible. Immediate postoperative manometry revealed an elevation of the average resting pressure by 8 to 10 mm Hg in the only animal tested in this group.

Postmortem examination of the three dogs with Endo GIA valve formation revealed staple row ischemia with only loose flaps of remaining tissue at 2 to 4 weeks. Because the tissue gap allowance was 0.35 mm for the stapler and the invaginated tissue was 10 mm in width before compression, we concluded that the resultant ischemia was caused by excessive tissue compression. Staple pull-out was suspected but not confirmed.

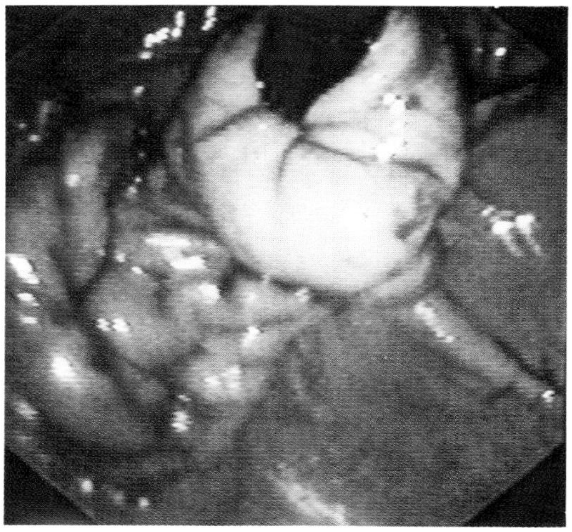

Fig. 22-7. An endoscopically created nipple valve.

Direct suturing of the nipple valve was attempted with both helical and conventional needles placed through a 10 mm reducer. The helical needle was insufficient in diameter to obtain a complete bite of invaginated esophageal and gastric tissue. In follow-up experiments not included in Table 22-1, even open suturing of invaginated full-thickness gastric and esophageal tissue was difficult. Full double-thickness penetration could only be guaranteed if the needle was viewed directly in the esophageal lumen.

The suture passer seen in Fig. 22-6 guarantees a full-thickness U-suture, but it was not always functional. The drive wheel mechanism required to push the suture through the instrument often needed repair, and among the seven animals in which this fixation method was tested, only one received a full complement of eight sutures. The nipple valves, as viewed endoscopically immediately after construction (Fig. 22-7), were satisfactory on gross inspection, and immediate postoperative manometry revealed an increase in average resting pressure of 10 mm Hg. Unfortunately, the valves invariably failed at 2 to 3 months because of suture pull-out. Postmortem evaluation revealed that the sutures were still tied in all but one animal. The limited number of sutures in some animals may have been a contributing factor, but in those animals receiving seven to eight sutures the same disruption occurred. The tension under which the sutures were tied varied, as evidenced by the size of the intact suture loops at postmortem examination. There did not, however, appear to be any corollary between tension on the suture and valve survival.

The suture-passing concept was abandoned because of these failures and a stapler was developed in the hope that multiple large staples would distribute the tissue tension load adequately for valve survival. In vitro studies were conducted to determine the optimal staple size and placement configuration. These tests determined that tension from invagination invariably sought out the most proximal staple regardless of its orientation to the axis of the esophagus or the number of staples seemingly at the same level. Because of this investigation, an improved fixation device has been identified; instrument and technique refinements should lead to completion of the phase II trial in the near future.

Because the endoscopic valve is constructed in a coaxial fashion (as in a Belsey fundoplication) with the stomach held to the esophagus in a longitudinal rather than a transverse orientation, contraction and relaxation occur along the same longitudinal axis. In contrast to the Nissen fundoplication, lines of relaxation and contraction of the esophagus related to the stomach are at right angles to each other. The Belsey 270-degree wrap has, however, proved to be an effective antireflux barrier. The competence of a Belsey-type valve in humans will depend on the length of the fundoplication and the amount of esophageal circumference surrounded by the wrap. A 4 cm long 270-degree Belsey wrap has been demonstrated in the past to function properly.[29]

It is apparent from our investigation to date that intraluminal pressures on a valve formed by invagination and secured by sutures or staples will be elevated. This increase in pressure along with the endoscopic resemblance to a nipple valve as constructed by Nissen fundoplication suggests but does not fully establish its competence. Durability of the valve has and still is our primary focus. A clinical protocol is under development, and when laboratory studies are complete, a pilot study will be implemented. We hope that an antireflux valve constructed in this manner will be appealing to clinicians and will allow the procedure to be performed on an outpatient basis.

ENDO-ORGAN HEMOSTASIS FOR UPPER GASTROINTESTINAL BLEEDING

Background

The mortality rate in patients with upper gastrointestinal bleeding due to ulcerations has not changed since the introduction of endoscopy.[30] Bleeding subsides spontaneously in 80% of patients.[31] In these patients the source of bleeding is often gastritis, Mallory-Weiss tears, erosion without angiodysplasia, or ulcers without evidence of a visible vessel. In the remaining 20% of patients, bleeding is severe and most often originates from ulcerations with a visible vessel. In approximately 20% of these patients, endoscopy fails to accurately localize the bleeding site because of impaired visualization secondary to abundant fresh and coagulated blood.[19] In the remaining 70% to 80% of patients in whom hemostasis could be achieved endoscopically, rebleeding rates of up to 30% are described[19] with an associated mortality rate of up to 40%. Emergency surgery (oversewing + truncal vagotomy + pyloroplasty or oversewing + antrectomy + truncal vagotomy) has resulted in a rebleeding rate of 1% and a mortality rate of less than 6% in studies when operation is performed early.[32] In the majority of studies the mortality rate for emergency operation is approximately 20%. This is secondary to delayed surgical intervention, which often results in prolonged hypotension and renal insufficiency.[30] In addition, intraluminal blood contributes to bacterial overgrowth in the upper gastrointestinal tract with consequent sepsis following duodenotomy or gastrotomy.

Suturing techniques comparable to those used during open surgery are potentially possible with endo-organ surgery without broaching the peritoneal cavity. It is hoped that postoperative septic complications will be reduced and earlier intervention encouraged because of the minimally invasive nature of the procedure.

Indications for Endo-Organ Surgery in Patients With Upper Gastrointestinal Bleeding

- Gastroduodenal ulcerations not controlled endoscopically
- Rebleeding after endoscopic therapy
- Unlocalizable gastric bleeding (Dieulafoy lesions)
- Bleeding gastric varices unresponsive to transjugular intrahepatic portal systemic stent

Indications

The indications for endo-organ surgery in upper gastrointestinal bleeding are the same as for open surgery. Surgical intervention should be initiated promptly in patients with active bleeding from gastric or duodenal ulcers that cannot be controlled endoscopically. Patients who have initially responded to endoscopic therapy but experience rebleeding may be considered for immediate endo-organ surgical intervention before numerous transfusions are required. The improved visualization provided by the endo-organ approach may benefit patients with Dieulafoy lesions, which are often difficult to localize. Patients with bleeding gastric varices unresponsive to transjugular intrahepatic portal systemic stent placement may be considered for an endo-organ approach as well.

Laboratory Studies

Whereas suturing in the stomach is easy to perform by an experienced laparoscopic surgeon, exposure presents a unique problem in the proximal duodenum. We have tested four techniques in anesthetized pigs to obtain adequate visualization in the duodenum. Two operative ports are placed anteriorly, one near the lesser curve just proximal to the incisura and the other near the greater curve at the junction of the gastric antrum and body.

Dilatation With a Balloon Prosthesis. A 35 mm diameter esophageal Regiflex balloon dilator normally used for esophageal pneumatic dilatation is introduced transorally into the stomach and guided into the duodenum by a grasper placed through one of the operative ports. The balloon is inflated to a pressure of 300 mm Hg for 5 minutes. Additional relaxation of the pylorus is achieved by administering 0.5 unit of intravenous glucagon.

Balloon Dilatation. This procedure was performed in two pigs. In the first pig the duodenum was adequately dilated for 30 minutes, but in the second, adequate access to the duodenum could be obtained for only 15 minutes.

Pyloric Dilator. After dilatation a three-pronged pyloric dilator is introduced through one of the operative ports, the pylorus is spread to an inner diameter of 2 cm for 5 minutes, and glucagon is given intravenously. Since one of the ports is now occupied by the pyloric dilator (Ethicon, Inc.), a third port needs to be introduced for suturing if the pyloric dilator is to be left in place. In three pigs the pyloric dilator prototype was introduced into the duodenum, deployed, and then removed after 5 minutes. Exposure was not adequate and suturing was tedious.

Transpyloric Technique. We have found that cautery scissors introduced through one operative port and a grasping forceps placed through an operating laparoscope in the second port permit sharp internal excision of the pyloric ring. The pyloric channel can thereby be opened to an inner diameter of 2 cm.

Attempts at pyloric resection in one pig did not improve exposure significantly. Only a relatively small portion of tissue was removed. This method requires further testing.

The grasping forceps, which was in fact used as a spreader rather than a grasper, provided fair exposure for posterior suturing of the duodenal bulb. This method was used in three pigs and was always preceded by 5 minutes of pyloric dilation with the pyloric retractor.

Suturing is currently the most efficient technique to achieve hemostasis. Two techniques can be applied: suturing by means of a standard laparoscopic needle holder and a grasper introduced through the operating laparoscope (Fig. 22-8) and suturing using the Endoscopic Suture Hook (Weck Endoscopy) (Fig. 22-9). Extracorporeal knot tying with a knot pusher is easier than intracorporeal tying. This limitation is a result of the limited view afforded by an operating laparoscope for intracorporeal tying.

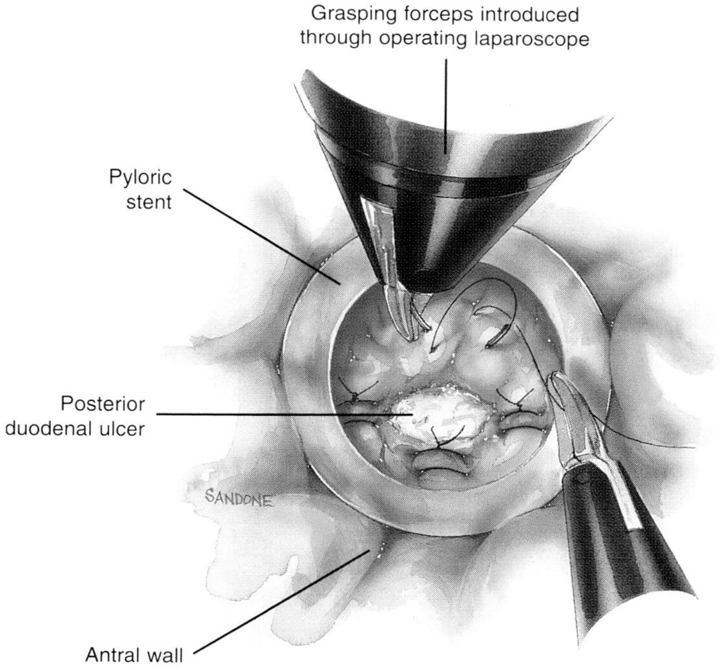

Fig. 22-8. Operative ports provide access and visualization of the first portion of the duodenum for suturing.

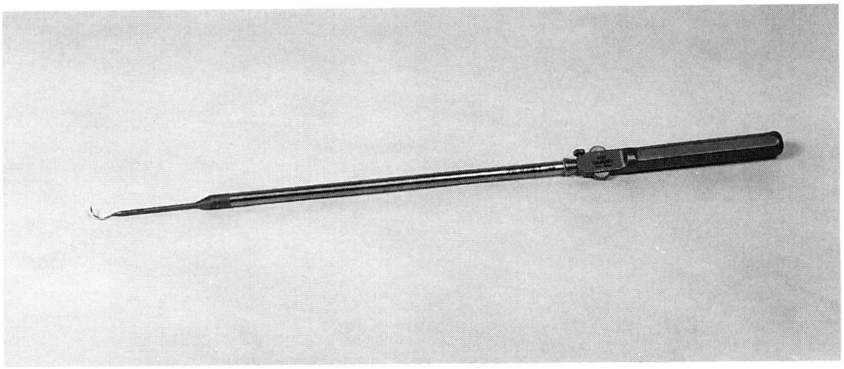

Fig. 22-9. Device for placement of sutures in the gastric or duodenal wall.

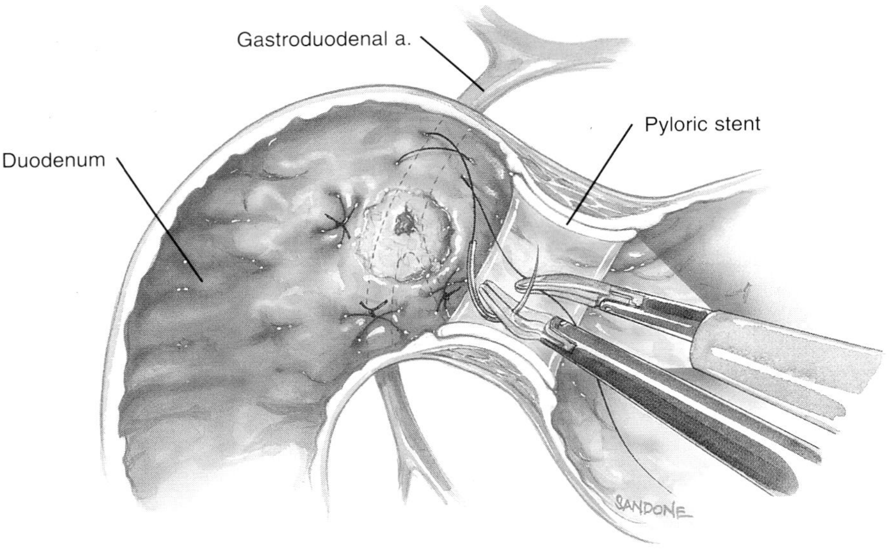

Fig. 22-10. Deep figure-of-eight sutures are used to occlude the gastroduodenal artery and its anastomotic branches.

Suturing using a needle holder and grasper and the suture passer is applicable in the stomach as well as in the proximal duodenum. For duodenal bleeding, the ligation technique described by Berne and Rosoff[20] is imperative. The gastroduodenal artery along with its branches is ligated with four stitches (Fig. 22-10). Deep placement of these four posterior duodenal sutures is currently being practiced in the laboratory.

Comments

Gastric bleeding, we believe, can be treated effectively by endo-organ surgery, as evidenced by our experience with excision therapy. However, endo-organ surgery for duodenal bleeding is more difficult, primarily because it requires efficient pyloric retraction. Instruments for this purpose are under development.

Early surgical treatment is essential. Endo-organ surgery is an alternative to open surgery that permits efficient suturing techniques for gastric and potentially duodenal bleeding secondary to peptic ulceration. Prompt intervention using this approach may reduce the need for additional transfusions, particularly in high-risk lesions.

ENDO-ORGAN GASTRIC EXCISION

Background

Gastric excision is performed for various disease processes. Benign mucosal or submucosal tumors and chronic ulcerations are the primary indications for limited gastric excision. Open laparotomy and gastrotomy are presently necessary to accomplish gastric excision. In 1984 Tada et al.[33] described an endoscopic strip biopsy technique for excision of early gastric cancer. Their technique involved injection of 5 to 10 ml of saline solution into the submucosal space and excision using an electrosnare. This is being used with increasing frequency in Japan.[33-35] The success of the endoscopic approach is limited by the size of the tumor, which should not exceed 2 cm, and its location. Only lesions of the gastric antrum can be satisfactorily resected with an endoscopic technique.[34] This technique has two additional disadvantages. Since endoscopic excision is performed with a snare cautery, the resection margins are burned, which impairs histologic evaluation of the resection margin. Complete excision may therefore be uncertain. In addition, when excessive tissue is grasped, perforation of the stomach may occur. Since suturing of the excision site is not possible, postoperative bleeding is a further possible complication.

Gastric excision by means of an endo-organ approach theoretically is not restricted by localization of lesions or their size. The risk of postoperative bleeding may be reduced, and suture closure of resection margins can be accomplished without difficulty. The risk of perforation is also minimized since excision can be performed under magnified endoscopic visualization, allowing for precise identification of all gastric wall layers. Endo-organ surgery of the stomach is not limited to mucosectomy. Full-thickness resection can be performed, thus extending the indications for this procedure.

Indications

Three disorders are amenable to endo-organ excision: benign mucosal, submucosal, or muscular tumors, benign gastric ulcers, and superficial gastric malignancies. Benign mucosal tumors that are symptomatic, precancerous, or histologically borderline are the primary indication for endo-organ excision. They can be cured by simple mucosectomy with minimal risk of perforation and postoperative bleeding. Included in this group are sessile polyps with recurrent erosion and bleeding, adenomatous polyps with or without dysplasia, and erosion with high-grade dysplasia.

Symptomatic benign muscular or submucosal tumors such as leiomyomas should also be considered for endo-organ excision. Large tumors with involvement of the serosa may require full-thickness excision. Benign tumors close to the cardia or pylorus with the potential for obstruction may be ideal because precise excision and closure can be accomplished and luminal patency assessed prior to completion of the operative intervention.

Excision of chronic gastric ulcers unresponsive to medical therapy is indicated occasionally. Since these ulcerations often include the entire gastric wall, full-

Indications for Endo-Organ Gastric Excision

Benign Lesions	Precancerous Lesions	Early Gastric Cancer
Polyps	Adenomatous polyps	Mucosal tumors
Chronic ulcerations	High-grade dysplasia	Tumors <2 cm
Leiomyomas		Lymphoma
		Leiomyosarcomas

thickness excision will be required. The most common locations of gastric ulcers are the gastric incisura and the prepyloric region. These sites are suitable for endo-organ full-thickness excision, which can be accomplished without technical difficulty.

Minimally invasive surgery in early gastric cancer has gained increasing attention in Japan. To date, tumors confined to the mucosa (stage IA) that show no evidence of retraction and are less than 2 cm in diameter can be recommended for endo-organ excision.[34] Under these circumstances, regional lymph node involvement occurs in less than 5% of patients; in larger tumors or tumors of the submucosal type lymph node, metastasis occurs in up to 20% of cases.[35-38] With endosonography, laparoscopic ultrasound imaging, and laparoscopic lymph node biopsies it may be possible to more accurately assess lymph node metastasis, which may in turn result in broadening the indications for endo-organ excision to include submucosal malignant lesions. Small lymphomas of the stomach may prove to be an additional indication for palliative full-thickness endo-organ excision before chemotherapy since they tend to perforate during medical treatment.

Laboratory Studies

Technique. A video endoscope (Olympus GIF-100) is passed into the stomach under general anesthesia (local anesthesia with sedation may be possible). After the optimal position is determined, two operative ports are placed in the stomach as described on p. 291. One port is used for the introduction of an operative laparoscope (Olympus OES II, 8-degree looking angle, 45-degree eyepiece, and 5 mm probe channel) and the other for additional laparoscopic instruments. To obtain optimal visualization, high-pressure insufflation of the stomach may be required. An insufflation pressure of approximately 8 mm Hg is necessary for mucosectomy and is achieved by a flexible endoscope introduced transorally or through a standard laparoscopic trocar placed in the operative port. A pressure of up to 20 mm Hg provides satisfactory visualization for full-thickness excision. The stomach can be fixed to the abdominal wall with two T-fasteners. This provides additional distraction of the stomach sidewalls when large pieces of full-thickness gastric wall are to be excised. Grasping forceps are then inserted through the working channel of the operating laparoscope. The gastric mucosa is grasped and sharply dissected from the muscle layer (Fig. 22-11). Bleeding sites can be cauterized. The excision edges are then sutured with interrupted 2-0 Prolene; we prefer a ski needle and an extracorporeal knot-tying technique. The full-thickness excision sites are also closed using interrupted 2-0 Prolene sutures (Fig. 22-12). A one-layer or a two-layer closure can be performed. When the gastric excision is completed, the ports can be replaced with a polyethylene 24 F feeding tube.

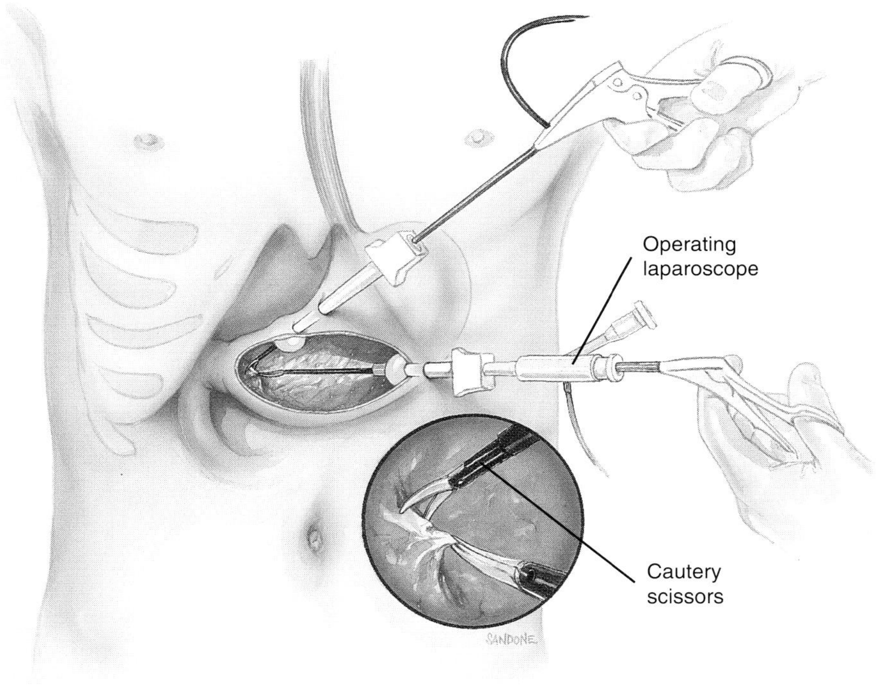

Fig. 22-11. Mucosectomy is performed using sharp dissection.

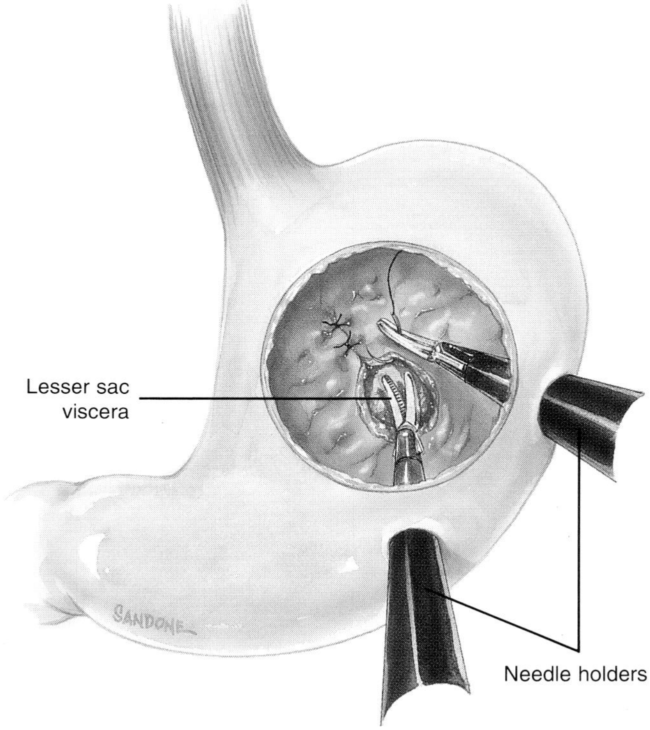

Fig. 22-12. Full-thickness excision is closed using an operating laparoscope with a grasping forceps and an additional port for a suture holder.

Results. Nine pigs were operated on. Postmortem inspection was used to confirm the accuracy of port placement and to determine the presence of intraperitoneal contamination or injury to adjacent viscera. In some animals, ports were placed in the posterior body because of gastric rotation by distention. The posterior positioning was not apparent at the time of placement. Orientation of ports was reasonably accurate in terms of maximum distance from the planned excision site. When the port was placed closer than 7 cm from the excision site, the procedure was tedious but excision could be accomplished.

A total of 10 mucosectomies (several pigs had multiple mucosectomies) were performed. Specimen sizes ranged up to 10 × 7 cm. Bleeding was limited and hemostasis was accomplished by cauterization. Suture ligation of bleeding sites was not necessary. Clots impaired the visualization by absorbing light, but suction and irrigation via the laparoscope were successful in improving light intensity.

Full-thickness gastric excision was performed in three additional experiments. In one pig (No. 5) the site of excision was the posterior antrum, which measured 3 cm in diameter. Two T-fasteners placed anteriorly and high-pressure insufflation (20 mm Hg) provided excellent exposure. Thorough cauterization of tissue edges was accomplished with cautery scissors and no bleeding was encountered. Full-thickness closure was performed with interrupted 2-0 Prolene and extracorporeal knot tying. In the second pig (No. 6) the site of full-thickness gastric excision was the posterior fundus and the excised piece of gastric wall measured 6 × 3 cm. T-fasteners were not used and exposure was accomplished only by high-pressure insufflation. Closure, performed as in pig No. 5, was satisfactory. Pig No. 7 had a 10 × 9 cm circumferential piece of antrum removed. Two T-fasteners were used and again exposure was satisfactory. The port placement was approximately the same as in pig No. 6. The full-thickness opening was first made posteriorly since sidewall collapse with a small-diameter defect did not create exposure problems. A running 2-0 Prolene suture was used for closure.

After the procedure the pigs were killed and postmortem examinations performed. No soilage, bleeding, or accidental damage to the small bowel, spleen, or liver was detected in any animals on inspection of the peritoneal cavity. All suture lines for animals with full-thickness excision were intact.

CONCLUSION

The endo-organ approach provides heretofore unavailable access to the stomach and duodenum. Large-diameter access ports permit introduction of instruments for ligation, cauterization, and tissue manipulation that once could not reach the intraluminal gastric environment, opening a range of therapeutic options.

The operative port is ready for clinical use; recent refinements will make it even easier to introduce and secure to the abdominal wall. Replacement of the port with a smaller caliber tube is technically simple and a kit is under development for that purpose. If immediate removal of the tube without replacement is considered appropriate, direct suturing through the abdominal wall port entry site can be accomplished. A retracting technique to elevate the stomach wall above the skin in thin patients has been developed for direct gastric suturing. For delayed removal, simple extraction can be performed and a dressing placed.

The endoscopic antireflux procedure is dependent on reduction of tension on the invaginated esophagus. Techniques are under investigation to accomplish this important aspect of the repair. A new fixation device that reduces the potential for tissue failure will soon be available. We believe this procedure has great potential and may revolutionize the surgical correction of gastroesophageal reflux disease. The procedure can be performed through percutaneous gastrostomies, therefore allowing gastroenterologists and surgeons to complete this procedure without patient hospitalization.

Patients with upper gastrointestinal bleeding requiring surgical intervention will unquestionably benefit from a minimally invasive procedure if it is effective and safe. Because laboratory experimentation has demonstrated the ease of suturing within the gastric lumen, patients with gastric ulcers will be excellent candidates for endo-organ hemostatic suturing. Instruments and techniques are currently under investigation for improved duodenal exposure and ligation of the gastroduodenal artery and its collateral vessels. Intraoperative Doppler confirmation of vessel occlusion may make this approach more effective than the open procedure for bleeding duodenal ulcers.

Endo-organ gastric excision of either gastric mucosa or full-thickness tissue is feasible. Benign and early gastric malignancies, although rare in this country, may be resectable using the endo-organ approach. Safety, convenience of operative ports, effective staging for superficial malignancies, and minimized risk of delayed gastric perforation are major factors in determining the benefits of this approach.

Precise lateral and deep margins of an early malignancy can be established by sharp dissection in contradistinction to the endoscopic cautery strip biopsy technique in which electrical damage to tissue compromises the assessment of histologic margins. In addition, a complete deep margin excision is possible because full-thickness muscular wall can be removed. Finally, endo-organ excision allows adequate deep tissue excision to be confirmed immediately by frozen section examination. If the lesion extends past the submucosal margin, an open procedure can then be performed.

Antral mucosectomy for peptic ulcer disease and full-thickness antrectomy have been performed in our laboratory. Further protocols will eventually be initiated in the laboratory to develop the technique and determine its effectiveness and safety in the porcine model.

REFERENCES

1. Dallemagne B, Weerts JM, Jehaes C, et al. Laparoscopic Nissen fundoplication: Preliminary report. Surg Laparosc Endosc 1:138-143, 1991.
2. Tytgat GN. Endoscopic therapy of esophageal cancer: Possibilities and limitation. Endoscopy 22:263-267, 1990.
3. Wetscher GJ, Hinder RA, Redmond EJ, et al. Laparoscopic highly selective vagotomy. Contemp Surg 44:153-159, 1994.
4. Stiegmann GV, Goff JS, Sun JH, et al. Endoscopic elastic band ligation for active variceal hemorrhage. Am Surg 54:105-108, 1988.
5. Spinelli P, Di Felice F, Pizzetti P, et al. Laparoscopic repair of full-thickness stomach injury. Surg Endosc 5:156-157, 1991.
6. Qian KD, Zhao CJ, Tang XQ, et al. The diagnosis and management of gastric polyps: Report of 198 cases. Presented at the First Shanghai International Symposium on Gastrointestinal Cancer. Shanghai, November 14-16, 1988, p 248.
7. Kawai K, Akasaka Y, Murakami K, et al. Endoscopic sphincterotomy of the ampulla of Vater. Gastrointest Endosc 20:148-151, 1974.
8. Siegel JH, Safrany L, Ben-Zvi JS, et al. Duodenoscopic sphincterotomy in patients with gallbladders in situ: Report of a series of 1272 patients. Am J Gastroenterol 83:1255-1258, 1988.

9. Silvis SE, Vennes JA. Endoscopic retrograde sphincterotomy. In Silvis SE, ed. Therapeutic Gastrointestinal Endoscopy. New York: Igaku-Shoin, 1984, pp 198-240.
10. Huibregtse K, Katon RM, Coene PP, et al. Endoscopic palliative treatment in pancreatic cancer. Gastrointest Endosc 32:334-338, 1986.
11. Soehendra N, Grimm H, Stenzel M. Injection of nonvariceal bleeding lesions of the upper gastrointestinal tract. Endoscopy 17:129-132, 1985.
12. Chung SCS, Leung JWC, Sung JY, et al. Injection or heater probe for bleeding ulcers. Gastroenterology 100:33-37, 1991.
13. Swain CP, Salmon PR, Kirkham JS, et al. Controlled trial of Nd:YAG laser photocoagulation in bleeding peptic ulcers. Lancet 1:1113-1117, 1986.
14. Afridi SA, Fichtenbaum CJ, Taubin H. Review of duodenal diverticula. Am J Gastroenterol 86:935-938, 1991.
15. Frimberger E, Classen M. A new pull-through trocar technique for percutaneous operative endoscopy. Endoscopy 23:338-341, 1991.
16. Way L. Personal communication, 1993.
17. Jennings RW, Flake AW, Mussin G, et al. A novel endoscopic transgastric fundoplication procedure for gastroesophageal reflux: An initial animal evaluation. J Laparosc Endosc Surg 2:207-213, 1992.
18. DeMeester TR, Bonavina L, Albertucci M. Nissen fundoplication for gastroesophageal reflux disease. Ann Surg 204:9-20, 1986.
19. Gostout ChJ, Wang KK, Ahlquist DA, et al. Acute gastrointestinal bleeding. J Clin Gastroenterol 14:260-267, 1992.
20. Berne CJ, Rosoff L. Peptic ulcer perforation of the gastroduodenal artery complex: Clinical features and operative control. Ann Surg 169:141-144, 1969.
21. Sedillot C. Operation De Gastrostomie, Pratiquee Pour La Permiere Fois Le 13 November. Gaz Med Strassbourg 9:566, 1849.
22. Ponsky JL, Gandevev MWL. Percutaneous endoscopic gastrostomy: A nonoperative technique for feeding gastrostomy. Gastrointest Endosc 27:9-11, 1981.
23. Ponsky JL, Aszodi A, Perse D. Percutaneous endoscopic cecostomy: A new approach to non-obstructive colonic dilatation. Gastrointest Endosc 32:108-111, 1986.
24. Haaga JR. CT-guided procedures. In Hagga JR, Alfidi RJ, eds. Computed Tomography of the Whole Body, vol 2. St. Louis: CV Mosby, 1988, p 1280.
25. Pope CE II. A dynamic test of sphincter strength: Its application to the lower esophageal sphincter. Gastroenterology 52:779-786, 1967.
26. Ellis FH, Crozier RE. Reflux control by fundoplication: A clinical and monometric assessment of the Nissen operation. Ann Thorac Surg 38:387-392, 1984.
27. McGouran RCM, Galloway JM. A laser-induced scar at the cardia increases the yield pressure of the lower esophageal sphincter. Gastrointest Endosc 36:439-443, 1990.
28. O'Sullivan GC, DeMeester TR, Joelsson BE, et al. The interaction of the lower esophageal sphincter pressure and length of sphincter in the abdomen as determinants of gastroesophageal competence. Am J Surg 143:40-47, 1982.
29. Stipa S, Fegiz G, Iascone C, et al. Belsey and Nissen operations for gastroesophageal reflux. Ann Surg 210:583-589, 1989.
30 . Jordan PH Jr. Surgery for peptic ulcer disease. Curr Probl Surg 28:265-330, 1991.
31. Stabile BE, Passara E Jr. Duodenal ulcer: A disease in evolution. Curr Probl Surg 21:1-79, 1984.
32. Branicki FJ, Coleman SY, Pritchett CJ, et al. Emergency surgical treatment for nonvariceal bleeding of the upper part of the gastrointestinal tract. Surg Gynecol Obstet 172:113-120, 1991.
33. Tada M, Shimada M, Yanai H, et al. A new technique of gastric biopsy. Stomach Intestine 19:1107-1116, 1984.
34. Haruma K, Sumii K, Inoue K, et al. Endoscopic therapy in patients with inoperable early gastric cancer. Am J Gastroenterol 85:522-526, 1990.
35. Sano T, Kobori O, Muto T. Lymph node metastasis form early gastric cancer: Endoscopic resection of tumour. Br J Surg 79:241-244, 1992.
36. Hioki K, Nakane Y, Yamamoto M. Surgical strategy for early gastric cancer. Br J Surg 77:1330-1334, 1990.
37. Maehara Y, Orita H, Okuyama T, et al. Predictors of lymph node metastasis in early gastric cancer. Br J Surg 79:245-247, 1992.
38. Ohta H, Noguchi Y, Takagai K, et al. Early gastric carcinoma with special reference to macroscopic classification. Cancer 60:1099-1106, 1987.

Chapter

23

Laparoscopic Feeding Gastrostomy and Jejunostomy

Thomas J. Watson, M.D. • Jeffrey H. Peters, M.D.

Providing long-term nutritional support poses some unique challenges. Patients frequently present in a malnourished, septic, or posttraumatic state and experience increased metabolic demands. In addition, various disease processes and surgical procedures can prevent the patient from consuming an adequate oral diet for prolonged periods of time. Under such circumstances the clinician must choose between a variety of enteral and parenteral nutritional supplements.

Recent studies in patients with a functional gut have affirmed the benefits of enteral nutrition over parenteral alimentation. Although isocaloric, isonitrogenous diets appear to provide the same nutritional benefits whether given enterally or parenterally,[1-4] research has demonstrated the relative nonnutritional benefits of the enteral route. Reports of infectious sequelae of total parenteral nutrition have been prevalent in the literature. Kudsk et al.[5,6] demonstrated that total parenteral nutrition in normal and malnourished rats was associated with higher mortality rates after septic peritonitis compared with enteral feedings. They subsequently found a higher rate of septic complications, especially pneumonia and abdominal infections, in severely traumatized patients fed parenterally compared with those fed enterally.[7] Similarly, Moore et al.[8] in a meta-analysis study of high-risk surgical and blunt trauma patients determined that parenterally nourished patients had a significantly higher incidence of infectious complications than those fed enterally. The Veterans Administration Cooperative Study revealed no difference in overall complication rates in a group of malnourished surgical patients who received preoperative total parenteral nutrition compared with controls.[9] Mild and moderately malnourished elective surgical patients given total parenteral nutrition, however, did experience a significant increase in pulmonary and wound infections.

The mechanisms by which total parenteral nutrition leads to an increased incidence of septic complications have yet to be fully elucidated. Much attention is being devoted to the role of the gastrointestinal tract as a guardian against microbial invasion and the role enteral substrates play in maintaining gut mucosal integrity. Involutional changes are observed in the gastrointestinal tract when nutrition is provided completely by the parenteral route. In most individuals these changes are of little clinical consequence and resolve once feedings are resumed.[10] In critically ill or septic patients, however, the functional and morphologic breakdown of the gastrointestinal mucosal barrier may have important implications. Experimental work supports the concept that systemic sepsis in such patients may result from bacterial translocation, the process whereby intraluminal enteric organisms cross this barrier to enter the bloodstream. In a series of animal experiments Deitch et al.[11-16] demonstrated that trauma, endotoxemia, an immunosuppressed state, and altered enteric flora secondary to bacterial overgrowth or oral antibiotics all promote bacterial translocation.

Enteral nutrition, on the other hand, may help to prevent translocation. Alverdy et al.[17] studied translocation in rats fed enterally and parenterally and found a higher rate of bacterial translocation to the mesenteric lymph nodes in the parenteral group. These results are consistent with those of a recent laboratory study suggesting that small amounts of tube feedings added to a total parenteral nutrition regimen could reduce the incidence of bacterial translocation to mesenteric lymph nodes and improve nitrogen balance.[18] Likewise, Inoue et al.[19] discovered that a single enteral feeding 12 hours after a significant burn suppressed yeast translocation in guinea pigs.

Equally important to the genesis of sepsis associated with total parenteral nutrition may be its immunologic effects. Working with parenterally nourished rats, Shou et al.[20] demonstrated impaired peritoneal macrophage microbicidal and splenocyte proliferative function, which were reversed by the administration of small volumes of oral feedings. The same group also demonstrated significant impairments in pulmonary macrophage function in rats following total parenteral nutrition.[21] Such defects were associated with an increased mortality rate after a pulmonary challenge. Secretory IgA has also been implicated as an important component of the gut mucosal defense system.[22,23]

The relative influences of total parenteral nutrition and enteral nutrition on intraluminal bacterial overgrowth, intestinal mucosal barrier function, bacterial and endotoxin translocation, host humoral responses, and cellular immune function are important considerations in choosing a mode of nutritional support. Further studies are needed to define how these factors interact to determine an individual's resistance to microbial proliferation.

Other benefits of enteral nutrition over total parenteral nutrition include the following:

1. Better utilization of nutrients[24]
2. Avoidance of central venous catheters with the attendant risks of pneumothorax, vascular or nervous injury, and infection[25]
3. A decreased incidence of metabolic complications such as hyper- or hypoglycemia
4. Fewer thrombotic events, both systemically and locally, at the site of insertion into peripheral or central veins
5. Less insult to hepatic function and morphology, especially steatosis[26-29]
6. A markedly decreased cost per patient (5 to 25 times less than total parenteral nutrition)
7. Ease of administration, especially for patients at home (no special facilities or trained personnel necessary)

As evidence accumulates confirming the superiority of enteral feeding over parenteral hyperalimentation, methods for establishing chronic enteral access become increasingly important.

RATIONALE FOR THE LAPAROSCOPIC APPROACH

Since its description in 1980, percutaneous endoscopic gastrostomy has gained wide acceptance as a technically simple, inexpensive, and well-tolerated method of establishing chronic enteral access.[30] The procedure is minimally invasive, avoids laparotomy, and is usually performed under local anesthesia. The stomach provides a reservoir for bolus feeding, and gastric alimentation may lessen the diarrhea associated with the jejunal route.

Percutaneous endoscopic gastrostomy, however, is not without its drawbacks. Anatomic barriers such as obstructing pharyngeal or esophageal neoplasms or strictures may make endoscopy impossible. Also, the stomach may be unsuitable as an access site in patients who have had an esophagectomy or gastrectomy. Likewise, a gastrostomy may be inadvisable in patients scheduled for esophagectomy since it may preclude the use of the stomach as an esophageal substitute. Since percutaneous endoscopic gastrostomy is a relatively blind procedure, intra-abdominal contents are not directly visualized, increasing the possibility of injuring hollow or solid viscera. Finally, it was anticipated that percutaneous endoscopic gastrostomy would decrease the incidence of aspiration pneumonia by eliminating the conduit between the stomach and pharynx, but this has proved unfounded. The risks of gastroesophageal reflux and aspiration are significant, occurring in 15% to 40% of patients.[31-35] The rate of these complications increases in certain high-risk groups such as those with a mechanically incompetent lower esophageal sphincter, gastroparesis, gastric outlet obstruction, or mental obtundation.

Duodenal and jejunal tubes placed through a gastrostomy have been used to administer feedings more distally in the bowel and have been recommended in aspiration-prone individuals.[36] Such tubes, however, may migrate,[36-37] are unreliable in keeping the feedings beyond the pylorus, and do not prevent aspiration. In fact, aspiration may occur in as many as 60% of patients following percutaneous endoscopic jejunostomy.[36] Nasoduodenal and nasojejunal tubes are also a poor alternative. They are uncomfortable for the patient, poorly tolerated over long periods of time, easily dislodged, and difficult to pass.

Surgical gastrostomies and jejunostomies are considered when less-invasive techniques are not appropriate. In recent years laparoscopic approaches have been developed for placement of gastrostomies and jejunostomies and may offer several advantages over open and endoscopic techniques.

LAPAROSCOPIC GASTROSTOMY

A surgical gastrostomy is required in patients who are candidates for long-term gastric feeding or decompression but who possess anatomic barriers to placement of a tube by the percutaneous endoscopic method. Such barriers may include obstructing pharyngeal or esophageal neoplasms or strictures, wired mandibles due to fractures, liver or colon overlying the stomach, intra-abdominal adhesions secondary to prior laparotomy, or an obese abdominal wall precluding endoscopic transillumination. Additionally, patients may be undergoing laparotomy or laparoscopy for another condition and need a gastrostomy placed concomitantly. Laparoscopic gastrostomy offers the obvious advantage over the traditional open technique of being less invasive. The laparoscopic procedures are also technically simple, easily tolerated, reliable, and require a short operative time.

Technique

All patients are given broad-spectrum intravenous antibiotics perioperatively. Either a general anesthetic or local anesthetic with intravenous sedation may be used. A nasogastric tube is passed if possible, and the bladder is decompressed with a Foley catheter. After the field has been prepped and draped, pneumoperitoneum is established to a pressure of approximately 15 mm Hg using a Veress needle inserted to the umbilicus. A 5 or 10 mm trocar is introduced, depending on the size of the laparoscope available. Alternatively, an open technique may be used by placing a Hasson trocar into the peritoneal cavity through a curvilinear infraumbilical incision. The laparoscope is inserted via this umbilical port and a 5 mm trocar introduced into the right abdomen under direct vision. The patient is placed in the reverse Trendelenburg position. A grasping forceps introduced via this second trocar is used to elevate the body of the stomach toward the anterior abdominal wall. If additional distention of the stomach is required, air may be introduced via the nasogastric tube.

A 7 cm, 18-gauge needle is pierced through the skin in the left subcostal region and into the stomach under direct visualization.[38] A J-wire is inserted via the needle into the stomach. The tract is dilated with 12 and 14 F dilators before a 16 F peel-away sheath is introduced. A 14 F Silastic balloon catheter is advanced into the stomach, the balloon inflated with 5 to 10 ml of water, and the peel-away sheath removed. The catheter is affixed to the skin after pulling the stomach up to the anterior abdominal wall. The abdomen is thoroughly examined for hemostasis and for leakage around the gastrostomy. The trocars are removed and the fascia at the umbilical site closed with interrupted absorbable sutures. The skin edges are reapproximated with a running subcuticular absorbable stitch.

A preferable technique uses T-fastener technology. T-fasteners provide four-point fixation of the stomach to the anterior abdominal wall, as described by Modesto et al.[39] A percutaneous gastrostomy kit is available (Ross Flexiflo R 18 F Introducer Gastrostomy kit with a Brown/Mueller T-fastener). A T-fastener needle is introduced percutaneously in the left upper quadrant and advanced through the anterior wall of the stomach under direct vision (Fig. 23-1). The stylet is inserted and the T-fastener is released. Three other T-fasteners are inserted 1 cm from the first to provide four-point fixation (Fig. 23-2). A J-wire is introduced into the stomach between these T-fasteners (Fig. 23-3). The gastrostomy tract is gradually enlarged over the J-wire using the dilators provided in the kit (graduated sizes up to 18 F). Countertraction on the stomach is provided by the T-fasteners while the tract is dilated. The gastrostomy tube is inserted over the J-wire into the stomach (Fig. 23-4).

The anterior gastric wall is approximated to the anterior abdominal wall by traction on the tube and the T-fasteners. The tube is sutured to the skin and the T-fasteners are secured by crimping the metal washer with a blunt-tip needle holder. The abdomen is examined, the trocars removed, and the wounds closed as previously discussed. The T-fasteners provide additional security in case the gastrostomy balloon ruptures or the tube dislodges.

Postoperative Management

Feedings are usually started 24 hours after surgery. We begin with full-strength formula at a rate of 15 ml/hr and then use a continuous-drip infusion that is gradually

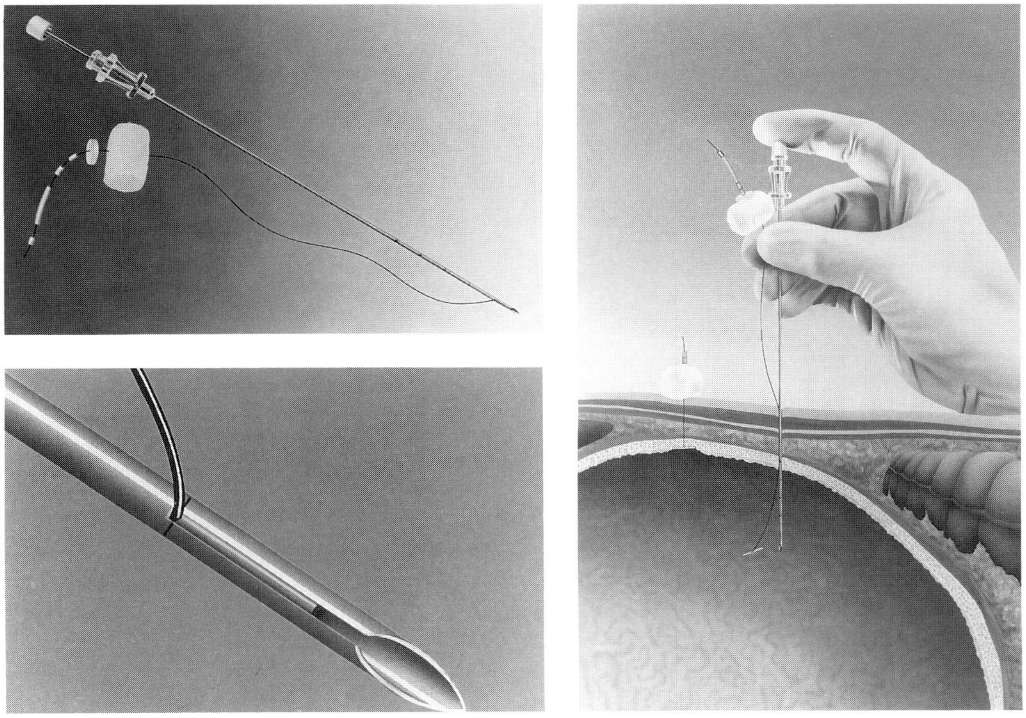

Fig. 23-1. A, T-fastener with insertion needle. **B,** T-fastener loaded into insertion needle. **C,** Insertion of T-fastener into gastric lumen. The stomach is insufflated via an intraluminal endoscope through a nasogastric tube.

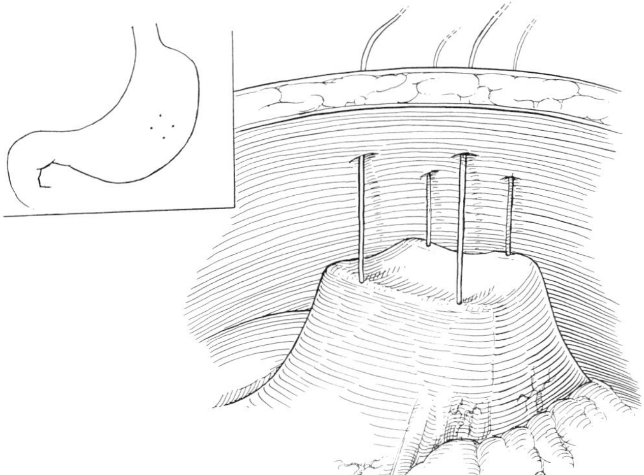

Fig. 23-2. Laparoscopic assisted placement of feeding gastrostomy using T-fastener technology. Four T-fasteners are placed under laparoscopic guidance into the gastric lumen.

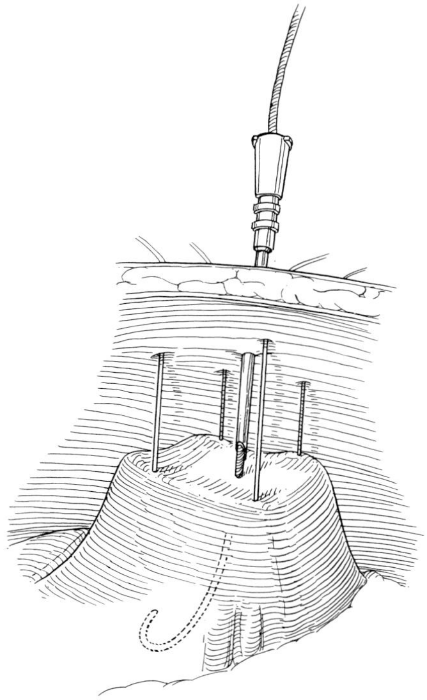

Fig. 23-3. A J-wire is placed into the gastric lumen after needle puncture between the T-fasteners. Correct placement of the needle and J-wire is guided by the laparoscopic image.

A

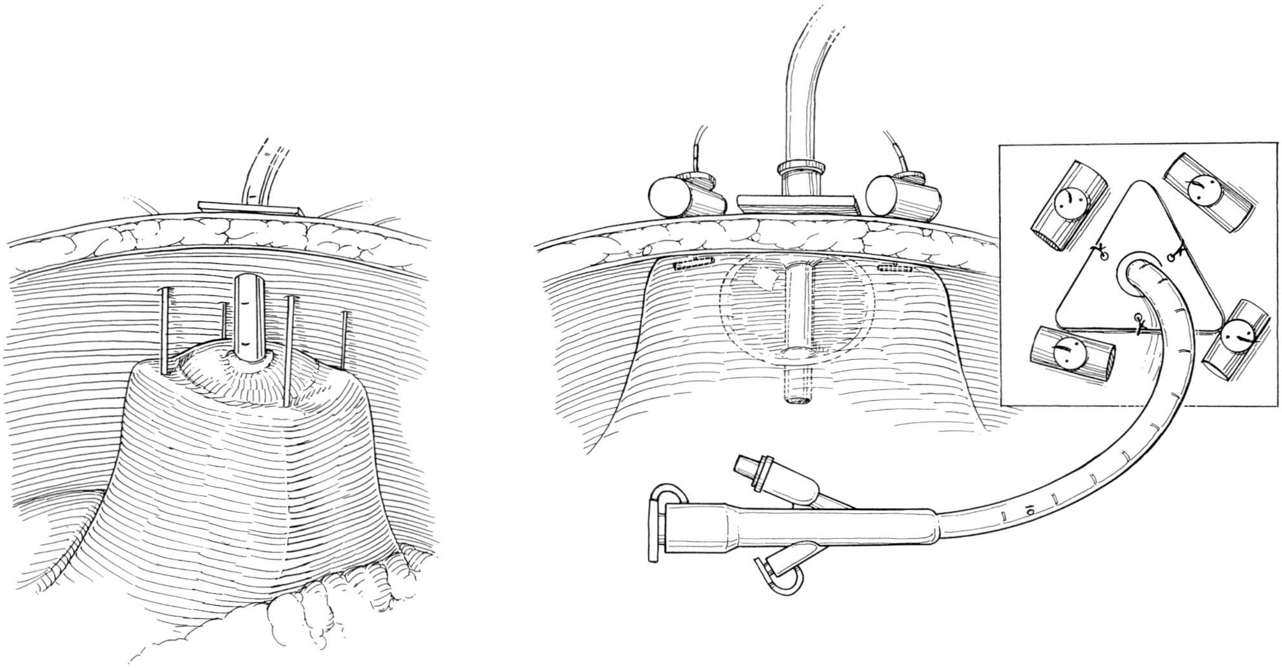

B

Fig. 23-4. A, The gastrostomy tract is successively dilated prior to placement of the final gastrostomy tube. **B,** Final appearance of the gastrostomy tube in place with the T-fasteners.

advanced in increments of 15 ml/hr/day until the goal rate is attained. Although a complete discussion of nutritional assessment and requirements is beyond the scope of this chapter, we typically administer 25 to 40 kcal/kg/day and 1 to 2 gm/kg/day of protein, depending on the nature and severity of the patient's underlying illness. Serum albumin and transferrin levels, patient weight, nitrogen balance, and overall clinical course are assessed to determine the adequacy of nutritional support. Once an oral diet is resumed, the level of supplementation is gradually tapered.

Patients who require continued enteral alimentation after discharge from the hospital are issued a portable pump (Ross Laboratories, Inc., Columbus, Ohio) that can be attached with a shoulder strap so that the patient can go about his daily activities. These pumps are reliable and easily maintained.

The stomach has the advantage of allowing bolus feeding if desired. Once a continuous infusion of feedings is tolerated, the patient can be slowly advanced to receive the same total daily volume in several discrete boluses. This method frees the patient from the burden of transporting and maintaining the feeding pump throughout the day and appears to be generally well tolerated.

Ambulatory patients may be discharged home on the day of surgery, although these procedures are more typically performed on an inpatient basis. The patients are provided instructions on the maintenance of the catheters and the advancement of tube feedings.

LAPAROSCOPIC JEJUNOSTOMY

A surgical jejunostomy is considered when the stomach cannot be used as a site for enteral access. The traditional open Witzel jejunostomy, which employs a 12 mm tube placed through a serosal tunnel, has not gained wide acceptance because of frequent and potentially serious complications such as intraperitoneal leakage, kinking of the tube or bowel, intestinal obstruction, and tube dislodgment. The incidence of these complications was reduced by the introduction of the intramural needle-catheter technique described by Delany et al.[40] A 14-gauge needle and a catheter from a central venous catheterization set are used.

The primary disadvantage of this technique is the small diameter of the tube, which frequently leads to clogging and sluggish flow. We use a commercially available needle-catheter jejunostomy kit that provides a larger lumen, allowing the use of more viscous formulas at a faster rate and clogging less frequently. The tube is also somewhat stiffer and therefore kinks less often. It may be easily replaced through an established tract should it become dislodged. The following technique of laparoscopic jejunostomy is a direct modification of our open procedure, as initially described by Roy and DeMeester.[41]

Technique

As with laparoscopic gastrostomy, all patients are given broad-spectrum intravenous antibiotics perioperatively. Laparoscopic jejunostomy, however, usually requires general anesthesia. A Foley catheter and nasogastric tube are passed for urinary and gastric decompression. After the field is prepped and draped, a 10 mm Hasson trocar is introduced into the peritoneal cavity through a curvilinear infraumbilical incision using an open technique. The incision is made larger than usual to allow evisceration of the small bowel. A Veress needle is not appropriate for this procedure because the bowel must be manipulated extracorporeally at the umbilical trocar site. Pneumoperi-

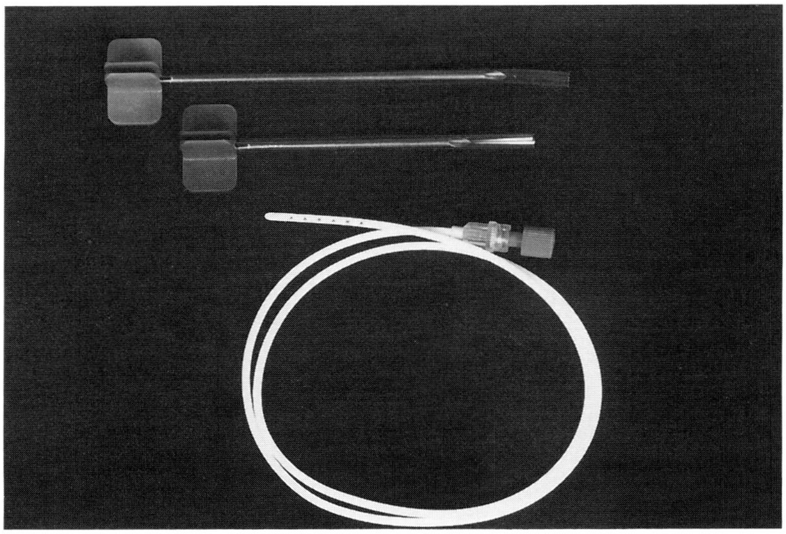

Fig. 23-5. Intestofix needle-catheter jejunostomy kit.

toneum is established to a pressure of approximately 15 mm Hg and the laparoscope inserted via this port. An additional 10 mm trocar is introduced in the left lower quadrant under direct vision, and a third is placed in the right lower quadrant.

As stated previously, we prefer a commercially available needle-catheter jejunostomy kit (Intestofix, Braun Melsungen AG, West Germany). The kit contains two breakaway needles and a flexible 12 F catheter (Fig. 23-5). The shorter needle is used to pass the catheter through the skin and the longer catheter to create an intramural tunnel within the jejunal serosa. The catheter is inserted into the peritoneal cavity in the left lower quadrant, tunneling it through the abdominal wall in a lateral to medial direction, and the breakaway needle is removed (Fig. 23-6). The Hasson trocar and laparoscope are removed and the tip of the catheter is brought out through the umbilical incision. This trocar and the laparoscope are then reinserted and pneumoperitoneum reestablished. The patient is placed in a reverse Trendelenburg position to allow the small bowel to fall toward the pelvis. The ligament of Treitz is located after lifting the transverse colon superiorly (Fig. 23-7). Sutures are placed to mark the proximal and distal bowel segments for later reference. A portion of proximal jejunum approximately 25 cm distally is grasped and 2 to 3 feet of small bowel at this site brought out through the umbilical incision. A pursestring suture of 2-0 chromic is placed on the antimesenteric border of the bowel. To create the intramural tunnel the serosa is pierced, the needle is held steady, and the wall of the bowel is advanced over it (Fig. 23-8). The tip of the needle should be visualized through the translucent serosa as the wall of the gut is pulled over the shaft. The length of the tunnel should be 12 to 15 cm, at which point the needle is angled in to pierce the mucosa. The catheter is threaded through the needle into the lumen for a distance of 1 to 2 feet. The needle is split and removed, and the pursestring is tied down. We verify the intraluminal position of the catheter by occluding the bowel proximally and distally and irrigating the catheter with saline solution.

The loop of jejunum is returned to the peritoneal cavity and the Hasson trocar replaced. Under direct vision the jejunum is affixed to the parietal peritoneum and the transversalis fascia with four silk sutures placed circumferentially around the cath-

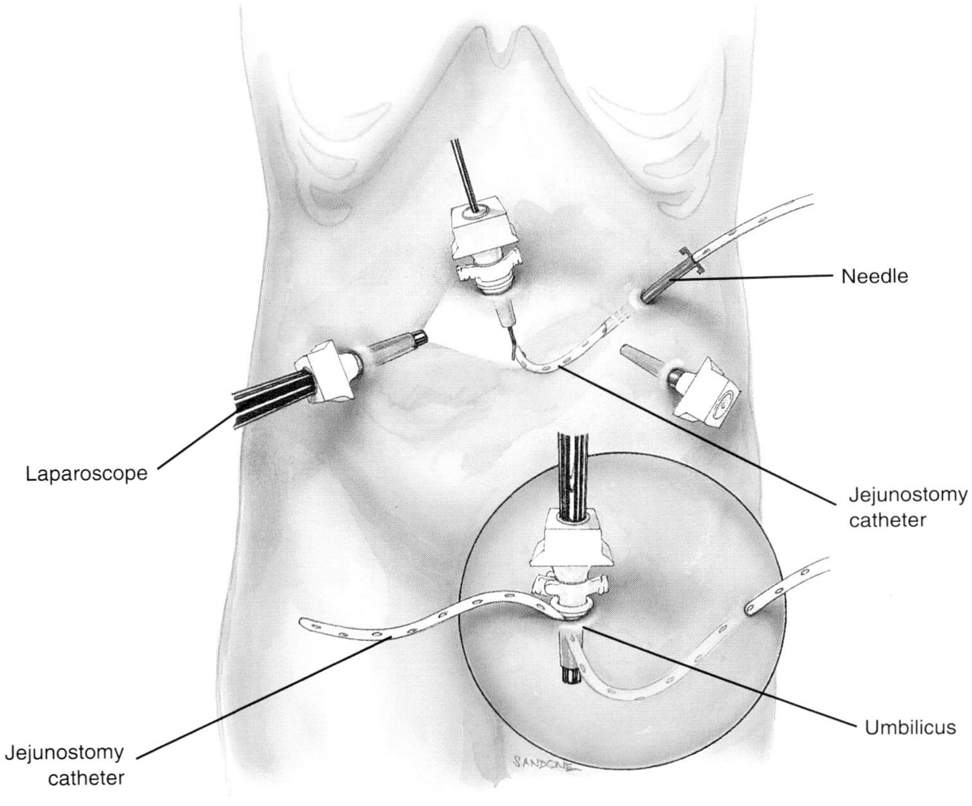

Fig. 23-6. Placement of needle-catheter jejunostomy through the abdominal wall of the left lower quadrant. Inset: The catheter is then pulled through the umbilicus and left beside the trocar.

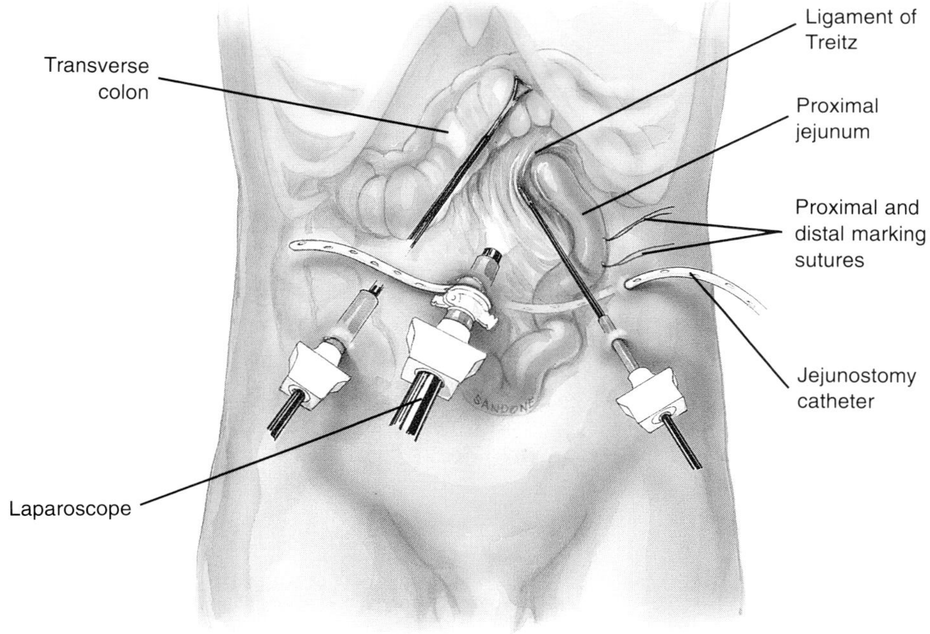

Fig. 23-7. Identification of the ligament of Treitz and the proximal jejunum. The transverse colon is held anteriorly and the ligament of Treitz identified. Colored sutures are placed into the jejunum to mark proximal from distal bowel, and 2 to 3 feet of jejunum is pulled out through the umbilicus.

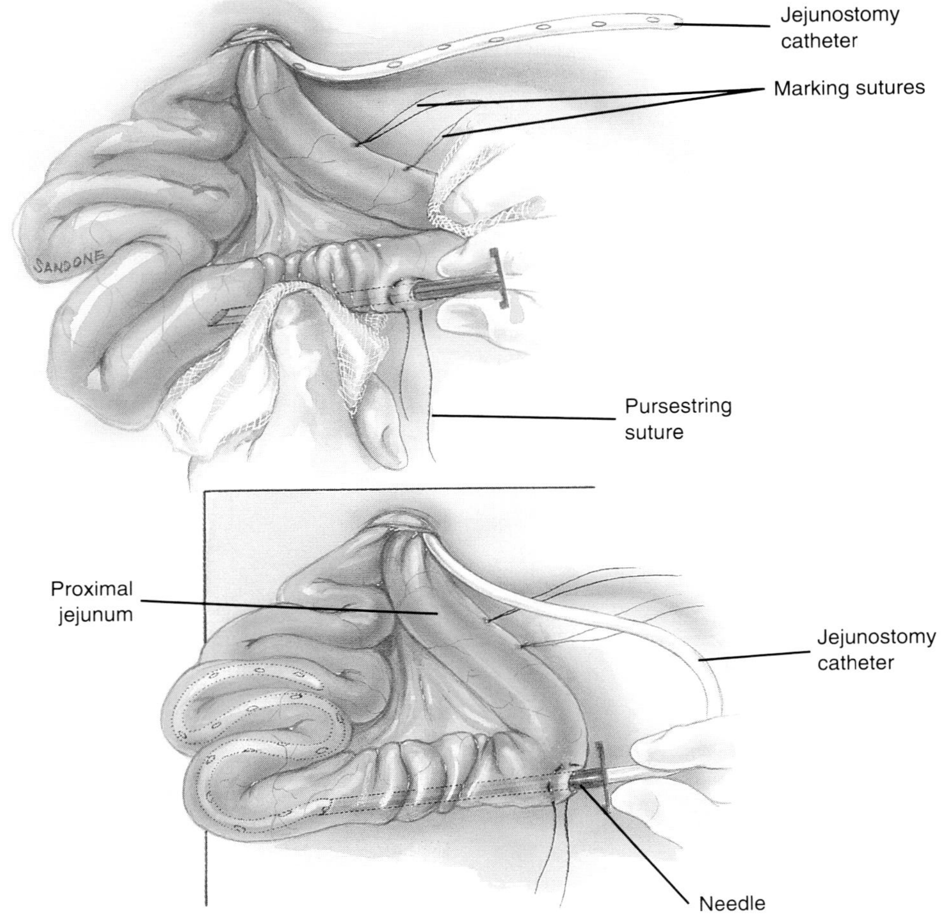

Fig. 23-8. Placement of the needle-catheter jejunostomy into the subserosal tunnel and jejunal lumen. Inset: The catheter is threaded approximately 1 to 2 feet into the jejunum.

eter (Fig. 23-9). Placing the first suture farthest from the laparoscope aids visualization. Care must be taken to ensure the proper orientation of the bowel proximally and distally to prevent iatrogenic volvulus and subsequent bowel obstruction. The trocars are removed and the fascia of the infraumbilical incision reapproximated with interrupted absorbable sutures. The skin edges are closed with running subcuticular absorbable sutures. The catheter is sewn to the skin surface with 2-0 polypropylene sutures using a 14 F red Robinson catheter slit along one end as a bolster. We have found it useful to affix the external portion of the catheter in a U configuration oriented transversely to prevent kinking when the patient bends forward.

If the commercial kit is not available, a small gallbladder trocar can be used to create the intramural tunnel. A 10 F infant feeding tube can be passed easily through the lumen of the trocar. We have found this an entirely satisfactory, if less elegant, alternative. The only caveat is that the feeding tube should be passed once through the trocar before the latter is inserted because the proximal flared end may require trimming to allow removal of the trocar after the tube is in place.

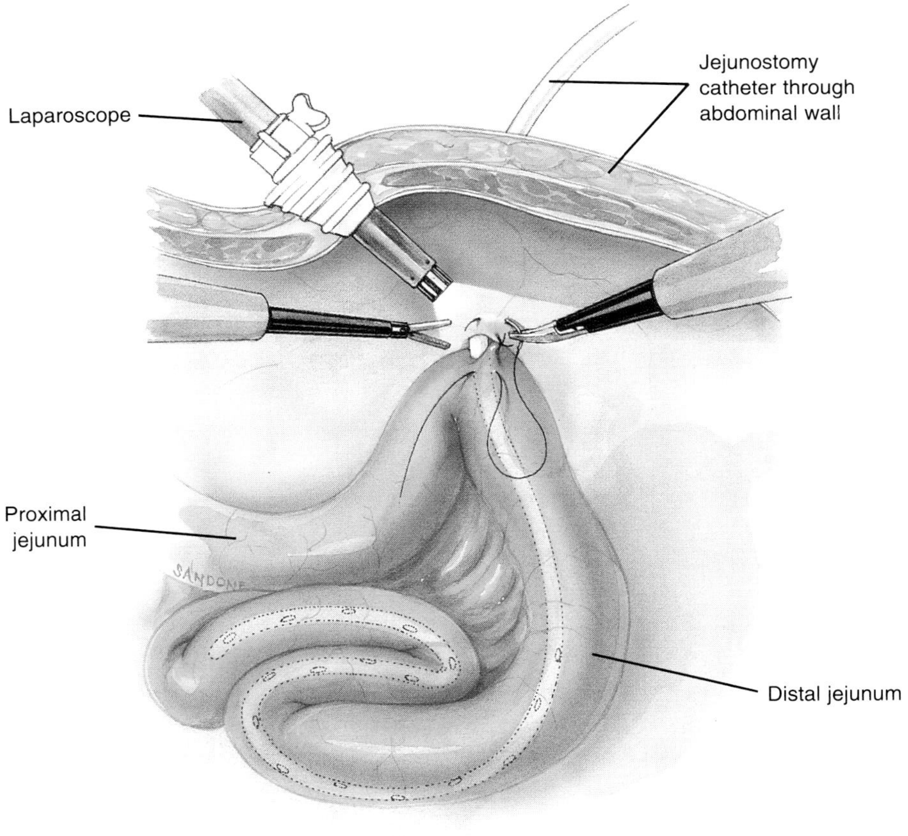

Fig. 23-9. Fixation of the proximal jejunum to the anterior abdominal wall.

Several other techniques of laparoscopic feeding jejunostomy tube placement have been reported in the literature. The technical elements are similar and include (1) laparoscopic visualization of the ligament of Treitz and proximal jejunum; (2) fixation of the jejunum to the anterior abdominal wall using intracorporeal,[42] extracorporeal,[43] or percutaneous[44] suturing techniques or T-fasteners[45]; and (3) advancement of an appropriate feeding tube into the jejunal lumen. The number of cases reported is small and data on complications and long-term function are sparse. These procedures resemble the open Witzel technique in certain key respects and consequently might suffer from the same pitfalls. None of the techniques appears to offer any distinct advantages over the method we have described herein.

Postoperative Management

Feeding is typically begun on the third postoperative day. Again, we start with full-strength formula at a rate of 15 ml/hr and using continuous-drip infusion gradually advance in increments of 15 ml/hr/day until the goal rate is attained. As oral consumption is resumed, the amount of supplementation is gradually tapered. Patients who require nutritional support after discharge from the hospital are issued a portable pump, as described earlier.

Any medications administered through the tube should ideally be in liquid form or at least pulverized thoroughly. Clogging of the catheters is prevented by routine irrigation with 15 ml of Coca-Cola, cranberry juice, or vinegar. We have found a 1 ml tuberculin syringe useful for applying pressure to the needle-catheter jejunostomy tubes should clogging occur. Diarrhea is common, especially shortly after placement. This may be controlled by adding Kaopectate or paregoric to the formula, by slowing the rate temporarily, or by switching to an isotonic formula. We have also found the intermittent administration of narcotic-based constipating agents such as diphenoxylate with atropine (Lomotil) or tincture of opium useful in difficult cases. Of course, antibiotic-induced diarrhea and pseudomembranous colitis are always important considerations and need to be ruled out. Rarely does diarrhea require interruption of feedings. If a catheter becomes dislodged or kinked after the first few days, a new one may be easily threaded under fluoroscopic guidance. Intraluminal positioning of the tube should be verified by an abdominal x-ray film after injecting a small amount of water-soluble contrast. The semirigid character of these tubes permits easy reinsertion.

COMPLICATIONS

Since laparoscopic gastrostomies and jejunostomies are relatively new procedures, there is little published data regarding perioperative complications and long-term follow-up. Edelman et al.[46] performed laparoscopic gastrostomy in six consecutive patients with no morbidity or mortality. Operative time averaged 18 minutes (range 10 to 25 minutes) and blood loss was estimated to be less than 10 ml. Two patients underwent the procedure on an outpatient basis. Our experience has been similar and we anticipate excellent long-term functional results.

To date only four series of laparoscopic jejunostomies in 32 patients with short-term follow-up have been reported in the literature.[42-45] Sangster and Swanström's series of 23 patients was the largest.[42] They report an operative time averaging 45 minutes and never exceeding 90 minutes. In none of the series has intraoperative organ injuries, bleeding, or the need to convert to an open procedure been reported. Other complications were few and included superficial skin breakdown or abscess about the tube, minor leakage around the tube, or dislodged tubes, which were easily replaced without the need for reoperation. Interestingly, no episodes of postoperative aspiration were reported.

Laparoscopically placed feeding tubes inevitably will entail some of the same problems encountered with those placed by an open surgical procedure. Of most concern after any form of enteral access is aspiration. As has been stated, percutaneous endoscopic gastrostomies are associated with a significant incidence of postoperative aspiration, most pronounced in certain high-risk groups. Published series have varied in their assessment of the exact risk, although reports that have focused specifically on the incidence of aspiration after either percutaneous endoscopic or open gastrostomy show a rate of 23% to 40%.[31,33-35] Whether jejunal tubes eliminate or even reduce this risk is unresolved to date. Several factors are pertinent to the problem. A large number of the patients assessed for feeding tube placement have underlying neurologic dysfunction such as mental obtundation, impaired swallowing, or a deficient gag reflex. As a result, many experience preoperative aspiration, especially of oropharyngeal secretions.[47] No form of enteral access can be reasonably expected to eliminate the risk of aspiration in such patients.

Table 23-1. Aspiration and mortality after open surgical jejunostomy

Study	No. of Patients	Aspiration (%)	Mortality at 30 Days (%)
Heimbach[48]	83	16	63
Matino[49]	54	9	33
Adams et al.[50]	73	12	40
McGonigal et al.[51]	100	N.A.	32
Weltz et al.[52]	100	8	21

Several series have addressed the incidence of aspiration after jejunostomy, although they have varied in their definition of what constitutes an aspiration event and the thoroughness with which such events have been sought (Table 23-1). Weltz et al.[52] report an 8% incidence of aspiration after open surgical jejunostomy, although they demonstrate that only 4% of such events can be directly attributable to the operative procedure, since the remaining patients aspirated prior to initiation of tube feedings in the postoperative period or had evidence of oropharyngeal secretion aspiration both preoperatively and postoperatively. Of note, feeding-related preoperative aspiration events in this series were completely eliminated in the postoperative period by placement of a jejunostomy.

Although direct comparison of series of gastrostomy and jejunostomy patients are difficult to assess in regard to the incidence of aspiration, the bulk of the available evidence supports jejunostomy as the feeding route of choice in patients at risk.

Another important consideration is the mortality associated with the various forms of enteral access. Again, a large percentage of the patients referred for feeding tubes have severe underlying medical problems and anesthesia can be a significant risk factor. An aura of pessimism regarding the placement of jejunostomies was created by Heimbach[48] in 1970 when he reported a 67% perioperative mortality in all patients and 80% in comatose patients. Other recent reports have shown significant, although smaller mortality rates (Table 23-1). While offering the advantages of a minimally invasive procedure, laparoscopic methods of feeding tube placement require abdominal insufflation with its inherent risks of hypercarbia, diminished venous return, and impaired ventilation. How these factors will influence morbidity and mortality awaits further study.

Small bowel obstruction,[33-35] intraperitoneal leak,[48,49] and tube dislodgment,[48,52,53] have been reported after open feeding tube placement and would also be expected to occur after laparoscopic placement, depending on the particular tube used and the manner in which it is placed. Other complications such as wound infections or dehiscences and postoperative ileus, however, might prove to be lower in the laparoscopic group.

CONCLUSION

Recent work has demonstrated the relative benefits of enteral alimentation compared with total parenteral nutrition in patients with a functional gastrointestinal tract. In addition, recent developments and improvements in laparoscopy have allowed new methods of feeding tube placement. Although percutaneous endoscopic gastrostomy generally is the procedure of choice for the establishment of chronic enteral access, surgical gastrostomies and jejunostomies are indicated in patients who are not candidates for percutaneous endoscopic techniques. Although comparative data between open and laparoscopic feeding tube placement are not yet available, the laparoscopic approaches would appear to offer several potential advantages such as less postoperative pain, improved cosmesis, a lower rate of wound infection, less postoperative ileus, a quicker recovery time, and a shorter hospitalization in ambulatory patients. The laparoscopic approaches, on the other hand, require more expertise and training than their open counterparts. Visualization of appropriate structures may be poor, and suturing techniques require practice to master. As with other laparoscopic procedures, unrecognized bowel perforation and intestinal volvulus are risks, and the effects of peritoneal insufflation must be considered. The risks inherent in placement of any form of feeding tube also need to be considered. Only by analyzing the results of large series of these procedures, including operative time, total hospital and physician costs, and complications rates, will their relative merit be determined.

Any reports of a new laparoscopic procedure must be assessed critically in regard to risks, benefits, alternatives, and costs. We believe that the laparoscopic procedures described are attractive alternatives for the establishment of chronic enteral alimentation.

REFERENCES

1. Bower RH, Talamani MA, Sax HC, et al. Postoperative *versus* parenteral nutrition. Arch Surg 211:1040-1045, 1986.
2. Fletcher JP, Little JM. A comparison of parenteral nutrition and early postoperative enteral feeding on the nitrogen balance after major surgery. Surgery 100:21-24, 1986.
3. Vernet O, Christin L, Schutz Y, et al. Enteral *versus* parenteral nutrition: Comparison of energy metabolism in healthy subjects. Am J Physiol 250:E47-E54, 1986.
4. Muggia-Sullam M, Bower RH, Murphy RF, et al. Postoperative enteral *versus* parenteral nutritional support in gastrointestinal surgery. A matched prospective study. Am J Surg 149:106-112, 1985.
5. Kudsk KA, Carpenter BA, Petersen S, et al. Effect of enteral and parenteral feeding in malnourished rats with *E. coli*-hemoglobin adjuvant peritonitis. J Surg Res 31:105-110, 1981.
6. Kudsk KA, Stone JM, Carpenter G, et al. Enteral and parenteral feeding influences mortality after hemoglobin-*E. coli* peritonitis in normal rats. J Trauma 23:605-609, 1983.
7. Kudsk KA, Croce MA, Fabian TC, et al. Enteral versus parenteral feeding. Ann Surg 215:503-513, 1992.
8. Moore FA, Feliciano DV, Andrassy RJ, et al. Early enteral feeding, compared with parenteral, reduces postoperative septic complications. The results of a meta-analysis. Ann Surg 216:172-183, 1992.
9. The Veterans Affairs Total Parenteral Nutrition Cooperative Study Group. Perioperative total parenteral nutrition in surgical patients. N Engl J Med 325:525-532, 1991.
10. Kotler DR, Levine GM. Reversible gastric and pancreatic hyposecretion after long-term parenteral nutrition. N Engl J Med 300:241-242. 1979.
11. Deitch EA, Maejima K, Berg R. Effect of oral antibiotics and bacterial overgrowth on the translocation of the GI tract microflora in burned rats. J Trauma 25:385-392, 1985.
12. Deitch EA, Winterton J, Berg R. Thermal injury promotes bacterial translocation from the gastrointestinal tract in mice with impaired T-cell-mediated immunity. Arch Surg 121:97-101, 1986.
13. Deitch EA, Bridges RM. Effect of stress and trauma on bacterial translocation from the gut. J Surg Res 42:536-542, 1987.
14. Deitch EA, Berg R. Endotoxin but not malnutrition promotes bacterial translocation of the gut flora in burned mice. J Trauma 27:161-166, 1987.
15. Deitch EA, Winterton J, Berg R. Effects of starvation, malnutrition, and trauma on the gastrointestinal tract flora and bacterial translocation. Arch Surg 122:1019-1024, 1987.

16. Deitch FA, Winterton J, Berg R. The gut as portal of entry for bacteremia: Role of protein malnutrition. Ann Surg 205:681-692, 1987.
17. Alverdy JC, Aoys E, Moss GS. Total parenteral nutrition promotes bacterial translocation from the gut. Surgery 104:185-190, 1988.
18. Illig KA, Ryan CK, Hardy DJ, et al. Differential effects of partial enteral nutrition (PEN) on gut function (in press).
19. Inoue S, Epstein M, Alexander JW, et al. Prevention of yeast translocation across the gut by a single enteral feeding after burn injury. JPEN 12(Suppl):5S, 1988.
20. Shou J, Lappin J, Minnard EA, et al. Total parenteral nutrition, bacterial translocation and host immune function. Am J Surg 167:145-150, 1994.
21. Shou J, Lappin J, Daly JM. Impairment of pulmonary macrophage function with total parenteral nutrition. Ann Surg 219:291-297, 1994.
22. Alverdy JC, Chi HS, Sheldon GF. The effect of parenteral nutrition on gastrointestinal immunity: The importance of enteral stimulation. Ann Surg 202:681-684, 1985.
23. Kagnoff MF. Immunology and allergic responses of the bowel. In Greene M, Greene HL, eds. The Role of the Gastrointestinal Tract in Nutrient Delivery. Orlando, Fla.: Academic Press, 1984, pp 239-257.
24. Allardyce D, Groves A. A comparison of nutritional responses from intravenous and enteral feedings. Surg Gynecol Obstet 139:179, 1974.
25. Ryan JA, Abel RM, Abbott WM. Catheter complications in total parenteral nutrition: A prospective study in 200 consecutive patients. N Engl J Med 290:757, 1974.
26. Sax HC, Bower RH. Hepatic complications of total parenteral nutrition. JPEN 12:615-618, 1988.
27. Ellis LM, Bryant MS, Copeland EM, et al. Postoperative enteral versus total parenteral nutrition immediately after partial hepatectomy: Effects on hepatic regeneration and function. Curr Surg 471:470-472, 1987.
28. Burgess P. Pathogenesis of hepatic steatosis [letter]. JPEN 16:399, 1992.
29. Keim NL. Nutritional effects of hepatic steatosis induced by parenteral nutrition in the rat. JPEN 11:18-22, 1987.
30. Gauderer MWL, Ponsky JL, Izant RJ Jr. Gastrostomy without laparotomy: A percutaneous endoscopic technique. J Pediatr Surg 15:872-875, 1980.
31. Cole MJ, Smith JT, Molnar C, et al. Aspiration after percutaneous gastrostomy. J Clin Gastroenterol 9:90-95, 1987.
32. Johnson DA, Hacker JF III, Benjamin SP, et al. Percutaneous endoscopic gastrostomy (PEG) effects on the lower esophageal sphincter (LES) and gastroesophageal reflux (GER). Gastrointest Endosc 32:144, 1986.
33. Burtch GD, Shatney CH. Feeding gastrostomy: Assistant or assassin? Am Surg 51:204-207, 1985.
34. Cogen R, Weinryb J. Aspiration pneumonia in nursing home patients fed via gastrostomy tubes. Am J Gastroenterol 84:1509-1512, 1989.
35. Hassett JM, Sunby C, Flint LM. No elimination of aspiration pneumonia in neurologically disabled patients with feeding gastrostomy. Surg Gynecol Obstet 167:383-388, 1988.
36. DiSario JA, Foutch PG, Sanowski RA. Poor results with percutaneous endoscopic jejunostomy. Gastrointest Endosc 36:257-260, 1990.
37. Wolfsen HC, Kozarek RA, Ball TJ, et al. Tube dysfunction following percutaneous endoscopic gastrostomy and jejunostomy. Gastrointest Endosc 36:261-263, 1990.
38. Edelman DS, Unger SW. Laparoscopic gastrostomy. Surg Gynecol Obstet 173:401, 1991.
39. Modesto VL, Harkins B, Calton WC Jr, et al. Laparoscopic gastrostomy using four-point fixation. Am J Surg 167:273-276, 1994.
40. Delany HM, Carnevale N, Garvey JW. Jejunostomy by a needle catheter technique. Surgery 73: 786-790, 1973.
41. Roy A, DeMeester TR. Perioperative management of carcinoma of the esophagus: The reduction of operative mortality. In Delarue NC, Wilkins EW Jr, Wong J, eds. Esophageal Cancer, vol IV. Trends in General Thoracic Surgery. St. Louis: CV Mosby, 1988, pp 101-113.
42. Sangster W, Swanström L. Laparoscopic-guided feeding jejunostomy. Surg Endosc 7:308-310, 1993.
43. Morris JB, Mullen JL, Yu JC, et al. Laparoscopic-guided jejunostomy. Surgery 112:96-99, 1992.
44. Albrink MH, Foster J, Rosemurgy AS, et al. Laparoscopic feeding jejunostomy: Also a simple technique. Surg Endosc 6:259-260, 1992.
45. Duh Q-Y, Way LW. Laparoscopic jejunostomy using T-fasteners as retractors and anchors. Arch Surg 128:105-108, 1993.

46. Edelman DS, Unger SW, Russin DR. Laparoscopic gastrostomy. Surg Laparosc Endosc 1:251-253, 1991.
47. Huxley EJ, Viroslav J, Gray WR, et al. Pharyngeal aspiration in normal adults and patients with depressed consciousness. Am J Med 64:564-568, 1978.
48. Heimbach DM. Surgical feeding procedures in patients with neurological disorders. Ann Surg 172:311-314, 1970.
49. Matino JJ. Feeding jejunostomy in patients with neurological disorders. Arch Surg 116:169-171, 1981.
50. Adams MD, Seabrook GR, Quebbeman EA, et al. Jejunostomy: A rarely indicated procedure. Arch Surg 121:236-238, 1986.
51. McGonigal MD, Lucas CF, Ledgerwood AM. Feeding jejunostomy in patients who are critically ill. Surg Gynecol Obstet 168:275-277, 1989.
52. Weltz CR, Morris JB, Mullen JL. Surgical jejunostomy in aspiration risk patients. Ann Surg 215:140-145, 1992.
53. Barber WH. Jejunostomy. Ann Surg 97:553-576, 1993.

Index

R